FAITH COMMUNITY NURSING EDUCATION

FOUNDATIONS OF

Faith Community Nursing Curriculum

PARTICIPANT

2014 REVISION

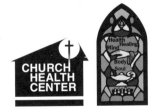

DEVELOPED BY
International Parish Nurse Resource Center
A Ministry of the Church Health Center
Memphis, TN

About the Church Health Center

The Church Health Center seeks to reclaim the church's biblical commitment to care for our bodies and our spirits. The Center's ministries provide health care for the working uninsured and promote healthy bodies and spirits for all. To learn more about the Center, visit www.ChurchHealthCenter.org. To learn more about our magazine on health ministry, *Church Health Reader*, visit www.chreader.org.

Faith Community Nursing Education
Foundations of Faith Community Nursing Curriculum: Participant 2014 Revision

Developed by
International Parish Nurse Resource Center
A Ministry of the Church Health Center
© 2014 Church Health Center

ISBN: 978-1-62144-047-5

Printed in the United States of America

Table of Contents

UNIT I: SPIRITUALITY

History and Philosophy
Sharon T. Hinton RN-BC, MSN, DMin

Health, Healing and Wholeness
Rev. Donna Smith-Pupillo, RN, BSN, MDiv

Spiritual Care
Annette Langdon, RN, BSN, MA

Prayer
Rev. Dr. Helen Wordsworth, RN, RM, RHV, MTh, DMin

Self-Care
Angela Sheehan MS, RN, NPP

UNIT II: PROFESSIONALISM

Ethical Issues
Jean Bokinskie, PhD, RN

Documenting Practice
Katora P. Campbell, RN, MSN, DrPH

Legal Aspects
Paulette Golden, MS, RN

Beginning Your Ministry
JoVeta Wescott, RN, MSHA

Communication and Collaboration
Faith Roberts, RN, MSN

UNIT III: WHOLISTIC HEALTH

Health Promotion
Myrna Harris Cassimere, RN, PhD

Behavioral Health
Rosalie T. Albright, RN, MSN, PMHCNS-BC, APRN

Transforming Life Issues: Family Violence
Anne Gifford, RN, MBA, MHS, MACE, D.Ed.Min.

Transforming Life Issues: Loss, Suffering and Grief
Anne Gifford, RN, MBA, MHS, MACE, D.Ed.Min

UNIT IV: COMMUNITY

Assessment
Pamela Deres, MS, RN, CNS

Accessing Resources
Judith Mouch, RSM, MSN, PHCNS-BC

Advocacy
Marabel Kersey, RN, MSN

Care Coordination
Beverly Siegrist, EdD, CNE

Introduction

The Title: Parish Nurse or Faith Community Nurse

Parish nurse is the historical term Rev. Dr. Granger Westberg chose as the name of this specialty practice. He did so as a theological choice for this professional ministry, because it connoted service not only to the congregation, but also to the wider community within the geographic area surrounding the physical location of the sanctuary. Just as the word *sanctuary* can mean both "church worship area" and "safe harbor," the word *parish* can mean "congregation" and "geographic area served by a congregation." Nowhere is this better illustrated than in Louisiana, where the geographic areas called *counties* elsewhere are *parishes* there; so parish nurses, in Louisiana, are called "church nurses" to avoid confusion with the county public health nurses.

Faith Community Nursing: Scope and Standards of Practice (2012, 2nd ed.) uses the term *faith community nurse* (FCN) to represent a registered nurse specializing in faith community nursing. This language is inclusive of all faith traditions. The FCN provides spiritual care in the faith community as well as in the broader community. The goals of the FCN are the protection, promotion, and optimization of health and abilities; the prevention of illness and injury; and the alleviation of suffering in the context of values, beliefs, and practices of a faith community, such as a church, congregation, parish, synagogue, temple, mosque, or faith based community agency (ANA/HMA, 2012, p.5).

Philosophy of Faith Community Nursing

Faith community nursing is a new specialty, but not a new concept.

"Parish nursing is rooted in the Judeo-Christian tradition, and the historic practice of professional nursing, and is consistent with the basic assumptions of many faiths that we care for self and others as an expression of God's love" (Church Health Center website, 2014).

The **philosophy of faith community nursing** encompasses four major concepts.

1. **Spirit.** The intentional care of the spirit sets the specialty practice of faith community nursing apart from other types of nursing. Continuing personal spiritual formation is an ongoing, essential component of practice and includes both self-care and hospitality through opening the heart to self and others.

2. **Roots.** The specialty practice of faith community nursing reclaims the historic roots of professional nursing, recognizing that similar aspects of health and healing are found in many faith traditions.

3. **Shalom.** The faith community nurse views health as an ongoing, ever-changing process that includes multiple aspects of a person, including spiritual, physical, psychological, and social.
   - Shalom is harmony and wholeness regardless of circumstance and serves as a foundation for understanding health.
   - A sense of well-being can exist in the presence of imbalance, and healing can occur in the absence of a cure.

4. **Community.** Faith community nursing practice focuses on a faith community.
   - The FCN is a member of the staff and works in conjunction with clergy and congregation to provide opportunities for the ongoing transformation of the faith community into sources of health and healing.
   - Through partnership with other community health resources, faith community nursing fosters new and creative responses to health and wellness concerns.
   - FCNs appreciate that all persons are sacred and must be treated with respect and dignity.
   - The FCN serves the community of faith, creates safe and sacred places of healing, and advocates with compassion, mercy, and dignity.

In addition to these core concepts, faith community nursing builds on these assumptions:

- Health and illness are human experiences.
- Wholistic health integrates spiritual, physical, psychological, and social aspects of the health care consumer to create a sense of harmony with self, others, the environment, and a higher power.
- Health may be experienced in the presence of illness or injury.
- Healing is the process of integrating the body, mind, and spirit to create wholeness, health, and a sense of well-being, even when the health care consumer's illness is not cured (ANA/HMA, 2012, p. 8).

Assumptions Regarding Faith Community Nursing Practice and the Curriculum

Practice

The **practice** of faith community nursing is a professional endeavor.

- The participant is a registered nurse with a current unencumbered license or a student in a baccalaureate nursing education program. The preferred minimum preparation for a registered nurse or advanced practice nurse entering the specialty includes a baccalaureate or higher degree in nursing with academic preparation in community or population-focused nursing. In the future, a baccalaureate degree in nursing will be required for certification in this specialized practice.
- Faith community nursing is considered a calling in which ministry shapes the practice.
- The practice of faith community nursing requires specialized knowledge and skills to implement faith community nursing professional standards.
- The practice of faith community nursing encourages a partnership model between faith community nurses, individuals, families, congregations, and communities across the life span.
- Faith community nursing contributes to the health of the faith community.
- Faith community nursing acknowledges *Faith Community Nursing: Scope and Standards of Practice* (ANA/HMA, 2012) as the guide for professional practice in the United States. Faith community nurses in other countries are accountable to their own specific professional standards of practice.

Curriculum

The **curriculum** that prepares FCNs to serve in this specialized ministry reflects certain assumptions.

- It focuses on core concepts of spiritual formation, professionalism, shalom as health and wholeness, and community, incorporating culture and diversity.
- It encourages individual spiritual growth.
- It is developed from a Judeo-Christian theological framework of care and is applicable to and respectful of other faith traditions.
- It is inclusive of sociocultural and geographic diversity including ethnicity, gender, lifestyle, sexual orientation and faith traditions.
- It includes various ways of thinking and knowing, such as the application of the nursing process of assessment, planning, implementation, and evaluation; a theological perspective is also emphasized.
- It develops the nurse for a leadership role in collaborative health ministry.
- It supplies the content to develop and sustain a faith community nursing practice.
- It fosters interprofessional collaboration.

Faith Community Nursing Curriculum Conceptual Model

Faith community nursing is recognized as a specialty nursing practice that combines professional nursing and health ministry. It emphasizes health and healing within the faith community and the larger community. The philosophy of this curriculum embraces four major concepts (Figure 1).

1. **The Spiritual Dimension**

   The spiritual dimension is the core of faith community nursing practice. It is described as the need for meaning, purpose and fulfillment in life, the hope or will to live, and belief and faith. The spiritual dimension is important for the attainment of an overall sense of health, well-being and quality of life. Crisis, illness, and hospitalization can affect spiritual well-being. Living out our beliefs and faith with self, others, and God or a higher power is core to faith community nursing practice.

2. Professionalism

Professionalism identifies parameters within which the FCN practices, including *Faith Community Nursing: Scope and Standards of Practice* (ANA/HMA, 2012, 2nd edition), *Nursing: Scope and Standards of Practice* (ANA, 2010), *Code of Ethics for Nurses with Interpretive Statements* (ANA, 2008), and state or country nurse practice acts. Other concepts deal with communication, collaboration, documentation and how to begin this ministry.

Faith Community Nursing Curriculum Conceptual Model
FiGURE 1

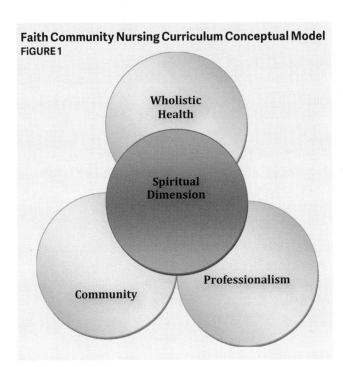

3. Wholistic Health

The FCN promotes shalom as a foundation for wholism, health and healing. Health promotion introduces the concepts of education, prevention and teaching and learning principles across the life span. Wholistic health includes addressing other life issues, such as suffering, grief and loss, and family violence.

4. Community

Community is a group with common interests, including the faith community, professional nursing community, geographic community, global community, demographic community, or other communities. Issues of diversity are considered within this model.

The four concepts serve as the organizational framework for content units within the Foundations of Faith Community Nursing Curriculum. Although modules have been assigned to one specific unit within the curriculum, content within each module may overlap with other modules in education and practice.

With a central focus on spiritual health and well-being, the FCN promotes health as wholeness within a faith community through the practice of nursing. While the spiritual dimension is central to faith community nursing practice, each of the other concepts within the model (Wholistic Health, Community, and Professionalism) interacts with one or more of the other concepts, in addition to interacting with the spiritual dimension in practice.

Contributing Authors

Rosalie T. Albright, RN, MSN, PMHCNS-BC, APRN
Faith Community Nurse
Coordinator, Faith Community Nursing Services
Community Service Department
Ephraim McDowell Health
Danville, Kentucky

Jean Bokinskie, PhD, RN
Faith Community Nurse
Director, Parish Nurse Ministry Program
Associate Professor, Nursing
Concordia College
Moorhead, Minnesota

Katora P. Campbell, RN, MSN, DrPH
Director, Faith Community Outreach
Church Health Center
Memphis, Tennessee

Myrna Harris Cassimere, RN, PhD
Academic Coordinator
The McFarland Institute—Congregational Wellness
Division
New Orleans, Louisiana

Pamela Deres, MS, RN, CNS
Manager of Health Ministries and Parish Nursing
St. Joseph Hospital
Nashua, New Hampshire

Anne Gifford, RN, MBA, MHS, MACE, D.Ed.Min.
Chaplain (Retired), Baylor Medical Center
Columbia, Missouri

Paulette Golden, MS, RN
Faith Community Nurse
Carrollton, Texas

Sharon T. Hinton RN-BC, MSN, DMin
Faith Community Nurse Specialist
Church Health Center/ International Parish Nurse
Resource Center
Memphis, Tennessee
Executive Director, Rural Nurse Resource, Inc.
Floydada, Texas

Marabel Kersey, RN, MSN
Faith Community Nurse/Faith Community Nurse
Educator
Des Moines Area Community College
Des Moines, Iowa

Annette Langdon, RN, BSN, MA
Advance Care Planning Liaison, Fairview Health
Services, Minneapolis, Minnesota
Adjunct Faculty, Concordia College
Moorhead, Minnesota

Judith Mouch, RSM, MSN, PHCNS-BC
Associate Professor
University of Detroit Mercy
McAuley School of Nursing
Detroit, Michigan

Rev. Donna Smith-Pupillo, RN, BSN, MDiv
Executive Director, Deaconness Parish Nurse
Ministries
St. Louis, Missouri

Faith Roberts, RN, MSN
Director, Community Parish Nurse Program
Carle Foundation Hospital
Urbana, Illinois

Angela Sheehan MS, RN, NPP
Faith Community Nurse
Director of Faith Community/Parish Nursing
St. Peter's Health Partners/St. Mary's Hospital
Troy, New York

Beverly Siegrist, EdD, CNE
Professor, School of Nursing
Western Kentucky University
Bowling Green, Kentucky

JoVeta Wescott, RN, MSHA
Executive Director
Kansas Parish Nurse Ministry, Inc.
Wichita, Kansas

Rev. Dr. Helen Wordsworth, RN, RM, RHV, MTh, DMin
UK Coordinator, Parish Nursing Ministries UK
22 The Rookery
Orton Wistow
Peterborough PE2 6YT

Special thanks to:
Members of Interfaith Partnership of St. Louis
for reviewing interfaith portions of the Health,
Healing and Wholeness Module. Dr. Bashir Bastani,
cardiologist and Muslim physician, reviewed
the material on Islam. Mr. Jack Sisk, executive
director of the Living Insight Center, reviewed
the Buddhism and Hinduism sections. Dr. David
Oughton, professor of theology and world religions
at St. Louis University, reviewed the material on
Judaism and did the general review.

Faith Roberts for the overview, explanation and
exercises on process dynamics.

Maureen Daniels for Guidelines for Teaching the
Foundations of Faith Community Nursing Course
Internationally.

Reviewers

Carol B. Bradford, MSN, RN
Faith Community Nurse
Parish Nurse Coordinator
Parish Nurse Ministry
Lourdes & Baptist Health Paducah Hospitals
Mayfield, Kentucky
Adjunct Faculty, School of Nursing
Western Kentucky University
Bowling Green, Kentucky

Maureen Daniels, RN, MN
Faith Community Nurse Specialist
Church Health Center/ International Parish Nurse
Resource Center
Memphis, Tennessee

Nancy L. Rago Durbin, MS, RN
Faith Community Nurse
Director, Parish Nurse Ministry & Parish Nurse
Support Network
Advocate Health Care
Park Ridge, Illinois

Sharon T. Hinton RN-BC, MSN, DMin
Faith Community Nurse Specialist
Church Health Center/ International Parish Nurse
Resource Center
Memphis, Tennessee
Executive Director, Rural Nurse Resource, Inc.
Floydada, Texas

Susan R. Jacob, PhD, RN
Education Consultant
Church Health Center/ International Parish Nurse
Resource Center
Memphis, Tennessee

Roberta Schweitzer, PhD, RN
Body-Spirit Wellness Center
Westfield, Indiana

Rev. Donna Smith-Pupillo, RN, BSN, MDiv
Executive Director, Deaconness Parish Nurse
Ministries
St. Louis, Missouri

Andrea M. West, RN, PhD
Faith Community Nurse
Rocky Mountain Parish Health Ministry Association
Denver, Colorado

Lisa Zerull, PhD, RN
Academic Liaison & Program Manager Faith-
Based Services
Winchester Medical Center/Valley Health
Winchester, Virginia
Editor, *Perspectives*
Church Health Center/International Parish Nurse
Resource Center
Memphis, Tennessee

Deborah Ziebarth, MSN Ed, PhD(c)
Manager of Research and Special Projects
Church Health Center/ International Parish Nurse
Resource Center
Memphis, Tennessee

Acknowledgments

The 2014 Foundations of Faith Community Nursing Curriculum represents the tireless work of many individuals. Dr. Susan Jacob led the efforts in her role as education consultant at the Church Health Center. The process began with a survey sent to faith community nurse educators asking them to identify areas of strength, weakness, and overlap of content in the 2009 edition of the curriculum. Five seasoned faith community nurse educators provided expert content review prior to the development of modules. A number of faith community nurses who attended the Westberg Symposium in 2013 and 2014 provided informal assessment of the curriculum, and input was also obtained from the Faith Community Nursing Advisory Team. Module authors revised the 2009 modules based on assessment results and latest evidence related to their topics. Two new modules, *Spiritual Care* and *Behavioral Health*, were developed based on feedback from faith community nurses. Module authors represent faith community nursing in a variety of roles, from educator to practicing faith community nurse.

Susan Martins Miller provided editorial guidance and expertise. Design work by Lizy Heard enabled us to provide modules that are uniform and visually appealing. Rachel Davis and John Shorb helped shepherd the project through its various phases. This curriculum revision could not have happened without their dedicated work and extensive knowledge.

We dedicate this 2014 Curriculum to faith community nurses who serve by tirelessly providing wholistic care in their faith communities.

Susan R. Jacob, PhD, RN
Education Consultant

Unit I
Spirituality

Unit I: Spirituality

History and Philosophy
of Faith Community Nursing

Unit I: Spirituality

History and Philosophy of Faith Community Nursing

Introduction

Learning Outcomes

Upon completion of this module, the participant will be able to:

1. Describe how the history and philosophy of health care and nursing provide a spiritual foundation for faith community nursing.
2. Analyze how the actions of Granger Westberg have contributed to the current conceptualization of faith community nursing.
3. Identify historic events that have contributed to the continued development of faith community nursing.
4. Relate the key aspects of the philosophy of faith community nursing practice to the development of a personal philosophy of this specialty practice.

Description

This module reviews the general history and philosophy of health care and nursing and then focuses on the specialty practice of faith community nursing. It emphasizes the multiple aspects of supporting the integration of health ministry into the life of the community of faith as well as the development of a personal philosophy of faith community nursing practice.

Hours: 2

Research

"Given the role that R/S [research on religion, spirituality, and health] could play in preventing illness, speeding recovery, and motivating individuals to care for one another in the community (thereby reducing the need for expensive health services), research in this area will be of critical importance in addressing the escalating health-care costs in the United States and countries around the world" (Koenig, 2011).

"Research conducted at the National Institutes of Health (NIH) and academic institutions has established a relationship between spiritual practices and health, thereby expanding the knowledge base for the specialty of faith community nursing" (ANA/HMA, 2012). In a review of 22 articles published between 2008–2013 Dandridge (2014) revealed that faith community nurses (FCNs) are providing a wealth of interventions to diverse populations, but they are not successfully evaluating outcomes.

Faith Tradition

"Nurses have long observed that when illness and brokenness occur, healthcare consumers—whether individually or with their family and friends—may turn to their source of spiritual strength for reassurance, support, and healing" (ANA/HMA, 2012).

"The primary focus of the FCN is the intentional care of the spirit, differentiating this specialty practice from the general practice of the registered nurse" (ANA/HMA, 2012).

The history of God and religions is passionate, intense, and important because it directly influences current beliefs just as current beliefs will influence the future. Our observations of the world are filtered by our unique "spatial, temporal, and social locations; by culture, history, status; by our occupational or other idiosyncratic concerns; and, especially relevant here, by the scholarly discipline within which our 'looking' takes place" (Scharen and Vigen, 2011, p. 119). Throughout history, faith and health have had a connected relationship of wellness and healing.

Key Terms

Faith community nursing: the specialized practice of professional nursing that focuses on the intentional care of the spirit as well as the promotion of wholistic health and prevention or minimization of illness within the context of a faith community.

Faith community nurse (FCN): a registered professional nurse who is actively licensed in a given state and who serves as a member of the staff of a faith community. The FCN promotes health as wholeness of the faith community, its groups, families, and individual members.

Faith Community Nursing: Scope and Standards of Practice (2nd ed., 2012): describes the unique scope of knowledge and the standards of practice and professional performance for a faith community nurse (FCN).

Health Ministries Association: a nonprofit organization whose mission is to encourage, support, and empower leaders in the integration of faith and health in their local communities (HMA website, 2014).

Wholistic: care based on an understanding that a health care consumer is an interconnected unity and that physical, mental, social, environmental, and spiritual factors need to be included in any interventions. The whole system, whether referring to a human being or a faith community, is greater than the sum of its parts. This is the preferred term when referring to the type of care provided by a faith community nurse.

Reflection

"The longer you look back, the farther you can look forward."
—Winston Churchill

"It is not the remembered, but the forgotten past that enslaves us."
—C.S. Lewis

"How shall we labor with any effect to build up the church if we have no thorough knowledge of her history? History is and must ever continue to be, next to God's word, the richest foundation of wisdom, and the surest guide to all successful activity."
—Philip Schaff

"Histories are a true school for learning how to order our lives."
—John Calvin

"History is a vast early warning system."
—Norman Cousins

"To be ignorant of what occurred before you were born is to remain always a child. For what is the worth of human life, unless it is woven into the life of our ancestors by the records of history?"
—Cicero

"It is said that we stand on the shoulders of those who have gone before us; in the stories of pre-Christian and early Christian caregivers are many shoulders on which to stand. There are many models of ministries of love and care for the sick that speak eloquently to us as nurses today."
—Sister Mary Margaret O'Brien

History and Philosophy
of Faith Community Nursing

Content Outline

OUTCOME 1

Describe how the history and philosophy of health care and nursing provide a spiritual foundation for faith community nursing.

The history of the practice of health and healing can be traced through both the pre-Christian and Christian eras.

Pre-Christian Era

In the **Stone Age**, health focused on physical needs and protection of self and others from danger. There is no evidence of formalized medicine or nursing.

From the **Age of Metal**, we find evidence of permanent shelters and domesticated animals. We also find the practice of dualism:
- an evil deity is responsible for illness
- a benevolent deity is responsible for health
- people are treated by a shaman (medicine man or woman), a priest-physician

In **early civilizations**, we begin to see developing ideas of health and medicine.

In **Egypt**, medicine was viewed as mystical and priestly.
- development of advanced knowledge of human anatomy and surgical procedures, including brain surgery
- worship of nature (animism)
- first physician was Imhotep, who lived some time between 1900 and 2800 BC, wrote the first medical textbook, and was later worshiped as a god of health
- kings and aristocrats used nurses to deliver babies and care for the sick (Ellis and Hartley, 2012)
- In Exodus 1:15–20, Shiphrah and Puah were midwives who delivered the baby Moses (Jacob, 2013)

In **Greece**, nursing was the responsibility of family members or slaves of the patient.
- Hippocrates, the father of medicine (460–370 BC), developed

treatments and medicines; emphasized the scientific method and patient-centered care
- worship of Asclepius (god of healing) and daughters: Hygeia (goddess of health) and Panacea (restorer of health)

In **Rome**, medicine consisted of natural and folk remedies.
- multiple Roman gods were offered libations for health and illness favors
- medical treatments adopted from other societies Romans conquered; for example, after the conquest of Corinth, Romans studied in Athens and learned skills of Greek healing

In **Israel**, people viewed God as the source of both health and disease.
- Mosaic Law provided foundations of public health nursing
- rules of nursing for those with contagious diseases
- hospitality and charity for anyone in need: "houses for strangers"
- first nurse recorded in history—Deborah is described as a nurse in the Old Testament (see Genesis 24:59 and 35:8); "appears at times as a combination servant, companion and helpmate" (Bullough and Bullough, 1969, p.14).

In **Babylonia**, the Code of Hammurabi (2067–2025 BC) was the first legal and civil measure for medicine.
- enrichment of drug therapy, concepts of hygiene, social medicine, and codifying responsibilities of physician and punishment for malpractice
- nurses were either slaves or domestic workers

In **India**, the Vedas, sacred book of Hinduism (1200 BC), was used to guide health care practices.
- Charak Samhita defined characteristics of a nurse (male): "Knowledge of the manner in which drugs should be prepared or compounded for administration, cleverness, devotedness to the patient waited upon and purity (both of mind and body) are the four qualifications of the attending nurse" (Frank, 1952, p. 58).
- country converted to Buddhism and Jainism
- King Ashoka started hospitals with male nurses in 300 BC
- the spread of Islam into India in the 7th and 8th centuries diminished nursing and medicine because of Islam's belief it was unsanitary to touch blood or morbid matter

HELPFUL RESOURCE
Choose a wide variety of nursing and medical history texts and articles from your local library. Include religious or denominational history representing the participants enrolled. Include a variety of photographs if possible. See the Additional References list at the end of the module for specific title suggestions.

Christian Era

Diakonal Ministry
Diakonia is Greek for "service": the serving, caregiving, and healing arm of the church; caring for the whole person.
- Ministry is composed of preaching, teaching, and healing or serving.
- *Diakonia* was Christ's service of walking among the people, healing diseases, and forgiving sins. Following the Servant

Christ, the early church took up the task of caring for and visiting the sick.

- The work was done by others so church leaders could preach and teach (Acts 6:1–6).
- In the New Testament, the office (deacon and deaconess) is held by men and women (Romans 16:1).

The **theological framework** for *diakonia* comes from following the example Jesus set in serving those in need.

- We approach service to others with the belief that with mercy and compassion others will know Jesus Christ through our example.
- Serving those in need actually is serving Christ (Patterson, 2003).

Early Deacons, Deaconesses, and Roman Matrons of the Third and Fourth Centuries

- Phoebe, the first deaconess, lived about 55 AD (Romans 16:1–2).
- St. Helena (Flavia Helena), a Roman matron, started the first *gerokomion*, or home for the aged.
- St. Paula, Roman matron, founded the first hospice for the pilgrims in Bethlehem.
- St. Marcella, Roman matron, was a scholar (O'Brien, 2003).

Arabian Empire

- Mohammed (570 AD) started the religion of Islam with the Koran.
- Arabs absorbed information from the countries they ruled.
- Translated Hippocrates to Arabic.
- Greeks and Romans met with the Pope about the increasing size of the Arabian Empire; Crusades resulted.

Crusades

- started in 1095 and lasted over 200 years
- formation of orders of men committed to battle and men committed to care for those wounded in battle
- Knights of St. Lazarus, one of five major orders rising from the Crusades, treated Templar knights who contracted leprosy
- The Knights Hospitaller (St. John's) and Knights of the Hospital of St. Mary's of Jerusalem also offered medical care

Deaconess Education and Ministries

In **Germany** in the early 1800s, Theodor Fleidner of Kaiserswerth, a pastor, was influential in developing a modern form of the diaconate. He established houses for people who were ill, developmentally disabled, transitioning from prison, or in any other need. He gathered women—deaconesses—to provide the care.

From **England**, Florence Nightingale (1820–1910) trained at Kaiserwerth and went to the Crimean War to care for British soldiers. Elizabeth Fry (1780–1845) started a prison ministry.

In the **United States**, immigrant churches imported the work of the deaconesses and Roman Catholic religious orders (1839–1889). Religious-based hospitals emerged.

Development of Nursing Standards and Education (1900–21st Century)

Nursing education has developed from the late 1800s when many hospitals established training programs to prepare nursing staff for their own institutions.

- These diploma programs varied based on the needs of the hospital, the availability of physicians and nurses for training students, and resources devoted to the training.
- It became apparent to many nurses that consistent minimum standards to practice across settings were necessary.
- These standards would provide for safety of the public and improve the mobility of nurses among institutions.
- Licensure became mandatory in all states in 1947.

In 1904 the first baccalaureate nursing program was established.

- Although a Bachelor of Science in Nursing (BSN) is not required for entry into professional nursing now, there has been a push for it to become the minimum degree for professional nursing since 1964.
- With coursework in nursing science, research, leadership, and nursing informatics, the BSN prepares nurses for professional roles. A BSN also provides the student with general education in math, humanities and social sciences.

In response to a nursing shortage after World War II, in 1952 associate degree programs were developed in community colleges. Currently the complexity of healthcare and acuity of patient needs are creating pressures on community colleges to join forces with universities to increase the percentage of baccalaureate-educated nurses.

Doctoral programs in nursing fall into two principle types: research-focused and practice-focused. Most research-focused programs grant the Doctor of Philosophy degree (PhD), while the practice-focused programs grant the Doctor of Nursing Practice (DNP).

Specialty certification occurs at the baccalaureate and advanced practice levels. The Health Ministry Association has been working with the American Nurses Association to seek certification for the specialty of faith community nursing.

OUTCOME 2

Analyze how the actions of Granger Westberg have contributed to the current conceptualization of faith community nursing.

Granger Westberg conceptualized parish nursing (later, **faith community nursing**) in the 1970s with the idea of **wholistic** care based on an understanding that a health care consumer is an

KEY TERM

A **faith community nurse** *is a registered professional nurse who is actively licensed in a given state and who promotes health as wholeness of the faith community, its groups, families, and individual members.*

KEY TERM

Wholistic *care is based on an understanding that a health care consumer is an interconnected unity of physical, mental, social, environmental, and spiritual factors.*

KEY TERM

Faith community nursing *is the specialized practice of professional nursing that focuses on the intentional care of the spirit as well as the promotion of wholistic health.*

"I realized that the nurse was the key member of the professional team" (Westberg, 1989, p. 27).

interconnected unity and that physical, mental, social, environmental, and spiritual factors need to be included in any interventions. The whole system, whether referring to a human being or a faith community, is greater than the sum of its parts. *Wholistic* is the preferred term when referring to the type of care provided by a **faith community nurse**.

A **faith community nurse** (FCN) is a registered professional nurse who is actively licensed in a given state and who serves as a member of the staff of a faith community.

- The FCN promotes health as wholeness of the faith community, its groups, families, and individual members through the practice of nursing as defined by that state's Nurse Practice Act in the jurisdiction in which the FCN practices.
- The FCN also adheres to the standards of practice set forth in the ANA/HMA *Faith Community Nursing: Scope and Standards of Practice* (2nd ed., 2012).

KEY TERM

Faith Community Nursing: Scope and Standards of Practice *(2nd ed., 2012) describes the unique scope of knowledge and professionalism for the specialty practice.*

Westberg's **first Wholistic Health Center** opened in Hinsdale, Illinois in 1973.

- Twelve more followed in diverse settings.
- Westberg observed the interactions of patients with the physician, chaplain, and nurse staff of the Wholistic Health Centers and realized the value of a nurse in the congregation.

Building on his observations and the historical roots of nursing, Westberg developed the parish nurse role.

- In 1983, Granger Westberg piloted parish nursing in Tucson, Arizona.
- By 1985, the model was adopted by Lutheran General Hospital (now Advocate Health Care) in Park Ridge, Illinois, where Westberg was working. Under the leadership of Rev. Larry Holst, the director of pastoral care at Lutheran General, the hospital sponsored a program with paid nurses in six churches representing multiple denominations.

Critical Thinking

What can the nurse learn from history and Granger Westberg's ideas that will assist in the development of a sound faith community nurse health ministry?

OUTCOME 3

Identify individual historic events that have contributed to the development of faith community nursing.

History of the International Parish Nurse Resource Center

Under the direction of Westberg, the **Parish Nurse Resource Center** and the **Health Ministries Association** were created.

In 1985, the **Parish Nurse Resource Center** began and was sponsored by Lutheran General Hospital (Advocate Health Care) under the direction of Ann Solari-Twadell.

In 1989, the **Health Ministries Association (HMA)** was created from the first Advisory Committee to the Parish Nurse Resource Center and incorporated as a nonprofit organization.

- The mission of the Health Ministries Association is to "encourage, support, and empower leaders in the integration of faith and health in local communities" (HMA website, 2014).
- Membership in HMA is open to faith community nurses, program coordinators, clergy, chaplains, faculty, lay health ministers, and health educators.
- The HMA sponsors a one-year mentor program for HMA members who have recently completed a Foundations of Faith Community Nursing course. For details, visit www.HMAssoc.org.

By 2002, the Parish Nurse Resource Center had become the **International Parish Nurse Resource Center (IPNRC)** and was sold to the Deaconess Foundation of St. Louis.

In 2011, the IPNRC joined ministry with the **Church Health Center** in Memphis, Tennessee.

"The Church Health Center cultivates relationships with individuals and congregations to encourage, educate, and equip people to build and sustain healing ministries. As an integral part of a healing ministry, faith community nursing is one of the best ways a congregation can promote health and wholeness. The mission of faith community nursing is the intentional integration of the practices of faith and nursing so that people can achieve wholeness in, with, and through the community of faith in which they serve" (Church Health Center website, 2014).

The Work of the IPNRC

The **IPNRC** provides education and resource support for faith community nurse coordinators. An FCN coordinator is an "RN who oversees, educates, and supports practicing faith community nurses while organizing, planning, and sustaining the viability of this health ministry within a congregation or a healthcare organization" (Church Health Center website, 2014).

Foundations of Faith Community Nursing Curriculum
One of the primary functions of the IPNRC is the development of the **Foundations of Faith Community Nursing Curriculum** based on the educational program originally designed by Westberg.
- The first basic preparation course was taught in 1991.
- The curriculum was published in 1997.
- The curriculum was revised in 2004, 2009, and 2014 to reflect the changing practice of faith community nursing.
- The Foundations of Faith Community Nursing curriculum is taught internationally by educational partners who offer coursework in their communities and online. For a complete listing, visit http://www.churchhealthcenter.org/findbystate.

World Forum
The IPNRC sponsors international faith community nursing through the mission of the World Forum, which promotes intentional care of the spirit by integrating faith and health in

KEY TERM
The **Health Ministries Association** *encourages, supports and empowers leaders in the integration of faith and health.*

Critical Thinking
How can you use the resources of the IPNRC, the HMA, and the Church Health Center to form your ministry as an FCN?

Critical Thinking
What impact does the development of the faith community nursing Scope and Standards of Practice and specialty certification have on your professional practice as a FCN?

wholistic nursing care locally, nationally, and internationally. Countries practicing faith community nursing in 2013 include: the United States, Australia, Bahamas, Canada, England, Ghana, Kenya, Korea, Madagascar, Malawi, Malaysia, New Zealand, Nigeria, Pakistan, Palestine, Scotland, Singapore, South Africa, Swaziland, Ukraine, Wales, Zambia and Zimbabwe.

Westberg Symposium

The IPNRC sponsors the Westberg Symposium annually. The first Westberg Symposium for parish nurses was held in 1987 with 74 participants attending. The 2014 Westberg Symposium had nearly 300 participants from the United States, Canada, Pakistan, Ukraine, and Australia.

Faith Community Nursing as a Specialty Practice

ASSUMPTIONS OF FAITH COMMUNITY NURSING

- *Health and illness are human experiences.*
- *Wholistic health integrates spiritual, physical, psychological, and social aspects of the health care consumer to create a sense of harmony with self, others, the environment, and a higher power.*
- *Health may be experienced in the presence of illness or injury.*
- *Healing is the process of integrating the body, mind, and spirit to create wholeness, health, and a sense of well-being, even when the health care consumer's illness is not cured. (ANA/HMA, 2012, p. 8)*

Faith community nursing was designated as a specialty practice by the American Nurses Association (ANA) in 1997.

- The *Scope and Standards of Parish Nursing Practice* was published in 1998 by the ANA in partnership with the HMA.
- In 2005, the standards were revised and the title changed to *Faith Community Nursing: Scope and Standards of Practice*, in order to accommodate all faith traditions and again in 2012 to reflect current practice.

The **American Nurses Credentialing Center (ANCC)** is working with HMA to develop a portfolio process for specialty recognition and eventually specialty certification for faith community nurses. According to the ANCC website, certification will be available beginning in 2014. Recognition and certification are optional and may also be available in some form from various religions and denominations. (http://www.nursecredentialing.org/FaithCommunityNursing)

OUTCOME 4

Relate the key aspects of the philosophy of faith community nursing practice to the development of a personal philosophy of this specialty practice.

Philosophy of Faith Community Nursing

Faith community nursing is a new specialty, but not a new concept.

Four major concepts comprise the **philosophy of faith community nursing**:

1. **Spiritual.** The intentional care of the spirit sets the specialty practice of faith community nursing apart from other types of nursing. Continuing personal spiritual formation is an

ongoing, essential component of practice and includes both self-care and hospitality, through opening the heart to self and others.

2. **Professionalism.** The specialty practice of faith community nursing reclaims the historic roots of professional nursing, recognizing that similar aspects of health and healing are found in many faith traditions.

3. **Wholistic.** The FCN views health as an ongoing, ever-changing process that includes multiple aspects of a person, including spiritual, physical, psychological, and social.
   - *Shalom* is harmony and wholeness regardless of circumstance and serves as a foundation for understanding health.
   - A sense of well-being can exist in the presence of imbalance, and healing can occur in the absence of a cure.

4. **Community.** Faith community nursing practice focuses on a faith community.
   - The FCN is a member of the staff and works in conjunction with clergy and congregation to provide opportunities for the ongoing transformation of the faith community into sources of health and healing.
   - Through partnership with other community health resources, faith community nursing fosters new and creative responses to health and wellness concerns.
   - FCNs appreciate that all persons are sacred and must be treated with respect and dignity.
   - The FCN serves the community of faith, creates safe and sacred places of healing and advocates with compassion, mercy, and dignity.

Implications for FCN Practice

Faith community nursing is designated as a specialty practice combining professional nursing and health ministry focusing on the intentional care of the spirit.

Preparation and Education

Specialty practice calls for additional educational preparation above the generalized education on spiritual care that is provided to all professional nurses as students.

- In addition to completing the Foundations of Faith Community Nursing course, ongoing continuing education is encouraged.
- Faith community nurses must be actively licensed registered nurses in the state in which they practice.
- Faith community nursing practice is regulated by the ANA's Scope and Standards of Practice for both registered nurses and faith community nurses, the nurse practice act of the state in which the nurse practices, the Nursing Code of Ethics,

Critical Thinking

How does the history and philosophy of faith community nursing apply to personal and professional spiritual care and development?

EDUCATION RECOMMENDATIONS FOR FCNS

Preferred baccalaureate or higher degree in nursing with academic preparation in community or population-focused nursing.

- *Experience as a registered nurse using the nursing process.*
- *Knowledge of the health care assets and resources of the community.*
- *Specialized knowledge of the spiritual beliefs and practices of the faith community.*
- *Knowledge and skills required to implement* Faith Community Nursing: Scope and Standards of Practice *(2nd ed., 2012, p. 11).*

and the policies established by the congregation or organization being served.

Actions and Tasks

The activities of the FCN are customized to meet the needs of those being served, but generally include:

- advocacy, education, and referrals for clients
- monitoring of the health and spiritual issues of clients
- providing emotional and spiritual support to clients and families
- actions derived from nursing diagnoses and assessments according to the Scope and Standards for registered nurses and faith community nurses
- any nursing care for which the nurse is licensed or has been declared competent to provide (If the nursing care is not a current skill of the nurse, then a referral to the appropriate caregiving service or emergency treatment is the appropriate action.)
- any care provided as a Good Samaritan in an emergency situation when other caregivers are not available

Actions and tasks that are *not* included in the FCN's scope of practice:

- treatments
- medications
- nursing care that must be directed or supervised by a physician's order; routine medical care that is the responsibility of agencies under the client's physician's direction such as home health and hospice

Standards of Professional Performance for Faith Community Nursing

The history and philosophy of faith community nursing provide the foundation to scope and standards of practice of faith community nursing.

Learning Activities

History and Philosophy of Health Care Ministry (Pre-class Assignment)

Instructions:
1. Choose a time period in history or a notable person in nursing history to research and read about. Prepare a short report including pictures, if applicable, to share with the other participants. Suggestions are found in Appendix A.
2. Visit the websites for the International Parish Nurse Resource Center (IPNRC), Health Ministry Association (HMA), Church Health Center, and your denomination, if applicable.
3. Begin preparing a personal philosophy of faith community nursing that you will further develop during the course.

Question:
What concepts are the strongest influences on your personal philosophy of faith community nursing?

Faith Community Nursing History

Instructions:
1. For this activity, assign participants to small groups and distribute books, articles, and other information related to the history of faith community nursing.
2. Designate 10 minutes for each group to create a presentation on one of the following topics: significant individuals in faith community nursing; significant events in faith community nursing; or significant research related to faith community nursing for the entire group. The presentation can be a report, a skit, or any other means of relating the history of their assigned topic.
3. Use the nursing history calendar for each day of your course to update the participants on historical nursing facts occurring on that date. See the following web site: http://www.aahn.org/nursinghistorycalendar.html

Question:
Which event or individual do you think most influenced the development of faith community nursing?

Group Roles

Instructions:
1. Break the group into small groups (or individuals if the class is small).
2. Assign each group to develop a list of potential actions or tasks and discuss how the listed items interact to provide wholistic care. Emphasize the importance of spirituality.
3. Provide poster paper and markers for each group. Encourage creative thinking for small groups or individuals to report to the group as a whole such as skit, dialogue, short story, or artistic interpretation.

Question:
Summarize how spirituality links the activities of an FCN.

Mind Map of Faith Community Nursing

Instructions:

1. Create a mind map with "Faith Community Nursing" in the center to encourage group assimilation of what the ministry might entail.

2. www.smartdraw.com offers a free download of mind mapping templates, or use a large poster board or white board.

3. Have the group brainstorm circles with words related to the roles, actions, or tasks of the FCN to connect and interconnect each circle.

4. Stop when the group is satisfied that each circle is connected.

Question:

What patterns do you see in the way parts of faith community nursing connect to each other?

Appendix A

Notable People in the History of Health and Healing

St. Marcella

St. Radegunde

St. Francis & St. Clare

Theodor Fliedner

St. Frances of Rome

Mother Mary Catherine McAuley

Florence Nightingale

St. Vincent de Paul

Dorothy Day

Knights of St. John

Dorothea Lynde Dix

Lillian Wald

Mary Brewster

Mary Adelaide Nutting

Deborah Patterson

St. Fabiola

St. Hildegard

Elizabeth Gurney Fry

St. Catherine of Siena

St. Helena

St. Francis de Sales

Clara Barton

Louisa May Alcott

May Ayres Burgess

Knights of St. Lazarus

Margaret Sanger

Minnie Goodnow

Mary Eliza Mahoney

Phyllis Ann Solari-Twadell

Granger Westberg

St. Paula

St. Matilda

St. Elisabeth of Hungary

St. Bridget of Sweden

Friederike Munster

Jeanne Mance

Mother Teresa

Dr. Anna Hamilton

Miss Annie Goodrich

Teutonic Knights

Mary Breckinridge

Linda Richards

Sojourner Truth

Jill Westberg

Appendix B
Time Line of Nursing History

Nursing History	Timeframe	General Historical Context
	Before Christ 6000	Earliest records.
	5000	Egyptian civilization.
	4000	Babylonian civilization.
	3000	Chinese civilization.
Deborah is identified as a nurse in the Old Testament book of Genesis.	1500	Early Greek civilization.
	1200	Veda of India and Persian sacred texts emerge.
	1100	Asclepius and early Greek medicine.
	900	Homer becomes a great Greek poet.
	700	Assyria is in power. Rome is founded.
	600	Chaldea is in power, followed by Persia. Buddhism is founded.
	500	Greece is the leader of the world. Confucius gains a following.
	400	The Golden Age of Greece and India.
	300	Egyptian civilization flourishes. Rome grows in power.
	250	King Asoka rules in India.
	150	Rome conquers Greece.
	55–51	Rome invades Britain (England) and Gaul (France).
	31 BC–14 AD	Caesar is emperor of Rome. Christ is born.
	Birth of Christ	
Phoebe is the first known deaconess.	1st century	Rome flourishes. Christianity begins.
	2nd century	Rome begins to decline.
	3rd century	Barbarians from the north invade the Roman Empire.

• Important Roman women take up nursing, hospital organization, and charitable work: Olympia, Macrina, Marcella, Fabiola, Paula, Helen, (mother of Constantine). St. Theodosia is skilled in medicine and surgery. • Emperor Constantine supports hospitals (300) • Fabiola opens a hospital in Rome (380).	4th century	Constantinople is the center of government, art and literature. Medicine declines.
	5th century	• Western Europe is Christianized. • Rome falls. • The Dark Ages begin. Art, literature and civilization decline. • The church becomes ascetic. • Mohammed founds a new religion. • Britain is Christianized.
• St. Hilda is Abbess of Whitby (614) • Hotel Dieu de Paris is oldest hospital in Paris. (650) • Benedictine monastery	7th century	• Monasteries increase greatly in number. • France, Italy and Spain become great powers.
	8th century	Arabs conquer Spain.
Early English hospitals form.	9th century	• Charlemagne comes to power. • Alfred is king in England. • Feudalism takes root in Europe. • Customs of knighthood form.
	10th century	• Constantinople becomes important center of art and commerce. • The church canonizes the first saints.
Knights of Lazarus form to care for men wounded in the Crusades.	11th century	• Spain is the seat of learning. • Popes enjoy a height of power. • The medical school at Salerno is prominent (1008). • The Normans conquer England (1066). • The Turks take Jerusalem from Christian control (1071). • The first Crusade begins (1095).
• Knights of St. John and Teutonic Knights form to care for men wounded in Crusades. • Hildegard, famous abbess • St. Clare nursing group (1100) • Second order of St. Francis • Benjines founded (1170) • St. Bartholomew's hospital opens in London.	12th century	• Commerce and industry flourish. • A middle class develops. • Some protest against church control. • The second and third Crusades occur.

	13th century	• Damascus, Alexandria and Baghdad become important centers. • Italy's great age of art and literature flourishes. • Marco Polo travels in Asia.
St. Catherine of Siena devotes herself to working with the poor and sick.	14th century	• Chaucer • Hundred Years War • The black death destroyed nearly half the population of Europe.
	15th century	• Feudalism declines. • Printing is invented. • Columbus and Vespucci explore the New World.
	16th century	• The Reformation ushers in the rise of Protestantism. • Henry VIII and Elizabeth rule in England. • Cortez conquers Mexico.
• Sisters of Charity in France (1600) • Revival of hospital nursing (1633) • Daughters of Charity is formed. • Augustinia Hotel Dieu in Quebec City, Canada (1639) • Jeanne Mance, Hotel Dieu in Montreal, Canada	17th century	• Colonists settle in the New World. • The Quakers become an important sect. • The great plague overtakes London. • The microscope is invented.
	18th century	• The Industrial Revolution begins with increased use of machinery. • The American Revolution separates the Colonies from England. • The French Revolution abolishes the monarchy. • John Wesley begins a movement that grows into Methodism.
	19th century	• Napoleon comes to power. • Missionary activity begins.
Sisters of Charity form in the US	1820	
Sisters of Mercy form in Dublin, Ireland	1831	
The Kaiserwerth School is founded in Germany to train nurses.	1836	
	1837	Victoria becomes Queen of England.
US imports work of deaconesses and Roman Catholic religious orders.	1838–1889	

Charles Dickens portrays Sairey Gamp as a nurse in his novel *Martin Chuzzlewit*.	1844	
	1846–1848	US goes to war against Mexico.
	1849	California and Australia experience gold rushes.
	1850	• Huge numbers of people emigrate to the US. • Missionary and temperance activity expand.
• The Pennsylvania Hospital is the first hospital in the US. • Florence Nightingale attends Kaiserwerth to train as a nurse.	1851	
Florence Nightingale nurses British soldiers at Scutari, Turkey.	1853–1856	Crimean War
The Florence Nightingale School of Nursing and Midwifery opens in St. Thomas Hospital, London	1860	
Dorothea Lynde Dix becomes superintendent of women nurses for all military hospitals.	1861	
	1861–1865	US Civil War
	1865	Japan opens to foreign trade.
	1870	Franco-Prussian war
• Linda Richards is the first trained nurse in the US. • Training School for Nurses attached to Bellevue Hospital opens, the first school in US to run according to Florence Nightingale's nursing principles.	1873	
Mary Mahoney is the first African American nurse to graduate from the New England Hospital for Women and Children in Boston.	1879	
Clara Barton establishes the Red Cross.	1881	
Lillian Wald and Mary Brewster establish Henry Street Settlement in New York.	1893	

The International Council of Nurses (ICN) is founded.	1899	
American Journal of Nursing publishes the first issue.	1900	
	20th century	
American Association of Nurses is established.	1911	
US Public Health Services is established.	1912	British passenger ship *Titanic* sinks in the North Atlantic.
	1914–1918	• World War I • Russian Revolution (1917)
Lavinia Dock writes much of the four-volume *The History of Nursing*	1921	
Sigma Theta Tau is founded. (In 1985 it becomes the International Honor Society for Nursing.)	1922	
The Goldmark Report criticizes inadequacies of hospital-based nursing schools and recommends increased educational standards.	1923	
	1929	US stock market crashes and Great Depression begins.
	1935	US Congress passes the Social Security Act.
	1937	War begins between China and Japan.
	1939–1945	World War II
The World Health Organization (WHO) is established.	1948	
Anna Cummings publishes a narrative, *In the Parish.*	1960	
	1950–1953	Korean War
	1954–1968	US civil rights movement is at its peak. Martin Luther King, Jr. is assassinated.
	1963	US President John Kennedy is assassinated.
	1969	US lands on the moon.
	1965	US Congress passes Medicare and Medicaid into law.

Journal of Christian Nursing launches.	1984	Indira Ghandi, prime minister of India, is assassinated.
Lutheran General Hospital pilots a parish nursing program.	1985	
The Parish Nurse Resource Center opens.	1986	Space shuttle *Challenger* explodes.
The first Westberg Symposium welcomes 74 participants.	1987	
	1989	The Berlin Wall comes down.
Granger Westberg publishes *The Parish Nurse.*	1990	
ANA designates parish nursing as a specialty practice.	1997	
Scope and Standards for Parish Nursing are established.	1998	
	21st century	
	2001	• Foreign terrorists attack US • US invades Afghanistan
	2003	Multinational invasion of Iraq
The IPNRC holds the first World Forum at the Westberg Symposium.	2004	
Faith Community Nursing: Scope and Standards of Practice (1st edition) is published.	2005	
	2010	US Congress passes Patient Protection and Affordable Care Act.
• IOM Report—*The Future of Nursing: Leading Change, Advancing Health* is released. • IPNRC becomes a ministry of the Church Health Center.	2011	• Coordinated multinational military operation begins in Somalia • Earthquake and killer tsunami strike Japan.
Faith Community Nursing: Scope and Standards of Practice goes into 2nd edition.	2012	

References

Required Textbook

American Nurses Association and Health Ministries Association. (2012). *Scope and standards of practice: Faith community nursing* (2nd ed.). Silver Spring, MD: Nursesbooks.org.

References

Bullough, V .L. & Bullough, B. (1960). The emergence of modern nursing (2nd ed). New York: MacMillan.

D'Antonio, P. (2010). *American Nursing: A history of knowledge, authority, and the meaning of work.* Baltimore: Johns Hopkins University Press.

Durbin, N. (2009). *Faith community nursing: Portfolio process.* Handout presented at a workshop, Dallas TX.

Ellis, J. & Hartley, C. (2012). *Nursing in today's world: Challenges, issues, and trends* (10th ed.). Philadelphia: Wolters Kluwer/Lippincott Williams & Wilkins.

Frank C. M. (1953). *The historical development of nursing.* Philadelphia: W. B. Saunders.

Jacob, S. (2013). The evolution of professional nursing. In Cherry, B. & Jacob, S. (Eds.). *Contemporary Nursing: Issues, trends, and management* (6th ed.). St Louis, MO: Mosby.

Koenig, H. (2011). *Spirituality and health research: Methods, measurement, statistics, and resources.* West Conshohocken, PA: Templeton Press.

O'Brien, M. E. (2003a). *Parish nursing: Healthcare ministry within the church.* Sudbury, MA: Jones and Bartlett.

O'Brien, M. E. (2003b). *Spirituality in nursing: Standing on holy ground* (2nd ed.). Sudbury, MA: Jones and Bartlett.

Patterson, D. L. (2003). *The essential parish nurse: ABCs for congregational health ministry* . Cleveland, Ohio: Pilgrim Press.

Scharen, C. & Vigen, A. (Eds.). (2011). *Ethnography as Christian theology and ethics.* London: Continuum International. p. 119.

Additional References

Davis, A. J. (2011). The charitable revolution: Why did the twelfth century bring a wave of new hospitals? *Christian History, 81,* 33–35.

D'Antonio, P. (2010). A*merican Nursing: A history of knowledge, authority, and the meaning of work.* Baltimore: John Hopkins University Press.

Hallett, C. (2010). *Celebrating Nurses: A visual history.* Hauppauge, NY: Barrons.

Hickman, J. (2006). *Faith community nursing.* New York, Lippincott Williams & Wilkins.

Hinton, S. (2013). *Preach, teach, and heal: Christian denominational administration of faith community nurse health ministry in the United States.* Unpublished Doctorate of Ministry Thesis, Saint Paul School of Theology: Kansas City, MO.

McNamara, J. W. (2014). *Stronger together: Starting a health team in your congregation.* Memphis, TN: Church Health Center.

Miller, T. S. (2011). From poorhouse to hospital: How the Christian hospital evolved from a house of charity that cared for the poor to the medical institution we know today. *Christian History, 82,* 16–23.

Morris, G.S., Miller, S. M. A new day for faith community nursing. *Journal of Christian Nursing 31*(2), 112–116. doi:10.1097/CNJ.0000000000000064

Peterson, W. (2002). *Granger Westberg verbatim: A Vision for faith and health.* St Louis: IPNRC.

Smucker, C., & Weinberg, L. (2009). *Faith community nursing: Developing a quality practice.* Silver Springs, MD: American Nurses Association.

Solari-Twadell, P. A. & McDermott, M., Eds. (2006). *Parish nursing: Development, education, and administration.* St Louis, Elsevier Mosby.

Tait, J. W. (2011). Healthcare and hospitals in the mission of the church. *Christian History, 81,* 18–19.

Westberg, G. (1990). *The parish nurse: Providing a minister of health for your congregation.* Minneapolis: Augsburg Press.

Online Resources

American Association for the History of Nursing: http:// www.aahn.org

Health Ministries Association: http://www.HMAssoc.org

International Parish Nurse Resource Center: http://www.churchhealthcenter.org/fcnhome

Religious and denominational websites

Wrap-Up and Evaluation

Measuring Competency

This chart can be used to assess the individual outcomes in this module.

- A copy of this chart is attached to the Participant Module, so that each participant can complete this short evaluation.
- Have participants read each outcome and then place an X in the box that best matches their opinion about the objective being met.
- Encourage each participant to write a short reflection about this module in the space provided at the bottom of this chart.
- Use this data to make any necessary changes.

Outcome	Not Met	Somewhat Met	Met
1. Describe how the history and philosophy of health care and nursing provide a spiritual foundation for faith community nursing.			
2. Analyze how the actions of Granger Westberg have contributed to the current conceptualization of faith community nursing.			
3. Identify historic events that have contributed to the continued development of faith community nursing.			
4. Relate the key aspects of the philosophy of faith community nursing practice to the development of a personal philosophy of this specialty practice.			
Reflection: *In one paragraph, write a reflection on this module.*			

Unit I: Spirituality
Health, Healing and Wholeness

Health, Healing and Wholeness

Introduction

Learning Outcomes

Upon completion of this module, the participant will be able to:

1. Examine historical concepts of health, healing and wholeness.
2. Examine theological/ conceptual perspectives that impact health, healing, and wholeness.
3. Examine the concepts of health, healing and wholeness from the perspectives of diverse faith traditions.
4. Integrate theological reflection into faith community nursing practice.
5. Use presence to promote health, healing, and wholeness in individuals, families, groups, and faith communities.

Description

Faith Community Nursing: Scope and Standards of Practice (2012, 2nd ed.) states that "healing, wholeness, and health are intricately connected and defined for the practice"(p. 55). This module examines historical and theological perspectives of health, healing, and wholeness from the perspective of diverse faith traditions. It also presents practices of theological reflection and presence.

Hours: 2.5–3

Research

A growing body of literature connects mind, body and spirit into the overall health and well-being of individuals. Koenig (2012) provides a comprehensive review of research on religion and spirituality and both mental health and physical health. "It is based on a systematic review of original data-based quantitative research published in peer-reviewed journals between 1872 and 2010, including a few seminal articles published since 2010. A large volume of research shows that people who are more Religious/ Spiritual (R/S) have better mental health and adapt more quickly to health problems compared to those who are less R/S. These possible benefits to mental health and well-being have physiological consequences that impact physical health, affect the risk of disease, and influence response to treatment" (p. 1).

Faith Tradition

Health, healing and wholeness are all part of the experience of living and worshipping in the Jewish tradition. In Bible times, daily routines included prayer and worship, keeping the laws, giving honor to God in thought and deed, and focusing upon life in the Promised Land. To be ill, to have sinned, or to be out of relationship with others or with God was to be separated from community—to be unclean. The unclean were not allowed in the temple and often were ostracized from the family and the community. To be healed not only meant physical or mental healing, but also being restored to community, including to the temple—spiritual healing. People sought the rabbi for counsel for body, mind and spirit. There was no delineation between treatment for body, mind and spirit as we now see in the Western world. To be whole meant being in right relationship to self, others, God, and the environment. From Judaism we get the concept of *shalom*, which means health, wholeness, harmony, and peace.

Key Terms

Healing: integrating body, mind and spirit to bring about an increase in wholeness, health, and sense of spiritual well-being (ANA/HMA, 2012, p. 55)

Health: the experience of wholeness, salvation or shalom (ANA/HMA, 2012, p. 55)

Presence: being with another, walking alongside another, traveling the person's journey

Theological reflection: discerning how God is present and involved in the situation (Bracke, 2013)

Wholeness: based on the understanding that a person is an interconnected unity and that physical, mental, social, environmental, and spiritual factors need to be included in any interventions (ANA/HMA, 2012, p. 58)

Reflection

"After this the Lord appointed seventy others and sent them on ahead of him in pairs to every town and place where he himself intended to go. ... Go on your way. See, I am sending you out like lambs into the midst of wolves. ... Whenever you enter a town and its people welcome you, eat what is set before you; cure the sick who are there, and say to them, 'The kingdom of God has come near to you.'"
—Luke 10:1, 3, 8–9

See Expanded Reflection *in the Learning Activities for deeper interactive reflection activity options.*

Health, Healing and Wholeness

Content Outline

OUTCOME 1
Examine historical concepts of health, healing, and wholeness.

Definitions of *Health, Healing and Wholeness*

Health

The World Health Organization (WHO) defines **health** as "complete state of physical, mental and social well-being and not merely the absence of disease." Health, including mental health, is related to the promotion of well-being, the prevention of (mental) disease and the treatment and rehabilitation of the disease process (http://www.who.int/topics/mental_health/en/).

A **medical model of care**, such as the American Medical Association, focuses on curing illness.

A **nursing perspective** offers three primary trains of thought.
1. Florence Nightingale said that health is to be free of disease and to be **able to use one's powers** to the fullest.
2. The American Holistic Nurses' definition of health states that health is the **harmonious balance** of body, mind, and spirit in an ever-changing environment.
3. *Faith Community Nursing: Scope and Standards of Practice* (2012, 2nd ed.) defines health as "the **experience of wholeness, salvation, or shalom**. The integration of the spiritual, physical, psychological, emotional, and social aspects of the healthcare consumer to create a sense of harmony with self, others, the environment, and higher power. Health may be experienced in the presence or absence of disease or injury" (p. 55).

From a **spiritual perspective**, faith traditions' definitions of healing, wholeness and health, and the faith community's role in healing, wholeness and health of its members often may be found on denominational or religious websites.
- "Physical health is not to be 'our chief end in this life,' only a possible byproduct of loving God and one's neighbor as oneself" (Westberg, 1999, p. 39).

- *Shalom* from the Old Testament is God's intention of health for the earth and its people; health, healing and wholeness in body-mind-spirit.

Healing

Faith Community Nursing: Scope and Standards of Practice (2012, 2nd ed.) defines **healing** as "the process of integrating the body, mind and spirit to bring about wholeness, health and sense of spiritual well-being, although the healthcare consumer's disease may not be cured" (p. 55).

Rev. Frederick W. Reklau gives the following "14 Theses on Healing (and Cure)," which delineates the difference between cure and healing from a Christian perspective.

1. Cure may occur without healing; healing may occur without cure.
2. Cure separates body from soul; healing embraces the whole. (Cure looks at what sort of disease a person has; healing looks at what sort of person has the disease—*derived from Hippocrates.* Cure categorizes; healing individualizes. Cure addresses disease; healing addresses illness.)
3. Cure isolates; healing incorporates. (Cure is technical; healing is relational.)
4. Cure costs; healing enhances.
5. Cure combats illness; healing fosters wellness. (Cure fixes; healing corrects. Cure is reactive; healing is proactive.)
6. Cure fosters function; healing fosters purpose.
7. Cure alters what is; healing offers what might be. (Cure controls; healing frees.)
8. Cure is an act; healing is a process. (Cure closes the past; healing opens the future. Cure is a goal; healing is a quest. Cure seeks to change reality; healing embraces reality. Cure takes charge; healing takes time.)
9. Cure acts upon another; healing shares with a sister, a brother. (Cure speaks; healing listens. Cure is produced by power; healing grows from surrender.)
10. Cure manages; healing touches. (Cure depends on dispassionate skill; healing depends on compassionate care.)
11. Cure seeks to conquer pain; healing seeks to transcend pain. (Cure is taunted by suffering; healing is taught by suffering.)
12. Cure ignores grief; healing assumes grief.
13. Cure encounters mystery as a challenge for understanding; healing encounters mystery as a channel for meaning. (Cure often issues from fear; healing usually issues from faith.)
14. Cure rejects death and views it as a defeat; healing includes death among the blessed outcomes of care.

Wholeness

Faith Community Nursing: Scope and Standards of Practice (2012, 2nd ed.) states that **wholeness** is "based on the understanding that a person is an interconnected unity and that physical, mental, social, environmental and spiritual factors need to be

> *"Physical health is not to be 'our chief end in this life,' only a possible byproduct of loving God and one's neighbor as oneself."*
> —Granger Westberg

KEY TERM

Healing *is integrating the body, mind and spirit to bring about an increase in wholeness, health, and sense of spiritual well-being.*

KEY TERM

Wholeness *is based on the understanding that a person is an interconnected unity and that physical, mental, social, environmental, and spiritual factors need to be included in any interventions* included in any interventions" (p. 58). Linguistically, Middle Eastern languages support this view of wholeness.

Salim, from the Arabic verb *salima*, which means "to be in peace, experience wholeness, state of well-being," includes most fundamentally a right relationship with God. Arabic speakers express the idea of "causing" such a right relationship by modifying the verb root *s-l-m* into *aslama*, whose noun form is *islam*, the condition of surrender to the fact that God is God and we are not. One who achieves this condition is a *muslim*, one who surrenders to God and is therefore in a state of wholeness, health, well-being.

The same *s-l-m* root is also at the heart of the Hebrew word *shalom*, which carries a similar meaning for a vision of the wholeness God intends for humans to experience. This word appears in the Old Testament more than 250 times, describing not only a spiritual connection to God, but a life of bodily health, contentedness, and social relationships.

Historical Perspectives

Before the Common Era, approaches to health and healing included these features:
- often relied on cultural and contextual spiritual practices for healing
- focused on relationships between creation and others
- used items from the local area to provide natural remedies
- often isolated ill people from the community

After the life and death of Christ, **Christians** ministered to the sick as an expression of God's love.

The **early church** ministered to the whole person. Family, community and faith were important concepts.

During the **Middle Ages**, the church and state increasingly functioned as one, and expressions of Christian care, such as hospitals, came into the mainstream. Monks offered herbal remedies along with spiritual care. Migrations and wars, such as the Crusades, precipitated better systems of care for the wounded, ill, and poor.

In the **seventeenth century**, philosopher René Descartes reintroduced Plato's ideas that the mind could know truth apart from the body. In the **eighteenth and nineteenth centuries**, an increase in the knowledge of anatomy and understanding of the human body bolstered the rise of medicine, further dividing spirit from body. At the same time, major religions experienced a proliferation of sects. The general separation of religious leaders from science contributed to division of care for the body and spirit.

In the **twentieth century**, technology rapidly advanced the knowledge of physiology. Care of the body resided with the health care system, and care of the spirit was the work of the faith community.

The **twenty-first century** has brought a swing back toward integrating faith and health. Faith communities are increasingly involved in promoting health and wholeness, with higher levels of individual responsibility for self-care.

OUTCOME 2

Examine theological/conceptual perspectives that impact health, healing, and wholeness.

Ideas About God

Humans have two ways of thinking about God. First is the **God concept**, which is intellectual in nature and formed by reason. Second is the **God image**, which is subjective, emotional and spiritual. The God image comes from within and outside the faith community.

The God concept:
- is central to how a person experiences and understands self, God and healing.
- is multifaceted and serves as a primary entry point into understanding one's relationship with God.
- must be understood by the FCN in order to interact appropriately.

These are common images of God.
- God is loving, caring, and compassionate. Words often used for this image are *shepherd*, *father*, *mother*.
- God is judgmental, distant, and critical. Words often used for this image are *judge* and *master*.
- God is *healer* and *creator*. These images acknowledge a wholeness of creation and that all creation is broken and in need of healing. Right relationships play a part in healing.
- Ideas about God may be fluid or stagnant over a lifetime, depending on experiences.

Thinking about God includes thinking about how humans relate to God and each other.
- Humankind and creation are defined by mortality and limits.
- Humans are creatures; we are not God.
- Both the Old Testament and the New Testament include passages about suffering and the need for healing, which ultimately comes from God.
- Humans bear the image of God (*imago Dei*). The Genesis account says that after commanding the earth to bring forth living creatures of every kind, God created humans in God's image and blessed them (Genesis 1:24–28). Humans reflect God's glory, and human worth is rooted in being made in God's image.
- Bearing God's image, humans live in community. Humans are relational, creative, and purposeful beings, just as God is relational, creative, and purposeful.

Critical Thinking
What is your personal definition of health?

Are there models in your community of health care that integrate faith and health? If so, describe these models.

Critical Thinking

How does the way you think about God affect your perspective on health, healing, and wholeness?

How does the FCN help connect being created in the image of God to a deeper understanding of wholeness?

- Communities of faith express these dimensions of the image of God through connection with each other, hospitality that welcomes others into the community, and an ethic of mutuality in the pursuit of wholeness. Right relationships play a part in healing.

Affirming the **goodness of God** in the midst of life, even in times of suffering, bears on attitudes toward health, healing and wholeness.

- The dynamics of joy encompass receiving both awfulness and awe-fullness in religious experience.
- When he sent the Pilgrims off on the Mayflower, Puritan pastor John Robinson said, "God has yet more light and truth to break forth out of his holy Word."
- A spiritual life of health and wholeness means living in a way that expresses this truth.
- Hope is grounded in God.
- God's *shalom* embodies peace, balance, well-being and harmony.

OUTCOME 3

Examine the concepts of health, healing and wholeness from the perspectives of diverse faith traditions.

Each faith tradition has particular beliefs, traditions, customs, rituals and prayers related to health, illness, healing and being in or returning to full right relationship with a higher power or community.

Places of worship include, but are not limited to:
- church
- assembly
- hall
- synagogue or temple
- tabernacle
- mosque
- shrine

The role of the FCN in health, healing, and wholeness includes the following thoughts.
1. The FCN promotes life, health and wholeness.
2. The FCN recognizes pain and suffering, along with the implications of stoicism.
3. The FCN promotes touch or avoidance of touch, as appropriate.
4. The FCN facilitates physical support, arranging care of family, home, pets, work, working fields, financial support in times of crisis.
5. The FCN arranges social supports, such as meals, child care, transportation.
6. The FCN provides emotional support, presence, visiting the sick, being present when individuals are near death.

7. The FCN participates in prayers, both formal and informal and in multiple settings.
8. The FCN provides healing services of anointing.

A faith community may use a variety of approaches to develop and implement a ministry of health, healing and wholeness.

- The role of the faith community in promoting health, healing and wholeness is exemplified by worship, service, disciplines of the faith, and belonging or relationships within the community.
- Depending on the faith tradition, transformation and salvation can be seen through baptism, repentance and forgiveness, or other rites, rituals and sacraments expressing a spiritual dimension of healing and wholeness.

The **beliefs of various faith traditions influence views on health and healing**. FCNs will benefit from basic information about topics such as prayers and practices related to illness, sin, forgiveness, pain and suffering, dying and death, and life after death.

Judaism

Judaism is the religion of the Jewish people with around **14 million individuals** (http://www.adherents.com/Religions_By_Adherents.html). It is one of the first recorded monotheistic faiths and one of the oldest religious traditions still practiced today. The values and history of the Jewish people are a major part of the foundation of other Abrahamic religions such as Christianity, Islam, and Bahá'ism.

Though monotheistic in theology, Judaism has seldom, if ever, been monolithic in practice. It differs from many religions in that its central authority is not vested in any person or group, but rather in its writings and traditions.

- Despite its variations, Judaism has remained tightly bound to a number of religious principles, the most important of which is the belief in a single, omnipotent, omnibenevolent, transcendent God, who created the universe and continues to be involved in its governance.
- According to traditional Jewish thought, the God who created the world established a covenant with the Jewish people, and revealed his laws and commandments to them in the form of the Torah.
- The practice of Judaism is devoted to the study and observance of these laws and commandments, as written in the Tanach (the Hebrew Bible), Talmud interpretations of the Torah, and the commentaries that followed throughout history.

Related to health, healing and wholeness, Judaic beliefs include:
- a mandate to heal
- God favors good over evil, life over death

HELPFUL RESOURCE

See also Appendix B, Prayers for Health and Healing from the Jewish Tradition.

- *mitzvah* (plural: *mitzvoth*) is a commandment, an obligation, a meritorious deed, a divine commandment
  - *pikkuah nefesh*, religious obligation to protect life or health
  - preservation of life and health is a mitzvah of highest order
- prayers for healing body and soul
- the Mitzvah of Bikkur Holim includes:
  - visiting the sick
  - taking away pain
  - sustaining one on one's sickbed
  - extends to non-Jews as well as Jews
- healing prayers include *Mi Sheberach, Aruch HaSchulchan* and *Amidah.*
- key themes surrounding *Mi Sheberach*
  - praise to God who has blessed us
  - send blessing on the sick ones
  - have mercy and restore to health and strength those who are sick
  - implore same for others who are stricken
  - grant the sick a complete recovery
  - may healing come speedily (For more information, see http://jewishhealing.org/aboutjh.html.)

Christianity

Christianity is a monotheistic religion centered on the life and teachings of Jesus of Nazareth as recounted in the New Testament. Christians believe Jesus to be the Jewish Messiah of the Old Testament, and thus refer to him as Jesus Christ.

With an estimated **2.18 billion adherents**, Christianity is the world's largest religion (http://www.pewforum.org/2011/12/19/ global-christianity-exec/ offers statistics on the world's Christians).

Christianity began in the first century as a Jewish sect and therefore shares many religious texts and early history with Judaism, specifically, the Hebrew Bible, which Christians call the Old Testament.

- Christianity is considered an Abrahamic religion, along with Judaism and Islam.
- The majority of Christians consider Jesus to be the incarnate Son of God.

Within Christianity, numerous distinct groups have developed with beliefs that vary widely by culture and place. Since the Reformation, Christianity is usually represented as being divided into three main branches.

- The **Roman Catholic Church** is the largest single body, with 50.1 percent of the world's Christians.
- **Eastern Christianity** represents Oriental Orthodox Churches, the Assyrian Church of the East, and the Eastern Orthodox

Churches (including Western Orthodox churches which preserve Latin practices while accepting Orthodox theology). Eastern Christianity includes 11.9 percent of Christians.
- **Protestantism.** Anglicans, Lutherans, Reformed, Evangelical, Charismatic, Presbyterians, Baptists, Methodists, Nazarenes, Anabaptists, Pentecostals, and others account for 36.7 percent of Christians. The oldest of these separated from the Roman Catholic Church in the sixteenth century Protestant Reformation, followed in many cases by further divisions. Some Protestants identify themselves simply as Christians, or "born-again" Christians. Others, particularly among Anglicans and Lutherans, identify themselves as being "*both* Catholic *and* Protestant."

Other denominations and churches, which self-identify as Christian but distance themselves from the above classifications, are 1.3 percent of Christians.
- African indigenous churches
- The Church of Jesus Christ of Latter-day Saints (also called Mormons)
- Jehovah's Witnesses

Traditional **Christian beliefs** and practices related to health, healing, and wholeness include:
- Scriptures include the Old Testament and New Testament, which teach the restoring love of God for all people.
- Every person is created in the image of God and is valuable to God.
- Jesus is the Son of God. The four gospels are accounts of Jesus' life. Jesus came to bring the healing kingdom of God.
- Jesus' life and teachings about love and fellowship are the basis of human relationships, including health, healing and wholeness.
- Sunday (Sabbath) commemorates the resurrection of Jesus and his defeat of death. It is a day of rest, worship, and sacraments to connect humans to God.
- Jesus prepared his disciples to be healing agents to carry on the work of God's kingdom.
- New Testament key concepts include illness and healing, disease and curing, and forgiveness as healing.
- Christian Scriptures encourage healing ministries, including prayer and anointing with oil.

HELPFUL RESOURCE
See Appendix C, Prayer for Health and Healing from the Christian Tradition.

Islam

Islam is a monotheistic religion founded by Muhammad with a sacred text known as the Qur'an. With approximately **1.57 billion adherents**, it is the world's second largest religion (http://www.pewforum.org/2009/10/07/mapping-the-global-muslim-population/).
- Followers of Islam are known as Muslims.

HELPFUL RESOURCE

See Appendix D, Prayers for Health and Healing from the Islamic Tradition.

- Muslims believe that God (Allah) revealed his word to humanity through many earlier prophets, and that Muhammad was the final prophet.
- Muslims believe the core message of Islam, which is submission to God, has been the essential message in the teaching of all God's prophets.
- The faith went through a period of rapid expansion after Muhammad's death in the seventh century, and its followers can be found all over the world today.

Islam beliefs include:
- There is one God, Allah.
- The Prophet, Muhammad, received revelations from God and recorded them in the Qur'an, the holy text of Islam.
- Muslims observe the Five Pillars.
  - *Shahadah*—profession of faith with prayers
  - *Salat*—ritual prayers
  - *Zakat*—using wealth to care for the poor
  - *Sawm Ramada*—month-long fast to cultivate patience and commitment
  - *Hajj*—a pilgrimage to Mecca at least once
- Humans face a judgment day and life after death.
- *Jihad* is the internal or external ways of striving or struggling and enduring hardship to do the will of Allah.
- Since life is a gift from Allah, disease, pain and suffering are manifestations of God's will. Pain and suffering are part of expiating sin.

HELPFUL RESOURCE

A helpful website for understanding world religions is www.pluralism.org/religion, part of the Pluralism Project of Harvard University

Like Judaism and Christianity, **Islam has multiple branches**. Upon the death of Muhammad, dispute arose about successors.
- The **Sunni** believed that Muhammad gave the community authority to choose its leaders. Today about 85 percent of the world's Muslims are Sunni.
- The **Shi'a** believed that Muhammad chose Ali, his cousin and son-in-law, to lead. Future leaders would descend from Ali and his wife, Fatimah. Most of the 15 percent of Muslims who are not Sunni belong to the Shi'a branch and come from the region of Iran and Iraq (http://pluralism.org/religion).

Hinduism

The roots of Hinduism date back 5,000 years. Hinduism is the third largest religion in the world with approximately **one billion adherents**. The majority live in India or adjacent countries, and there are about two million in the United States (http://www.mamandram.org/tools/world-hindu-population.html).

Hinduism includes numerous schools of thought and has no single governing organization, no identified founder, and no single sacred text. The Four Vedas, from around 1400 to 900 BC, are the earliest sacred literature of Hinduism.

Hindu **beliefs and practices** include the following.
- Virtually all Hindus believe there is only one God, or Divine, which is infinite, incomprehensible, formless and nameless, although Hindus give it a name so as to be able to refer to it—Brahman. The plurality of gods usually associated with Hinduism must be understood in relation to the one God or one Reality.
- Hindus relate to God through worship and devotion. Individuals typically choose one or more forms for their particular focus but understand many manifestations of God are real. Some Hindus prefer to relate to God through meditation rather than worship. Hindus believe each person is entitled to his or her own relationship with God, and that all faiths can lead to God.
- God creates and continually sustains the universe within itself, so God is neither distant nor even separate from us; therefore, everyone and everything is sacred.
- Hindus have a code of conduct in *dharma*. The ten essential rules for observance of dharma are: patience, forgiveness, piety or self-control, honesty, control of senses, reason, knowledge or learning, truthfulness, absence of anger and sanctity.
- God has given humans life in order that we may learn to dissolve away our sense of separation from God and attain release from the cycle of rebirth. We are given as many lifetimes as it takes to accomplish this, and all of us will do so. Death is only the end of a chapter of a long book that always has a happy ending.
- Rebirths are governed by the system of karma, whereby people reap what they sow. Each action has a consequence. We may be reborn into a heavenly or hellish realm, but those are temporary conditions. Karma determines much of what we experience, but not everything.
- Pain and suffering are seen as a result of past actions. Future lives are influenced by how one faces illness, disability, or death. Liberation from the cycle of rebirth and redeath is the goal of existence.
- Some believe in faith healing; others believe that illness is God's punishment for sins.
- Prayer for health is considered a low form of prayer; stoicism is preferable.

Buddhism

Buddhism is a religion and philosophy focusing on the teachings of the Shakyamuni Buddha (Siddhartha Gautama), who probably lived in the fifth century BC. Buddhism spread throughout the ancient Indian subcontinent in the five centuries following the Buddha's death, and propagated into Central, Southeast, and East Asia over the next two millennia.

Today, Buddhism is divided into **three primary traditions**: Theravada, Mahayana, and Vajrayana. Buddhism continues to

CHARTER OF COMPASSION

"The Charter for Compassion is a cooperative effort to restore not only compassionate thinking but, more importantly, compassionate action to the center of religious, moral and political life. Compassion is the principled determination to put ourselves in the shoes of the other, and lies at the heart of all religious and ethical systems" (http://charterforcompassion. org/the-charter#sthash.shmxsZB8.dpuf).

The Charter for Compassion is a document that transcends religious, ideological, and national differences. Supported by leading thinkers from many traditions, the Charter activates the Golden Rule around the world. It is translated into 30 languages and is based on Karen Armstrong's book Twelve Steps to a Compassionate Life *(2010). Over 80 cities have adopted the charter in an effort to bring wholeness to their communities. See Appendix F for more information.*

Critical Thinking

What challenges do you face in providing spiritual care to individuals from diverse faith communities?

Do you think your community would be interested in the Charter of Compassion? Why or why not?

attract followers worldwide, and, with **488 million adherents**, it is considered a major world religion (http://www.pewforum. org/2012/12/18/global-religious-landscape-buddhist/).

A **Buddha** is considered to be a person who discovers the true nature of reality through years of study and investigation of the various religious practices of his time and meditation.
- This transformational discovery is called *bodhi* or "enlightenment."
- Any person who has, without the instruction of others, become awakened to the principles of the dharma, or the truth of what the Buddha taught, is called a Buddha.
- The Shakyamuni Buddha is said to have been only the latest of many of these; there were other Buddhas before him and there will be others in the future.

- According to the Buddha, any person can follow his example and become enlightened through the study of his words and putting them into practice, by leading a virtuous, moral life, and purifying his mind.
- In general, the aim of Buddhist practice is to end all kinds of suffering in life; people suffer because they always want more.
- Siddhartha Gautama, the Buddha, believed that life is unsatisfactory when conditioned by a mind full of greed, hatred and delusion. An unclear mind produces suffering and bad karma, leading to repeated rebirths in unsatisfactory worlds.
- Buddhism has Four Noble Truths.
  - Life is suffering.
  - Suffering is due to grasping and desire.
  - There is a way out.
  - The way is the Eightfold Path.
- One transcends this existence through the Eightfold Path.
  - right understanding
  - right thought
  - right speech
  - right action
  - right livelihood
  - right effort
  - right mindfulness
  - right concentration
- Illness is the result of karma (law of cause and effect), an inevitable consequence of actions in this or a previous life. Healing and recovery are promoted by awakening to the wisdom of Buddha, which results in spiritual peace and freedom from anxiety.

OUTCOME 4

Integrate theological reflection into faith community nursing practice.

Theological reflection is discerning how God is present and involved in a situation. It is a process by which we explore how God is present in our experience so that we are able to be hearts that beat God's presence with another human being. It helps the work of the FCN stay focused on God and the work of the spirit in spiritual care (Bracke, 2013).

Core questions for the work of the FCN include:
- What is the church or faith community?
- What is the ministry?
- What is the ministry of the FCN?
- What is health or healing?
- What is the good or right thing to do in this situation?

How one answers these questions depends on how one answers the core questions about God or Jesus.

Here is one **four-step process** for theological reflection.

1. **Develop a clear case on which to reflect and discover**. The best cases are recent and involve FCNs. Most of the FCN's work is messy and complex, so spend some time becoming clear about the complexity of the situation. This is sometimes referred to as the "thickness" or "messiness" of the situation.

2. **Examine the situation using the acronym VOTER** (Browning, 1996).
   - **V—Vision.** Discern the big picture concerns in the situation: What is the vision of health? The vision of the church? The vision of the FCN? The vision of a hospital or even the vision or image of God?
   - **O—Obligations.** How do the people in this situation understand the obligations of themselves, others and you? For instance, someone who views God as all-powerful might imagine God has an obligation to cure a son's cancer. Or if you view an FCN as a patient's advocate, then you have an obligation to speak up when you think a patient is not receiving the best care available.
   - **T—Tendency or Need.** What do you and others involved in the situation need? For instance, someone being told bad news may tend to go into denial. Or someone who feels threatened may tend to strike back verbally, if not physically. Or someone losing something important (a loved one to death, independence, or some ability) will likely grieve the loss.
   - **E—Environmental or Social.** In what context does this occur? For instance, for one situation you might ask if there is a stable family environment, or is it significantly dysfunctional? In other situations, you might ask about

KEY TERM

Theological reflection *is discerning how God is present and involved in a situation.*

See the Self-Care Module for more on reflection.

the community support services available. Or you might ask about the congregational context and what the faith community is willing or able to do.

- **R—Rules or Roles.** This is about how those involved in a situation understand the rules of the game. These are often expressed as "should" or "ought to." *The spiritual leader should come visit me. You should be willing to go to the pharmacy to pick up my prescriptions. A good doctor would come to my house.* Usually behind the articulation of such spoken or unspoken rules is a vision and sense of obligation.

At the end of the reflection about the complexity of the situation, think about questions like these.
- What is going on here really?
- What are the issues?
- What are the conflicts and tensions in this situation?
- Do you have a better understanding of what is bothering you about the situation? About the issues you need to address spiritually with the person or persons?

3. **Discern how you see God is present in the situation.** Begin thinking about who God is and what God is doing. For instance, here are two readily identifiable ways to reflect on God's activity.

God disrupts order. God turns things topsy-turvy. It seems that God is putting an end to what has been, so there can be a new beginning. The way things have been seem to stand in God's way or frustrate God's purpose, and God will not tolerate the status quo any longer.
- Examples of this way of envisioning God are found in the stories of the flood, the Exodus, and Israel's exile to Babylon in Hebrew Scriptures.
- In the New Testament, we see disruption in Jesus' proclamation of God's coming reign, Jesus' confrontation with the religious leaders of his time, or Paul's reflection on everyone being a new creature in Christ with the ministry of reconciliation (2 Corinthians 5).
- In this model, God is the One who saves, liberates and redeems.

God establishes order. In this way of thinking of God, God brings order to chaos and establishes zones of safety and security in the world. Where the world seems chaotic, and where life seems impossible, God brings order and works toward well-being.
- Examples of seeing God as establishing order are the stories of creation, David, Solomon, and many of the Psalms (such as Psalm 23) in the Hebrew Scriptures.
- In the New Testament we see a new order in Jesus' Beatitudes (in the Gospels of Luke or Matthew), the stilling of the storm (Mark 4 and parallel passages), or Paul's assurance

---

Critical Thinking

What is your experience with theological reflection?

How can the FCN's theological reflection enhance provision of spiritual care that promotes health, healing and wholeness?

that nothing can separate us from God's love (Romans 8:31 and following).

God may act in different ways in different situations.

- Sometimes God's judgment is that order needs to be disrupted because the way things are will not further God's purposes.
- At other times, God's judgment is that God's world purposes will be better served if order is restored and conditions of safety and security prevail.
- While a new creation, a new heaven and new earth, and peace in all the cosmos seem to be God's ultimate end, to move toward that end, it seems that God finds it necessary to disrupt things. Most of us do not like to imagine God doing this, but God's acting in this way is the central claim of the scriptural witness.

In some situations it is also important to **ask how others think of God** or Jesus.

- Sometimes there is conflict in a situation because people have different understandings of God or Jesus, or of the church, or of what serving God involves.
- When you discern that the root of the conflict is a theological disagreement, it is important to try to understand how those involved in the conflict understand these matters differently.
- However, you should not expect that people in such a conflict will explicitly articulate their views of God, Jesus or other theological issues. You may have to discern what is implicit and what is explicit as you uncover the heart of the matter.

4. **Draw a conclusion.**
   Think through these questions.
   - What is the overall view of this situation and what is going on?
   - What is the FCN's role in this situation?
   - What needs to be done next in this situation?
   - What are the issues of faith and health related to this situation?
   - How might you want or need to be in your role as an FCN in this situation?
   - What did I learn that will change this situation or similar situation next time?

OUTCOME 5

Use presence to promote health, healing, and wholeness in individuals, families, groups, and faith communities.

Presence is being with another, walking alongside another, traveling the person's journey.

OUTCOMES OF THEOLOGICAL REFLECTION

The desired outcomes of theological reflection are:
1. *Deeper awareness of God's presence in our daily lives.*
2. *Deeper acceptance of an individual's human freedom, acceptance of others' values and beliefs, and believing that true presence will enhance quality of life.*
3. *Cultivation of a belief and practice that respects human-universe interconnections to provide healing.*

KEY TERM

Presence *is being with another, walking alongside another, traveling the person's journey.*

HELPFUL RESOURCE

See Appendix E, Presence: The Heart of Faith Community Nursing.

HELPFUL RESOURCE

See the Communication and Collaboration Module and Spiritual Care Module for more on a ministry of presence.

Critical Thinking

What challenges does the FCN face in providing presence to individuals and groups in the faith community?

Compare and contrast your comfort level with providing health teaching to an individual diagnosed with diabetes and providing presence for an individual with a terminal illness.

- Parse (1999) defined *presence* as being with another and valuing the other's human dignity and freedom to choose within situations. Her theory is called Human Becoming Theory.
- Borysenko (1987) defined *presence* as "holy moments" where you stop *doing* as a professional and are just *being* with another human being. You travel with the person on a journey, with respect, not judgment. You love and appreciate the person for where he or she has been and who he or she is at this moment.

Presence and active listening are distinct concepts.
- Active listening includes paying attention, showing you are listening, providing feedback, deferring judgment and responding appropriately.
- Margaret Wheatley (2009, p. 92–94) says, "One of the easiest human acts is also the most healing—listening to someone. Simply listening. Not advising or coaching, but silently and fully listening. ... Our natural state is to be together. Though we keep moving away from each other, we haven't lost the need to be in relationship. Everybody has a story, and everybody wants to tell their story in order to connect. If no one listens, we tell it to ourselves and then we go mad. In the English language, the word for *health* comes from the same root word as *whole*. We cannot be healthy if we are not in relationship. And whole is from the same root word as *holy*. Listening moves us closer, it helps us become more whole, healthier, and more holy."

Standards of Professional Performance for Faith Community Nursing

The FCN must have specialized knowledge of the spiritual beliefs and practices of the faith community in order to focus on intentional care of the spirit in promoting health, healing, and wholeness. However, there is no specific professional standard designated for health, healing, and wholeness.

Learning Activities

Expanded Reflection

Instructions:
1. Choose Option 1 or Option 2 for an expanded reflection time at the beginning of the module.
2. Read the selected passage.
3. Use the points or questions provided to guide the discussion of the passage.

Questions:
1. What is your favorite healing story from the Bible and why?
2. How would you like to experience God's healing in your life in the future?

Option 1
Read Luke 10:1–11, where Jesus sends out pairs to preach the good news and heal the sick. Make these points.
1. We must take to heart what Jesus thinks about healing and do what Jesus did, including healing.
2. Healing announces the kingdom of God (Luke 10:9).
3. In the book of Acts, early church stories are full of healing.
4. Jesus calls us to care about what he cares about.
5. Wellness is a pursuit of the wholeness God wants for us.

Option 2
Select one of the Hebrew Bible passages about healing listed in Appendix A to read aloud. Then for one minute, sit in quiet reflection. Ask participants to offer a word or phrase that struck them in this reading (no explanations needed). Then read the selection again. Allow one minute of silent reflection. Ask again for a word or a phrase that struck them. As this response wanes, consider asking one or more of the following questions.
1. What is happening in this reading?
2. Describe the situation from the viewpoint of each of the characters. What does each character want or hope to gain? What is the obstacle? Who can or does help?
3. What kind of healing is evidenced?
4. What is the role of the faith community in this story?
5. Where is God in all this?

Creative Art of Health, Healing and Wholeness

Instructions:
1. Provide white paper, markers, colored pencils, magazines, scissors, glue sticks and tape.
2. After introducing the concepts of health, healing and wholeness, ask: What image comes to mind when you think of those words?
3. Encourage the participants to use the art supplies to make a picture, and then share in a small group.

Question:
What insight about health, healing and wholeness is coming into focus for you?

Exploring Images of God

Instructions:
1. Ask participants to form small groups.

2. Assign various Scripture passages on healing from Appendix A.

3. Ask participants to explore the stories and consider the impact of ways of thinking of God. With which way of thinking about God do they resonate? Which one bothers them or seems strange to them? What effect would it have on their care of others if they have the image of God as judge? Or of God as love?

Question:
How does a person's or a community's way of thinking about God affect an understanding of healing, health and wholeness?

Faith Traditions Panel Discussion or Role-Play

Instructions:
1. Consider having a panel of three spiritual leaders representing diverse faith traditions, such as Muslim, Jewish and Christian.

2. Or, assign the participants into small groups and ask them to role-play the following situations.

1. You are an FCN who is going to visit an elderly woman from a Protestant congregation who has entered hospice. Prior to your arrival at the home, her son has called to tell you that his sister and her husband, who are practicing Muslims, have arrived from Iran. How do you include them in your care? How will you be sensitive to their beliefs? Have one participant be the elderly woman, another the daughter, another the son-in-law, and one the FCN.

2. A young woman in a Catholic faith community just had a baby. The family gathered at the hospital to celebrate the birth. The young woman's in-laws are Jewish. The FCN makes a visit. Have one participant be the young woman, another her husband, two participants the in-laws, and one the FCN.

3. You are the FCN who is active with the interfaith circle that helped the community adopt the *Charter of Compassion* (see Appendix F). The group is planning a health and wholeness program to address the needs of the youth in the community. Have each participant represent his or her own faith community as you plan a program on health issues for youth for the greater community, which has diverse faith traditions. The group can choose one health issue to address.

Case Studies for Theological Reflection

Instructions:
1. Read aloud one or both of the following case studies about discovering the process of theological reflection, combining perceptions about God, and God's activity.

2. Ask participants to form small groups and discuss the questions that follow the case.

CASE 1
Joe

This case was provided by Rev. Dr. John Bracke, retired professor of Old Testament Studies at Eden Seminary, St. Louis, Missouri.

Joe is a member of St. Mark's Church where I serve as the FCN. I met Joe—a spry, small, friendly man in his eighties—in passing at the church on a few occasions. Sometimes he would have me take his blood pressure at the faith community's coffee hour, which I do on the first Sunday of each month. Joe joked with me and engaged in casual conversation. About five weeks ago, Joe was hospitalized with serious heart problems that finally resulted in open heart surgery to replace a defective valve. The pastoral staff called on him in the hospital, and I also visited him regularly.

Joe's recovery from surgery was much slower than expected, and the hospital staff was not sure why. Some days he would seem to be doing well—eating, walking the hall with some assistance, lucid, and in good spirits. But on other days, he was lethargic, ate little, refused to walk, and even groused about getting up to sit in a chair. Unfortunately, Joe's ups and downs continued as the time for his discharge approached.

Joe was a widower. His wife of 50 years died three years earlier. Joe had two adult children, but neither lived in the vicinity. His son had flown to town at the time of Joe's surgery but had to return to his home after a few days. His daughter then arrived but could only stay 48 hours. I met them both; they seemed to be nice folks who cared for their father. Joe lived in a modest home not far from his faith community. I never had occasion to visit Joe in his home, but the spiritual leaders had. They described the home as relatively well kept, but of a design that had the bedrooms on one level, the kitchen and living areas on another, and the laundry on a third. It did not seem likely to the spiritual leaders that Joe could live in his home, even with assistance, given his condition. From their description of the situation, I concurred.

As the time for Joe's discharge approached, the hospital staff was very concerned about his living arrangements after his discharge. The hospital social worker told Joe his medical team thought he must go to a rehabilitation facility for at least a period of recuperation and therapy to see if he could regain his strength. After hearing this, Joe insisted with some vehemence that he wanted to go home. During one visit with me, he said he "would rather die than go to one of those homes." The nursing staff had heard him say something similar. The last time I visited Joe in the hospital, the nurse caring for Joe informed me that the decision had been made that Joe would be transferred to a rehabilitation facility. The hospital social worker was in contact with Joe's children, who agreed to this plan. The nurse also indicated that after some time for rehabilitation, another decision would need to be made—whether Joe would be able to return home or if he would need long-term care.

While there was clarity about the next steps in Joe's treatment, neither of his children were able to come to town to help with the transition. Each talked to Joe on the phone but met the same resistance Joe had been expressing. When the spiritual leader called the children to discuss the situation, it was agreed that on the day of Joe's transfer, I and the one spiritual leader whom Joe liked a great deal would be at the hospital and then follow up with Joe at the rehabilitation facility within a few days.

As I write this, Joe has been in the facility almost three weeks. I called on him there the day after his transfer and have had two subsequent visits; the spiritual leader has also seen him three times. We have both had the same experience in our visits. Joe seems, if anything, weaker and probably regressing. He complains of fatigue, is not eating well, is withdrawn, and when not withdrawn is angry. The health care team thinks he will likely need to go back to the hospital soon for further evaluation. They are becoming increasingly concerned. Joe is very discouraged about his progress and very down. Even worse for me, however, is that Joe blames me (and the spiritual leader) for why he could not go home. He said to me that he thought I was his friend and on his side, but now he knows I was a traitor who conspired with the spiritual leader, the hospital staff, and his children to "put him away." He told the spiritual leader something similar. Together the spiritual leader and I have called both the son and daughter, who plan on coming to town in the next few days to confer with the medical staff of the facility about their father's condition. They hope they will be able to calm their father down. The spiritual leader and I have made Joe's children aware that their father blames both us and them for his being in the rehabilitation facility.

However, I'm mostly concerned about how I can minister to Joe now. I think my visits upset him more than comfort him. He is clearly angry with me.

Discussion questions:
1. Did I handle this situation well?

2. Might I have done something differently?

3. At this time, I don't think that I represent the caring and healing presence of God for Joe as he struggles with his health issues. What role, if any, can I (and the spiritual leader, who also feels badly about this situation) play in Joe's continuing care?

CASE 2
Maggie

The FCN visits Maggie, a 65-year-old woman who recently had a successful hip replacement. The surgery went well without complications. Maggie is on some new medications; she is not able to say what they are or what they are for, but she does say that they do help her with her blood and bowels. She lives alone, except for her cat, Max, who has been her constant companion for the nine years since her husband died. Her two children, a son and daughter, live out of town but keep in contact with her by phone and visits. She has been active in her faith community for a number of years, singing in the choir, helping with meals served to families at wakes, and being a part of the women's group.

Now she is staying at Rest Haven Rehabilitation and Nursing Home until she is able to navigate the stairs in her house and take care of herself at home. During the FCN's visit, Maggie cries, saying she has not seen Max since before the surgery 20 days ago. She is anxious about not being able to go back to her part-time job in a card shop. She says she is staying awake at night worrying over these issues.

Maggie tells you that she feels lonely. She says that she misses her faith community and her friends there. She has been praying and using her daily devotional guide as she has done for years. However, now she says she realizes that her relationship with God could be stronger. She expresses a desire to deepen her relationship and learn meditation. She says, "I know God loves me, and I know that God is with me, but how do I know what God's will is for me now at this time?"

Discussion questions:
1. What are some problems the FCNs see and hear from Maggie?
2. What would be your plan for her?
3. What spiritual understandings can help the FCN in providing care for Maggie?

Experiencing Presence

Instructions:
1. Have participants pair up.
2. Ask one partner to relate an experience to the other. This can be any experience, based on the preference of the speaker. The second partner should not speak, but only offer presence.
3. Then the second partner relates an experience while the first offers presence.
4. Have each person reflect on experiencing the presence of the other.

Questions:
1. How did the person give you comfort?
2. What actions by the person were helpful?
3. How will practicing presence impact your ministry?

References

Required Textbook

American Nurses Association and Health Ministries Association. (2012). *Faith community nursing: Scope and standards of practice*. (2nd ed.). Silver Spring, MD: Nursesbooks.org.

References

Armstrong, K. (2011). *Twelve steps to a compassionate life*. New York, NY: Anchor Books.

Borysenko, J. (1987). *Minding the body, mending the mind*. Reading, MA: Addison-Wesley.

Browning, D. (1996). *Fundamental practical theology: Descriptive and strategic proposal*. Minneapolis, MN: Fortress Press.

Chase-Ziolek, M. (2005). *Health, healing & wholeness: Engaging congregations in ministries of health*. Cleveland, OH: Pilgrim Press.

George, L. K., Larson, D. B., Koenig, H. G., McCullough, M. E. (2000). Spirituality and health: What we know, what we need to know. *Journal of Social and Clinical Psychology 19*, 102–116.

Hickman, J. (2006). Holistic health and the faith community. In *Faith community nursing*. Philadelphia: Lippincott Williams & Wilkins.

Holtz, K. and Matthews, M. (2012). *Dust and breath: Faith, health and why the church should care about both*. Grand Rapids, MI: William B. Eerdmans.

Koenig, H. (2008). *Medicine, religion and health: Where science and spirituality meet*. West Conshohocken PA: Templeton Science and Religion series.

Koenig, H. (2012). Religion, spirituality, and health: The research and clinical implications. *ISRN Psychiatry, 2012*, 1–33. doi:10.5402/2012/278730

Morris, G. Scott and Miller, S. (2013). *Faith and health in the Bible*. Memphis TN: Church Health Center.

Parse, R. R. (1999). *Illuminations: The human becoming theory in practice and research*. Sudbury, MA: Jones and Bartlett.

Reklau, F. (1993) *Thesis on Healing (and Cure)*. Winfield, IL.

Westberg, G. (1999) A personal historical perspective. In Solari-Twadell, P. A. and McDermott, M. A. (Eds.). *Parish nursing: Promoting whole person health within faith communities* (pp. 35–41). Thousand Oaks, CA: Sage Publications.

Wheatley, M. (2009) *Turning to one another: Simple conversations to restore hope in the future*. San Francisco: Berrett-Koehler.

Additional References

Chase-Ziolek, M., & Holst, L. E. (1999). Parish nursing in diverse traditions. In P. Solari-Twadell & M. McDermott (Eds.). *Parish nursing: Promoting whole health within faith communities*. Thousand Oaks, CA: Sage Publications.

Chase-Ziolek, M. & Iris, M. (2002). Nurses' perceptions on the distinctive aspects of providing nursing care in a congregational setting. *Journal of Community Health Nursing, 19*, 173–186.

Delgado, C. (2005). A discussion of the concept of spirituality. *Nursing Science Quarterly, 18*(2), 157–162.

Eiberg, A. Eight possible ways in which prayer may "work." In *NCJH Training Manual for Bikkur Cholim*. New York: UJA Federation of New York. www.ncjh.org/downloads/PrayerEightWays.doc

Flam, N., Offel, J. and Eiberg, A. Acts of loving kindness. In *NCJH Training Manual for Bikkur Cholim*. New York: UJA Federation of New York. Available at www.ncjh.org/downloads/BikurWhatIs.doc

Freeman, D. L., & Abrams, J. Z. (Eds.). (1999). *Illness and health in the Jewish tradition: Writings from the Bible today*. Philadelphia: Jewish Publishing Society.

George, L. K., Larson, D. B., Koenig, H. G., McCullough, M. E. (2000). Spirituality and health: What we know, what we need to know. *Journal of Social and Clinical Psychology 19*:102–116.

Johnston Taylor, E. (2006). Spiritual formation for the ministry of parish nursing practice. In Solari-Twadell, P. A. & McDermott, M. A. (Eds.). *Parish nursing: Development, education, and administration* (pp. 37–51). St. Louis, MO: Elsevier Mosby.

Koenig, H. G., McCullough, M. E., & Larson, D. B. (2001). *Handbook of religion and health*. New York, NY: Oxford University Press.

Koenig, H. G., King, D. E., & Carson, V. B. (2012). A history of religion, medicine, and healthcare. In *Handbook of Religion and Health* (2nd ed.). New York, NY: Oxford University Press.

Macrae, J. (1995). Nightingale's spiritual philosophy and its significance for modern nursing. *Image: Journal of Professional Nursing Scholarship 27*, 8–10.

Martin, J. P. (1989). Eastern spirituality and health care. In Carson, V. B., *Spiritual dimensions of nursing practice*. Philadelphia: W. B. Saunders.

Morriarty, G. and Hoffman, L. (Eds.) (2008) *God image handbook for spiritual counseling and psychotherapy: Research, theory and practice (monographic separates from the Journal of Spirituality and Mental Health)*. Routledge, UK: Taylor and Francis.

O'Brien, M. E. (2008). *A sacred covenant: The spiritual ministry of nursing*. Sudbury, MA: Jones and Bartlett.

Parse, R. R. (1990). Parse's research methodology with an illustration of the lived experience of hope. *Nursing Science Quarterly, 3*, 9–17.

Parse, R. R. (1992). Human becoming: Parse's theory of nursing. *Nursing Science Quarterly, 5*, 35–42.

Peterson, W. M. (Ed.) (1982). *Granger Westberg verbatim: A vision for faith & health*. St. Louis, MO: International Parish Nurse Resource Center.

Reklau, F. (2010). *Partners in care: Medicine and ministry together*. Wipf & Stock.

Sasso, S. (1994) *In God's Name*. Woodstock, VT: Jewish Light.

Shelly, J. and Miller, A. (2006). *Called to care: A Christian theology of nursing*. Downers Grove, IL: InterVarsity Press.

Smith, H. (1994) *The illustrated guide to the world's religions: A guide to our wisdom traditions*. New York, NY: Harper Collins.

Stone, H. and Duke, J. (2013) *How to think theologically* (3rd. ed.). Minneapolis, MN: Fortress Press.

Vandecreek, L. & Mooney, S. (Eds.). (2002). *Parish nurses, health care chaplains, and community clergy: Navigating the maze of professional relationships.* New York: Haworth. Sections I–III, pp. 1–112.

Way, P. (2005) *Created by God: Pastoral care for all of God's people.* St. Louis, MO: Chalice Press.

Westberg, G. (1987). *The parish nurse: How to start a parish nurse program in your church.* Park Ridge, IL: International Parish Nurse Resource Center.

Wylie, L. J. & Solari-Twadell, P. A. (1999). Health and the congregation. In Solari-Twadell, P. A. & McDermott, M. A. (Eds.). *Parish nursing: Promoting whole person health within faith communities* (pp. 25–33). Thousand Oaks, CA: Sage Publications.

Online Resources:

Check your denomination's website for perspectives on healing, health, wholeness, shalom and salvation.

Bible Gateway: BibleGateway.com: a site that allows you to download the NET Bible for free
http://www.myfreebible.org/

CAIR (Council on American-Islamic Relations) Research Center, *A Health Care Provider's Guide to Islamic Religious Practices*:
https://virtuecenter.s3.amazonaws.com/files/2013-02-19-14/health_care_guide.pdf

Music: http://www.shainanoll.com/music/songs-for-the-inner-child/

National Center for Jewish Healing: www.jbfcs.org/NCJH

Religious Beliefs and Healthcare Decisions:
http://www.advocatehealth.com/beliefs

World Council of Churches: http://www.oikoumene.org/en

World Health Organization: http://www.who.int

Youtube—short videos on faith traditions: http://www.youtube.com/results?search_query=Faith+traditions

Wrap-Up and Evaluation

Measuring Competency

This chart can be used to assess the individual outcomes in this module.

- A copy of this chart is attached to the Participant Module, so that each participant can complete this short evaluation.
- Have participants read each outcome and then place an X in the box that best matches their opinion about the objective being met.
- Encourage each participant to write a short reflection about this module in the space provided at the bottom of this chart.
- Use this data to make any necessary changes.

Outcome	Not Met	Somewhat Met	Met
1. Examine historical concepts of health, healing and wholeness.			
2. Examine theological/conceptual perspectives that impact health, healing, and wholeness.			
3. Examine the concepts of health, healing and wholeness from the perspectives of diverse faith traditions.			
4. Integrate theological reflection into faith community nursing practice.			
5. Use presence to promote health, healing, and wholeness in individuals, families, groups, and faith communities.			
Reflection: *In one paragraph, write a reflection on this module.*			

Appendix A

Scriptures of Healing from the Hebrew Bible and the Christian New Testament

Part 1: Stories of Healing

HEBREW BIBLE

"I am the Lord who heals …":
Exodus 15:26

God forgives and restores:
Isaiah 57:18; 58:8

Infertility healed:
Genesis 18:11–14; 21:1–2; 20:17–18; 25:21; 30:22–23

Widow's son revived:
1 Kings 17:17–24

Shunammite boy raised:
2 Kings 4:28–37

Naaman's leprosy healed:
2 Kings 5:1–19

Hezekiah's life extended:
2 Kings 20:1–11

Hezekiah prays for healing of the people:
2 Chronicles 30:16–23

Psalmist asks God for healing:
Psalm 30:2; 103:3; 107:18–20; 147:3

God's words are healing:
Proverbs 3:7–8; 4:20–22

Calls for national healing:
2 Chronicles 7:13–14; Hosea 6:1

CHRISTIAN NEW TESTAMENT

Jesus' ministry of healing to crowds:
Mark 1:29–34; Luke 4:44, 6:17–19

Jesus heals "many":
Matthew 4:24–25, 12:15–16, 14:34–36, 15:29–31; Mark 3:7–12, 6:53–56; Luke 4:38–41; John 6:22–25

People with leprosy:
Matthew 8:1–4; Mark 1:40–45; Luke 5:12–16, 17:11–19

Peter's mother-in-law:
Matthew 8:14–15; Mark 1:29–31; Luke 4:38–39

Various diseases:
Matthew 8:16–17; Mark 1:32–34; Luke 4:40–41

Man possessed by demons:
Matthew 9:32–34; Mark 5:1–20; Luke 8:26–39

Man with paralysis:
Matthew 9:1–8; Mark 2:1–12; Luke 5:17–26; John 5:1–9

Jairus's daughter:
Matthew 9:18–19, 23–26; Mark 5:21–34; Luke 8:40–56

Hemorrhaging woman:
Matthew 9:20–22

People who were blind:
Matthew 9:27–31, 20:29–34; Mark 8:22–26, 10:46–52; Luke 18:35–43; John 9:1–41

Individuals who were mute:
Matthew 9:32–34, 12:22–24; Mark 7:31–35; Luke 11:14

Man with a withered hand:
Matthew 12:9–14; Mark 3:1–6; Luke 6:1–11

Canaanite woman:
Matthew 15:21–28; Mark 7:24–30

Man who was deaf:
Mark 7:31–37

Boy with a demon:
Matthew 17:14–21; Mark 9:14–29; Luke 9:37–43

Widow's son:
Luke 7:11–17

Woman unable to stand:
Luke 13:10–17

Man with dropsy:
Luke 14:1–6

Man who could not walk:
John 5:2–27

Lazarus raised:
John 11:1–44

Man begging at temple:
Acts 3:1–10

Apostles heal "many":
Acts 5:12–16

Peter heals Aeneas with paralysis:
Acts 9:32–34

Peter restores Tabitha:
Acts 9:36–40

Paul heals on the island of Malta:
Acts 28:7–9

Paul's healing prayer:
1 Thessalonians 5:23–34

Anointing for healing:
James 5:13–16

Part 2: Passages that Shape Healing Ministry

HEBREW BIBLE

Created in God's image:
Genesis 1:26; 2:7

Answer God's call in time of need:
Esther 4:1–17

Find God in stillness:
Psalm 46:10

God's healing wholeness:
Isaiah 58:6–9; 61:1–3

"Here I am. Send me."
Isaiah 6:8–9

The weary renew their strength:
Isaiah 40:31

Caring for those in need:
Ezekiel 34:1–4

CHRISTIAN NEW TESTAMENT

Salt and light to the world:
Matthew 5:13–16

Abundant life:
John 10:10

Commission to heal the sick:
Matthew 10:5–8; Mark 3:15, 6:7–13; Luke 9:1–2, 10:1–9

True rest:
Matthew 11:28–29

Where two or three are gathered:
Matthew 18:19–20

Love for God, neighbor and self:
Matthew 19:19, 22:39; Mark 12: 31–33; Luke 10: 27–29

Parable of the Good Samaritan:
Luke 10:29–37

Laying on hands for prayer:
James 5:13–16

Health in body and spirit:
3 John 2

Creation redeemed:
Revelation 21:1, 3–5; 22:1–2

Appendix B

Prayers for Health and Healing from the Jewish Tradition

The Eternal will deliver him in the day of evil
The Eternal preserve him and keep him alive, let him be called happy
    in the land;
And you will not deliver him unto the greed of his enemies.
The Eternal will support him upon his bed of illness
May you turn all his lying down in his sickness.

Heal us O Lord and we shall be healed, save us and we shall be saved;
for You are our praise. Grant a complete healing for all our wounds; for
You are God, the Sovereign, the faithful and compassionate Healer.
Blessed are You O Lord, Who heals the sick of the people Israel (Talmud.
Avodah Zarah 8; Brachot 34).

May it be your will, O Lord my God and God of my ancestors, that You
send quickly a complete healing from the heavens. May it be a cure of
both soul and body for this ill one, _____ son/daughter
of _____ among all the other sick of Israel (from *Mishnah
Brurah*).

May the One who blessed our forefathers Abraham, Isaac, and Jacob,
and our foremothers Sarah, Rebecca, Rachel, and Leah, bless and heal
this person, _____ the son/daughter of _____. May
the Holy One, blessed be God, be merciful and strengthen and heal
him/her. Grant him/her a complete and speedy recovery—healing of
body and healing of soul. And let us say: Amen (*Mi SheBerackh* prayer).

Blessed are You, Lord our God, Ruler of the Universe, who has formed
the human being with wisdom, and has created in us a multitude of
openings and cavities.
    It is obvious and known before Your glorious Throne that if but one
of these were open [that should be closed], or one were closed [that
should be open], we would be unable to stay alive and stand before
You. Blessed are You, who heals all flesh and does wonders (*Asher Yatzar*
prayer).

Appendix C

Prayer for Health and Healing from the Christian Tradition

Health and Well Being

To you, O Lord God,
covered by the splendor of light and
alone worthy of our adoration,
we, the people, lift our petitions.
Congratulations, Lord,
for your most magnificent creation: the human body.

And Lord have mercy when it starts to fall apart.
Over the years we come to realize that
every faculty we enjoy,
every disease we don't have,
and every miracle we assume will recur
in body and mind
become incredible blessings once they are threatened.
The truth is, our health has been so good
we forget to thank you for it.
So when the stresses and strains of life overtake us,
our Father,
or accident, diseases, or a thousand things,
it is then we are startled and ask for explanations.
Actually, we don't need explanations, Lord,

since we remember the good old days,
nothing less than miracles will do.
First and foremost we petition you
for the nearness of Jesus
who helped people care about themselves
as much as He did.

We especially commend to your Son, Christ the Healer,
those ravaged by pain
and fighting for life, at home, and in hospitals.

We ask for the miracle of new sight
to see matters differently,
a new flame in the heart to keep hope burning,
and the miracle of wisdom
to know what to hope for.

We ask for the miracle of ministry,
so that we attend to another's aches and pains
before our own are cured.

We ask for the miracle of a sense of humor,
so that we can regale friends with our symptoms
without boring them to death.
We ask for the miracle of courage and willpower
so that we don't accept death
one minute before its time.

And lastly we pray for the miracle of breath and Spirit;
I pray that you, Holy Spirit, will move
gently as a breeze
among us just now.

Breathe into the dust of our being
the breath of life again.
Through Christ our Lord, Amen.

Robert James St. Clair, Prayers for People Like Me
(Berkley, CA: BIBAL Press, 1989)

Appendix D

Prayers for Health and Healing from the Islamic Tradition

FROM THE QUR'AN
Prayer on bearing difficulty
On no soul does God place a burden greater than it can bear. Each gets every good that it earns and suffers every ill that it earns. Pray: Our Lord, Condemn us not if we are heedless or fall into error. Our Lord, Lay not on us a burden like that which you did lay on those before us. Our Lord, Lay not on us a burden greater than we have the strength to bear. Blot out our sins and grant us your forgiveness. Have mercy on us, you who are our Protector (Qur'an 2:286).

Prayer attributed to Abraham
Lord, grant me wisdom and associate me with the upright. Grant me a reputation for truthfulness among my descendants. Make me among those who inherit the Garden of Delight. Forgive my father [for his idolatry], for he has been among those who have gone astray. Do not put me down on the day of Resurrection, the day when neither riches nor prosperity will be of any use except for those who come before you with a sincere heart (Qur'an 26:83–89).

Prayer attributed to Moses
Lord, expand the core of my being for me and make my life's mission easy for me. Untie the knot in my tongue that they may understand what I say. Appoint me an assistant from among my people, my brother Aaron, to accompany me in my mission, that together we might give you glory and be ever-mindful of you; for you are aware of us at all times (Qur'an 20:25–35).

PRAYERS ATTRIBUTED TO MUHAMMAD
When visiting the sick
Banish this illness, O Lord of humankind, and bring healing, for it is You who heal. Apart from your healing there is no healing, a healing that leaves no trace of illness.

Say: I seek refuge in the Lord of Daybreak from the evil of what He has fashioned, from the evil of darkness when it envelops, from the evil of those who engage in consorting with evil, and from the evil of the envious one when his jealousy is manifest (Citing Qur'an chapters 113 and 114).

Say: I seek refuge in the Lord of humankind, the King of humankind, the God of humankind, from the evil of the conniving tempter who insinuates suggestions into the hearts of humankind …

In the name of God, may the dust of our land mingled with saliva heal the patient with our Lord's permission.

In the name of God, I seek refuge in the efficacy and power of God from the fearful evil of what I discover in myself. (Repeat seven times.)

In the name of God, I proclaim you protected from whatever might harm you, from the harm any being might bring … May God heal you. In the name of God I proclaim you protected.

I entrust you to the perfect words of God from every evil.

I implore God the Magnificent, Lord of the Splendid Throne, to bring you healing.

Our Lord who are in Heaven, may your name be sanctified. Yours is the command both in heaven and on earth. As your mercy prevails in heaven, so let your mercy prevail on earth. Forgive us our sins and shortcomings. Send down mercy from your mercy and healing from your healing for this ailment.

O God, allow me to live, so long as life is better for me, and let me die when death is best for me.

Prayers for gifts and blessings

O God, please see how I implore from you goodness through your knowledge, capability through your power, and blessing from your endless generosity. Indeed, it is you who are all-powerful, not I; it is you who know, not I, for you have full knowledge of all that is hidden to me.

O God, if in your knowledge what I ask is for the good of my faith, my sustenance, and for the outcome of my life, then please make it so for me, make it easy for me, and bless me with it. But if in your knowledge, what I ask is injurious to my faith, my sustenance, and for the outcome of my life, then deflect it from me and me from it. Make my lot only the good and let me be content with that.

Glory to God, Lord of the Universe. I implore from you all that leads to securing your mercy and pardon, benefits of every act of uprightness, and protection from every sinful deed. Leave no sin of mine unforgiven, no anxiety unrelieved, and no pleasing deed unfulfilled, O you who are the most merciful of any who show mercy.

When death approaches

Behold, we are God's and to God do we return. O God, reward me in my suffering and grant me a gift greater than this suffering.

O God, forgive [add name] and elevate his/her condition among those who are truly guided. Let one of his/her survivors fill his/her place after he/she is gone. Lord of the Universe, forgive us and him/her, and make his/her place of repose spacious and illumined. [A response to the Islamic tradition that part of the suffering of death is the experience of the "construction of the grave."]

Adapted and revised by John Renard, SJ (Professor of Theological Studies, St. Louis University, from the Arabic texts included in Farid, A. H. (1974 repr.). Prayers of Muhammad. *Lahore: Sh. Muhammad Ashraf.*

Appendix E

Presence: The Heart of Faith Community Nursing
By Randi Friedl

Faith community nursing is a highly visible way for churches to develop collaborative partnerships with other health care institutions and play an instrumental role in promoting health, healing, and wholeness among the congregation and the community. The faith community nursing movement has exceeded all expectations, as this is a deep "calling" for the faith community nurse. The discernment is very real as registered nurses go deep into their souls to practice this ministry. Using key elements of both the faith community nursing practice and the "Human Becoming Theory" by Rosemarie Rizzo Parse, presence is infused into the core of the faith community nursing curriculum. Joan Borysenko (1987) described presence as "holy moments" where you stop *doing* as a professional and are just *being* with another human being. You travel with the person on the journey, respect the person and do not judge, and love and appreciate where he or she has been and who the person is at this moment. **Presence** is defined by Parse as being with another and valuing the other's human dignity and freedom to choose within situations.

Background on Presence
Now in the twenty-first century, national attention has been directed toward the crisis in the health care system. Lack of access to primary care, spiraling health care costs, the expanding elderly population, and the refocus from disease care to true health care is beginning to gain attention. Health education and health promotion are being noticed as many now are not going to their primary care doctors due to no insurance or lack of coverage. Many elective surgeries are being delayed. People's choices have had to change due to the financial crises many are in and also the lack of understanding in this nation to reflect the reality of individuals' needs. Presence is not a tool, but an art of traveling with others and assisting them in both healing and wholeness.

For the discipline of faith community nursing to advance, it must continue to build a scientific knowledge base. It is this knowledge base that guides the human-human process and separates faith community nursing from other health-related disciplines. Human-human means a human-to-human relationship in the human-human process. Parse (1992) stated that nurses who value the Human Becoming Theory live the theory of true presence with others. Faith community nurses who develop skills in using presence are more likely to come to the practice arena comfortable with themselves, humble and competent, and available to all persons of different faith backgrounds, as there is no judgment. Presence is available to us at all times in being with another human. As the network of faith community nursing grows, the public will become more aware of the uniqueness in the discipline of faith community nursing.

Parse's Human Becoming Theory
Rosemarie Rizzo Parse's Human Becoming Theory is a set of beliefs and values concerning the human-universe-health process that is lived moment to moment. According to Parse (1992), "Humans are viewed as open beings co-created, becoming with the universe, recognized by patterns, and freely choosing between situations" (p. 36). This theory is grounded in the belief that each individual is an expert in his or her own life.

Wholeness: Experiencing a physical crisis can have great value to an individual if approached as a learning experience about oneself and what the body is trying to teach the person having a form of disease. Engebretson (1996) explained that the Western medical tradition in its dualistic approach has stripped illness of its meaning and context, leaving behind only clinical descriptions of disease.

One of the primary functions of religion is to provide explanatory models of life's purpose and meaning. As the faith community nurse continues to educate on wholeness, the patient can then be a conduit to educate the health care system and begin to be a voice for themselves and their families. Wholeness is defined as the harmonious functioning of a person's body, mind and spirit (Djupe et al., 1990).

Granger Westberg (1987) stated that the chief ingredient that either keeps people well or makes them sick, is a person's outlook on life, which is basically his or her "faith stance." To eliminate this chief ingredient from the discussion of a person's health is to do that person a disservice. Thus, faith community nurses must be advocates for wholeness.

Human Becoming Theory: Parse (1992) identified the goal of nursing as the quality of life as perceived by the person. Since there is no specific or expected outcome, and since human interrelationships are not predictable, each person must be guided by his/her values. According to the Human Becoming Theory, nursing practice is guided by a theoretical foundation that states the human is a free agent and meaning giver, choosing rhythmical patterns of relating while reaching for personal hopes and dreams.

The Human Becoming Theory is composed of three dimensions which occur all at once in practice:

1. Illuminating meaning: This process explores the personal meanings people give to their experiences.
2. Synchronizing rhythms: This process involves the human-human dwelling with the situation and the nurse going with the person as he/she uncovers new meanings.
3. Mobilizing transcendence: This process occurs when their hopes and dreams move with them (Parse, 1987).

Bunkers and Putnam (1995) explored the relationship between faith community nursing and Parse's Human Becoming Theory. They developed a nursing theory based on a model of health ministry entitled, "Living Parse's Theory of Human Becoming in the Parish Community." In their model, Bunkers and Putnam compared the eight beatitudes to Parse's Human Becoming Theory. By weaving together constructs from theology and nursing, they created a conceptual framework through which further research can be conducted.

Quality of Life: According to the Human Becoming theory, the focus of nursing is the lived experience of the person and quality of life from the person's perspective. Parse (1994) stated that the most valuable conclusion to be drawn from all the research is that the quality of life cannot be quantified. Parse dared ask the question, "Who can judge the quality of one's life?" (p.16).

The essence of life differs from one person to another; therefore, Parse answers her own question by stating that the quality of life can be judged only by the person living the life.

Presence: It is by being truly present with the person, listening to what the person has to say or not to say, and traveling with the person on the journey which makes a difference in their quality of life. True presence as practiced by the faith community nurse means making oneself available in an authentic way to the human (Parse, 1994). Presence is defined as an attentive, loving "being with" another, and a "valuing of the other's human dignity and freedom to choose within situations" (Parse, 1995).

Parse (1990) explained that during presence the nurse approached the person and family as a nurturing gardener rather than a "fix it" mechanic. Experiencing true presence with a person places the emphasis upon the human-human relationship as a traveler with the person, as the person chooses options to change patterns of health. Persons who have witnessed presence have said they experience feelings of dignity and that their own values are honored.

True presence is a non-routine, unconditional, loving way of "being with" in which the nurse witnesses the blossoming of others. The nurse needs to become centered in preparation for true presence. The centering in oneself produces a calming effect through quiet contemplation, leaving the nurse open to the possibilities in the human-human process. The full attention of the nurse is with the person or families as they move beyond the present moment. The person is appreciated as the captain of his or her own ship, as one knowing the way (Parse, 1995).

So the main difference between active listening or empathetic listening and presence is being calm, centered, and truly present with no judgments. Nursing practice guided by the Human Becoming Theory focuses on "being" with people in true presence. Such presence is in accordance with the Christocentric model that Christ taught and lived. True presence is an interpersonal art grounded in a strong knowledge base reflected in the belief that each person knows the way somewhere within one's self (Parse, 1992).

Humans are not static machines but dynamic individuals. They relate to the universe in intricate and personal ways. With a clearer understanding of human existence, nurses are able to be with individuals in ways that respect and inspire individuals as they make personal choices in living health.

Appendix F

Charter for Compassion

A call to bring the world together ...

The principle of compassion lies at the heart of all religious, ethical and spiritual traditions, calling us always to treat all others as we wish to be treated ourselves. Compassion impels us to work tirelessly to alleviate the suffering of our fellow creatures, to dethrone ourselves from the center of our world and put another there, and to honor the inviolable sanctity of every single human being, treating everybody, without exception, with absolute justice, equity, and respect.

It is also necessary in both public and private life to refrain consistently and empathically from inflicting pain. To act or speak violently out of spite, chauvinism, or self-interest, to impoverish, exploit or deny basic rights to anybody, and to incite hatred by denigrating others—even our enemies—is a denial of our common humanity. We acknowledge that we have failed to live compassionately and that some have even increased the sum of human misery in the name of religion.

We therefore call upon all men and women: (1) to restore compassion to the center of morality and religion; (2) to return to the ancient principle that any interpretation of scripture that breeds violence, hatred or disdain is illegitimate; (3) to ensure that youth are given accurate and respectful information about other traditions, religions, and cultures; (4) to encourage a positive appreciation of cultural and religious diversity; and (5) to cultivate an informed empathy with the suffering of all human beings—even those regarded as enemies.

We urgently need to make compassion a clear, luminous, and dynamic force in our polarized world. Rooted in a principled determination to transcend selfishness, compassion can break down political, dogmatic, ideological, and religious boundaries. Born of our deep interdependence, compassion is essential to human relationships and to a fulfilled humanity. It is the path to enlightenment and indispensible to the creation of a just economy and a peaceful global community.

This charter was created by Karen Armstrong and presented to the Parliament of the World's Religions in Melbourne, Australia on December 6, 2009.

Appendix G
The Golden Rule According to the Major World Religions

HINDUISM: "Whatever you consider injurious to yourself, never do to others. This is the essence of dharma." (*Mahabharata*, Udyoga Parvan 39, 71)

BUDDHISM: "Hurt not others in ways that you yourself would find hurtful." (*Udana-Varga* 5, 18)

JAINISM: "In happiness and suffering, in joy and grief, regard all creatures as you would regard your own self." (*Mahavira*)

SIKHISM: "Be not estranged from another for God dwells in every heart." (Guru Granth Sahib)

CONFUCIANISM: "Is there one maxim which ought to be acted upon throughout one's life? Surely it is the maxim of loving-kindness: do not do to others what you would not have them do to you." (*Analects: Sayings of Confucius* 15, 23)

TAOISM: "Regard your neighbor's gain as your own gain, and your neighbor's loss as your own loss." (*Tai Shang Kan Ying P'ien*)

ZOROASTRIANISM: "That nature alone is good which refrains from doing to another whatever is not good for its own self." (Dadistan-i-Dinik 94, 5)

JUDAISM: When Rabbi Hillel was asked to teach the entire Torah while standing on one foot, he replied: "What is hateful to you, do not do to your fellow men and women. That is the entire Torah; all the rest is commentary." He then added: "Now go and study." (Talmud, Shabbat 3id)

CHRISTIANITY: "Treat others the way you want them to treat you. This is the Law and the Prophets." (Jesus of Nazareth, Matthew 7:12)

ISLAM: "No one of you is a believer until he desires for his brothers and sisters that which he desires for himself." (*Hadith* of Muhammad)

BAHA'I FAITH: "He should not wish for others that which he does not wish for himself, nor promise that which he does not fulfill." (*Gleanings* of Baha'u'llah)

NATIVE AMERICAN: "Great Spirit, grant that I may not criticize my neighbor until I have walked a mile in his moccasins."

Provided by Dr. David Oughton, faculty in theology at St. Louis University and board member of Interfaith Partnership in St Louis, MO. Used by permission.

Unit I: Spirituality
Spiritual Care

Spiritual Care

Introduction

Learning Outcomes

Upon completion of this module, the participant will be able to:

1. Distinguish between spirituality and religion.
2. Integrate faith and health to provide spiritual care to individuals, families, groups, and communities.
3. Use a framework for spiritual assessment to discern spiritual needs.
4. Identify resources for continuous personal spiritual growth and self-care.

Description

This module focuses on the intentional care of the spirit in the practice of faith community nursing. It explores spirituality along with means of spiritual assessment and provision of spiritual care for individuals, families, and communities. Because spiritual care flows from the provider, the module also emphasizes the need for faith community nurses (FCNs) to understand their own spirits and the importance of tending to one's own spiritual journey.

Hours: 2

Research

"There is mounting evidence from randomized clinical trials and prospective studies that religious beliefs and practices have positive effects on coping and on speeding remission from emotional disorders, such as anxiety and depression. By improving coping, giving hope, and fostering a sense of meaning and purpose during difficult life circumstances, religious beliefs have the potential to impact not only mental health, but physical health as well" (Koenig, p. 172). This affirms the work of FCNs in providing spiritual care with the potential of effecting healthy outcomes for individuals, families, and communities.

Faith Tradition

The gift of salvation in the Christian tradition relates to the whole person and is understood as healing, wellness, peace, forgiveness, and shalom. The Scriptures encourage Christians in the practices of prayer, worship, and care of others and the earth. The spiritual care an FCN might offer in this tradition includes caring presence, prayer, encouragement through Scripture, and the support of the broader faith community. The Psalms are a great resource, as they relate to human struggles and emotion through stories, prayers, laments, and praise.

Key Terms

Spiritual care: "the practical expression of presence, guidance, and interventions, individual or communal, to support, nurture, or encourage an individual's or group's ability to achieve wholeness; health; personal, spiritual, and social well-being; integration of body, mind, and spirit; and a sense of connection to self, others and a higher power" (ANA/HMA, 2012, pp. 57–58)

Spirituality: a universal dimension about relationships and meaning within every person— religious, atheist, or humanist (Carson & Koenig, 2008)

Religion: an organized system of beliefs, ceremonies, and rules used to worship a god or a group of gods

Reflection

Take a deep breath; encourage a moment of silence or prayer. Read aloud this English translation of a Japanese version of Psalm 23.

The Lord is my Pace-setter, I shall not rush;
He makes me stop and rest for quiet intervals.
He provides me with images of stillness, which restore my
serenity.
He leads me in ways of efficiency
through calmness of mind,
and His guidance is peace.
Even though I have a great many things
to accomplish each day,
I will not fret, for His presence is here;
His timelessness, His all importance,
will keep me in balance.
He prepares refreshment and renewal
in midst of my activity,
By anointing my mind with His oils of tranquility.
My cup of joyous energy overflows;
surely harmony and effectiveness
shall be the fruits of my hours,
for I shall walk in the pace of my Lord
and dwell in His house forever.

Source: Toki Miyashina in Psalm 23: Several Versions Collected and Put Together, *K. H. Strange, ed. (1970). Edinburgh: St. Andrew's Press.*

Provide a period of silence for reflection. Ask participants to reflect on a time when they received spiritual care. Ask who cared for their spirits and how. What was helpful? What was not?

Spiritual Care
Content Outline

OUTCOME 1
Distinguish between spirituality and religion.

Religion and spirituality are two related yet distinct terms associated with faith.

Spirituality is a "universal dimension within every person—religious, atheist, or humanist" (Carson and Koenig, 2008). MacKinlay and Trevitt (2007) say, "The concept of spirituality is about core meaning and connectedness, and it is from this that we respond to all of life. Anger, hate, love, forgiveness and hope come from this core."

There are many definitions and descriptions of spirituality.
- Spirituality is the umbrella concept with "religion being one way to express spirituality" (MacKinlay and Trevitt, 2007).
- "Spirituality is about relationships and meaning, whereas religion reflects our attempts to structure and codify spirituality" (Carson & Koenig, 2008).
- Spirituality is "intangible" and "highly personal" (Taylor, 2002).
- Spirituality is that part where you find hope, meaning, and passion.

O'Brien (2011) suggests three characteristics of spirituality.
- unfolding mystery
- harmonious interconnectedness
- inner strength

Ways that people understand spirituality (Martinson) may include the following.
- mystery of being human—awe of life
- core of our being—deep, basic values and commitments being lived out
- meaning-making—seeking the significant
- sense of purpose—pursuing what matters
- transcendence—looking beyond or outside of self
- openness to God—seeking and receiving truth from a higher power

KEY TERM
Spirituality *is a universal dimension within every person—religious, atheist, or humanist.*

- faith—believing or a gift of grace
- hope—looking forward with anticipation
- peacefulness—living with serenity
- vitality—peak existence, life is exciting, meaningful

In contrast, **religion** may be defined as an organized system of beliefs concerning the cause, nature, and purpose of the universe, along with ceremonies and rules used to worship a god or a group of gods.

A religious person usually accepts a certain moral code and set of beliefs. For instance, a Christian believes Jesus is God's Son and observes baptism and communion. A Muslim believes Allah is God and observes Ramadan and prayers (*Salat*).

Based on these definitions, the major difference between religion and spirituality is one of *believing* versus *being*. Religion's focus is the content of one's belief and the outward expression of that belief; spirituality's focus is the process of becoming more attuned to unworldly affairs. It's possible to be religious without being spiritual and spiritual without being religious (Schreiber and Brockhopp, 2012).

KEY TERM

Religion *is an organized system of beliefs concerning the cause, nature, and purpose of the universe.*

Critical Thinking

What is your understanding of spirituality?

What are some of your most valued religious practices?

OUTCOME 2

Integrate faith and health to provide spiritual care to individuals, families, groups, and communities.

Spiritual care is "The practical expression of presence, guidance, and interventions, individual or communal, to support, nurture, or encourage an individual's or group's ability to achieve wholeness; health; personal, spiritual, and social well-being; integration of body, mind, and spirit; and a sense of connection to self, others and a higher power (ANA/HMA, 2012, pp. 57–58).

This definition shows the FCN's role in the process of spiritual care. **Practical expressions** of spiritual care include:
- presence
- guidance
- interventions

Spiritual care is offered to individuals or groups with the **purpose to enhance** their experience of:
- support
- nurture
- encouragement

Spiritual care increases the **ability to achieve hopeful outcomes** of:
- wholeness
- health
- personal, spiritual, and social well-being
- integration of body, mind and spirit
- a sense of connection to self, others and a higher power

Faith Community Nursing: Scope and Standards of Practice reminds us that, "The **primary focus of the FCN** is the intentional

KEY TERM

Spiritual care *is the practical expression of presence, guidance and interventions to nurture connection to self, others and a higher power.*

Conceptual models can serve as a guide for the FCN in the delivery of spiritual care. See Appendix A for the following selected conceptual models.

- *Wholeness Wheel*
- *Model for Healthy Living from the Church Health Center*
- *Model of Spiritual Care*
- *New Conceptual Model*

care of the spirit" (ANA/HMA, 2012, p. 8). The FCN integrates faith and health, tending to the spirit in all areas of the FCN practice with individuals, families, groups, and communities.

The role of the FCN is about **healing rather than cure**. For the FCN coming out of acute care settings where the focus on the physical is so automatic, it will take effort to change the primary focus to the spiritual focus.

Dr. Alan Wolfelt's *Companioning* expresses the concept of presence and providing spiritual care.

- Companioning provides a good example of an action that can facilitate healing.
- Companioning is the art of bringing comfort to individuals by becoming familiar with their stories, experiences and needs.
- To companion others who are experiencing difficult situations, therefore, is to break bread literally or figuratively, as well as listen to their stories. This process may involve give and take of the story: "I will tell you my story and then you tell me yours." Companioning involves sharing in a deep and profound way.
  Source: *Jewish Spiritual Companion for Medical Treatments: Resources for Patients, Family Members, Friends, Clergy and Health-Care Professionals*, published by Twin Cities Jewish Healing Program and the National Center for Jewish Healing (2007).

The **provision of spiritual care** includes these points.

- Spiritual care **flows out of who we are**, what we believe, and where we are in our own spiritual journeys.
- The more we have addressed **our own struggles**, pain, and dark sides, the more open we are to hear and stand with others in their times of difficulty and suffering.
- Life is messy. For example, the FCN may be visiting a woman in the hospital who spills out her confused relationships, some with men and some with women. The establishment of a therapeutic nurse-client relationship will facilitate the individual's disclosure of situations like this that might be causing guilt, regrets, pain, and sorrow. Spiritual care is about being **willing to be with someone** in the midst of muckiness— like the Precious Moments picture "Blessed are the pure in heart" of a sweet girl smelling a flower while being in the middle of a mud puddle.
- Ask yourself the question: **Am I willing to get dirty?**
- Our **willingness to be stretched**, to experience discomfort, of being out of our comfort zone, opens us to growth and greater ability to care for whomever God places in our path.
- Spiritual care is about taking our shoes off. We are **standing on holy ground** because God is present. We need to prepare, pray, and let God take the lead.

Forms of Spiritual Care

The FCN may offer spiritual care in many ways. He or she should be creative and discerning. Terminology from the Nursing

Intervention Classification (NIC) below may generate thoughts about pertinent actions that can be carried out in the provision of spiritual care.
- presence
- active listening
- coping enhancement
- counseling
- decision-making support
- emotional support
- hope instillation
- spiritual support
- referral (Burkhart, 2002, p. 30)

Primary Spiritual Care Interventions

Ministry of presence includes these elements.
- Presence is the **primary tool** of the FCN in providing spiritual care (Smucker, 2009).
- Presence is about **being with rather than doing for** or fixing; this may take some getting used to for many nurses, who are used to being busy, always assessing, thinking about what needs to be done.
- Presence requires **letting go** of what we are used to and learning to value just being.
- Experience the moment with another and allow **room for the sacred**—ushered in with you and within you.
- "Just to be is a blessing. **Just to live is holy**" (Abraham Joshua Heschel).
- Presence is about **open acceptance**, compassion, and comfort; holding no judgment.
- It comes with a **sense of humility**, understanding that this is about the other person and it is a gift to be allowed to enter into another's journey.
- It is a non-anxious presence with a sense of inner peace, strength.
- Presence is not always easy. Sometimes the hardest thing is to show up, especially when you think you have nothing to offer, but the ministry of presence offers a great deal.

Active listening is being open, aware, and attentive to the individual, oneself, and God or a Greater Wisdom.
- "Listening is a precious gift that you give people and a powerful tool for change. Helping people to thoughtfully reflect on their situation may lead to life-changing insights" (Smucker, 2009, p. 40).
- Do not underestimate the power of presence and listening.

Appropriate **therapeutic touch** can reduce the sense of aloneness.
- Therapeutic touch communicates **comfort** and compassion.
- It is important to ask for **permission** before offering touch.

Use **Scripture and sacred readings**.
- Ask, "What scripture or sacred text might be meaningful?"
- One way to personalize Scripture is to insert the person's

Critical Thinking
What are the concepts involved in preparing to provide spiritual care?

What thought processes lead you to recognize spiritual needs?

HELPFUL RESOURCE
See Health, Healing and Wholeness Module for more information on presence.

name. For example, using Deuteronomy 31:8: It is the Lord who goes before you, (name); he will be with you, (name), he will not fail you or forsake you, (name); do not fear or be dismayed.

- Choose scriptures for specific needs.

Various faith traditions offer many resources of **prayers and rituals**. (See Prayer Module for more information.) Here are some examples of simple rituals.

- Say a benediction before leaving a home visit
- Make the sign of the cross (with or without oil) on the forehead or hands of the person you minister to.
- Use the words from baptism along with the sign of the cross. For instance, in the Lutheran tradition: "(Name), child of God, you have been sealed by the Holy Spirit and marked with the cross of Christ forever." This takes on new meaning in different situations; at the end of life, the word *forever* stands out with hope of eternal life.

HELPFUL RESOURCE

See Appendix C, Scripture Resources for Spiritual Care.

We live in a noisy world with constant busyness. Therefore, it may take practice to grow in your ability and comfort with **silence**.

- Silence offers space for the client, for self, and for the Holy One.
- Sometimes just lingering a bit after a comment or question will invite deeper reflection, revelation, and sharing.

Acknowledge **lament**.

- In times of suffering, there is a time for complaining! Real life is not Disney World.
- Lamenting acknowledges the significance of the pain or difficulty.
- It offers permission to be sorrowful and not put on a happy face.
- It gives language for relating to God in times of suffering.
- The Psalms are a good source of lament. For example, in the case of chronic illness, Psalm 13: "How long, O Lord? Will you forget me forever?"

Scientific research has shown that **laughter** may have both preventive and therapeutic values. Laughter has shown different physiological and psychological benefits (Mora-Ripoll, 2011).

Use **reminiscing, storytelling, and journaling.**

- FCNs can wander with those they care for and deepen their story by exploring feelings, attitudes, expectations, and thoughts.
- The FCN may help another share a story through journaling, painting or storytelling.
- Stories reflect who people are, affirming their gifts and their value in being.

Be ready with an **appropriate referral**. It is important to have awareness of limitations and use resources within the faith community and local area.

- counselors
- spiritual leaders
- support groups

Just as there is ministry of presence, the **ministry of absence** allows for healthy boundaries and fosters confidence in the client's ability to cope. When the FCN leaves, he or she is sending a message that the individuals have strength and ability in themselves.

Relaxation techniques include a number of practices, such as progressive relaxation, guided imagery, visualization, and deep breathing exercises. The goal is to consciously produce the body's natural relaxation response, characterized by slower breathing, lower blood pressure, and a feeling of calm and well-being.

Meditation can result in a state of greater calmness, physical relaxation, and psychological balance. Practicing meditation can change how a person relates to the flow of emotions and thoughts.

The arts can be a vehicle for providing spiritual care to those who are hurting. Music, poetry, visual arts or icons may be nurturing to individuals and groups in unique ways that we cannot comprehend.

> **THREE REMINDERS FOR SPIRITUAL CARE**
> - *Be prepared to hear anger, confession, sorrow, and shame.*
> - *The more we are aware of our own darkness, the more open we will be to stand with others in theirs.*
> - *Pay attention to spiritual "nudges" to call or visit someone.*

Spiritual Care in Specific Situations

FCNs are likely to encounter some specific needs among congregation members.

Homebound, dementia, and long-term care. Individuals who have dementia, are homebound, or are in long-term care have special needs. In these situations the FCN ministers to the family or caregivers as well as the identified person. The FCN may be the only person coming to visit; for family who live at a distance, this can bring great comfort.
- The FCN serves as a connection to the faith community.
- The FCN should involve others from the faith community, such as spiritual leaders and lay visitation ministers. Artwork created by children and prayer shawls made by ministry volunteers can be shared with clients and families to increase their connection with the faith community.
- Similarities Between a Home Visit and a Service of Worship in Appendix D illustrates the potential of the home visit to be spiritual in nature, and therefore, therapeutic.

Crisis and tragedy. The FCN may or may not be involved in the immediate crisis, but often is the one to offer ongoing spiritual care during recovery. This can occur in communities where there are mass shootings or natural disasters such as tornadoes or mud slides, as well as in experiences of personal tragedy.
- A supportive community and trustworthy information are essential to recovering a sense of "normal."
- FCN spiritual care interventions at time of crisis may include

HELPFUL RESOURCE
See Appendix E, Spiritual Care During Crisis, for more information on disorientation and reorientation, as well as a story of an FCN's spiritual care during crisis.

presence, prayer, touch, and a prayer shawl—all part of God's love and comfort.
- Ongoing care includes assessing for elements of recovering well from crisis and offering continued support as needed.

Other specific needs or situations include:
- divorce
- serious diagnosis
- grief
- loss of job
- caregiving

Spiritual Care for Families, Groups and Communities

Families sometimes need to process together in order to move toward healing.
- Example: Moving out of a familiar home can be a very difficult transition. Rituals can help in facilitating a smooth transition.
- Example: A special service of remembrance and healing was created for a family two years after the death of their youngest child. This child had been developmentally disabled but was a joy to the whole family, which included three teenage siblings.

HELPFUL RESOURCE
See Appendix G, Ritual of Thanksgiving, to use during a transition to a new home.

Within every faith community, it can be confusing for members to know how to respond to issues they don't personally understand or experience. FCNs can help bring healing through promoting acceptance in faith communities and the greater community. Some of these groups are:
- veterans and their families
- people with physical disabilities and their families
- lesbian, gay, bisexual and transgender individuals
- people struggling with mental illness
- people and families dealing with cancer, unemployment, dementia, obesity or addiction
- couples experiencing infertility

Potential resources for offering healing to individuals with specific struggles include the following.
- Support group that intentionally addresses spiritual aspects along with general support.
- Educational opportunities for individuals, families, staff, leadership, and the faith community about the specific issues.
- Training of lay caring minsters (such as health promoters, Stephen Ministers or BeFrienders) with awareness and sensitivity to specific needs.
- Naming specific difficulties in newsletter articles or in prayers offered during worship services (without identifying individuals); this raises awareness and lets the individuals with specific struggles know that they are not alone, but rather are part of a supportive, caring community.

Critical Thinking
How would you go about providing spiritual care to a terminally ill individual in your faith community?

What identifiable spiritual needs do you see in your community?

Just like individuals and families, **faith communities experience painful times** and need ways to heal. While the FCN may not be the one to lead a healing response, he or she can initiate or support such efforts.

- Some of these difficult times may result from conflict and discord, changes in staff, unethical behavior, grief, or severing ties with a faith community.
- Possible interventions may include prayer service or prayer vigil, guided small group conversations, large group meeting to hear and allow expression of feelings.

Spiritual needs might be evident in the **community surrounding the faith community**. The FCN can be one to raise awareness and encourage the faith community to be a place of healing and hope. For example, in response to the tragic death of a nine-year-old child, one faith community opened its doors and had a community service with candle lighting for the family, school friends, teachers, and others.

OUTCOME 3

Use a framework for spiritual assessment to discern spiritual needs.

Preparing to Provide Spiritual Care

Some ways to prepare include the following.

- Use personal prayer or centering prayer before an encounter.
- Reflect on who is steering the tandem prayers that open oneself for God's service.
- Consider potential resources for each encounter—what might you need to bring with you?
  - Scripture, holy texts
  - devotional or other pertinent reading
  - questions or wonderings
  - prayer shawl, care basket, holding cross, or other tangible item

Assessing for Spiritual Care

Remember that assessing for spiritual care is completed over time, not with a clipboard but more like discovering pieces of a puzzle during each encounter.

Assessment tools can offer a framework for listening; the FCN should resist viewing them as forms to be completed.

IMPORTANCE OF FORGIVENESS

Research supports that forgiveness is healthy for our whole being (Dorn et al., 2014). There are no quick fixes—forgiveness can take years, depending on the experience.

- *Forgiveness is a process that begins by turning in the direction of healing. If needing to forgive, an individual may move from "I can't forgive; Go, you forgive" to "I want to forgive; help me to forgive" to finally "I forgive." An individual seeking forgiveness may move from "I can't be forgiven" to "I desire to be forgiven; help me to receive forgiveness" to "I trust God and receive God's love and forgiveness."*
- *The practice of forgiveness is supported by the community of faith through such actions as corporate and individual confession and absolution.*
- *The FCN can support forgiveness by informally hearing confession and sharing God's love through Scripture and prayer.*
- *The FCN might encourage an individual to write a statement such as: "I wish to be forgiven for the times I have hurt my family, friends, and others; and, I wish for my family, friends, and others to know that I forgive them for when they may have hurt me in life."*
- *Many resources on forgiveness are available through various faith traditions.*

Critical Thinking

What challenges might you
have in assessing spiritual
needs of individuals, families
or communities?

What are your concerns
about providing spiritual
care to individuals, groups,
and your faith community?

Acronyms, such as FICA or HOPE can guide listening and help frame questions for discerning needs. (See Appendix H, Spiritual Assessment Acronyms: FICA and HOPE.)

- While an FCN may assume some of the answers while interacting with members of the faith community, it is helpful to be aware of these assumptions and to keep an open mind about a person's particular beliefs, values, and practices.
- The determination of spiritual needs and resources, evaluation of the impact of beliefs on health care outcomes and decisions, and discovery of barriers to using spiritual resources are all outcomes of a thorough spiritual assessment. (See Assessment Module for additional spiritual assessment tools.)

Good **questions that invite reflection** and discovery are particularly helpful. (See Appendix I, Questions for Spiritual Assessment.) Through listening and observation, FCNs can identify **Nursing Diagnoses** related to spiritual needs. (See Documentation module.)

- Basic, universal spiritual needs include meaning and purpose, love and belonging, forgiveness and reconciliation, sense of community, connection to holy, and hope (Bauer, 2012).
- Terminology for specific spiritual needs from North American Nursing Diagnosis Association (NANDA) include these words.
  - anxiety
  - fear
  - loneliness
  - caregiver role strain
  - spiritual distress
  - spiritual well-being
  - decisional conflict
  - hopelessness

OUTCOME 4

Identify resources for continuous personal spiritual growth and self-care.

The FCN must commit to lifelong learning in nursing, spiritual growth, and the beliefs and practices of the faith community.

- Nurturing one's own spirit is essential to being able to nurture another's.
- Research supports that the spiritual care of nurses increases their sense of well-being and "improves the quality of services provided to their patients" (Batcheller, Davis, and Yoder-Wise, 2013, p. 310).

Identifying personal need for renewal and refreshment is essential to faith community nursing. The FCN can use a process of self-spiritual assessment to recognize personal needs. The following may be signs of spiritual emptiness or exhaustion.

- crabbiness and irritability
- not wanting to make eye contact with others (who might want a listening ear)

- loss of sense of humor, especially about self
- self-absorbed (not open to feel concern for others with difficulties)
- no zest for life
- feeling tired in the morning; insomnia
- prayer time is a chore
- it's hard to sing or praise God
- finding yourself being critical or unforgiving
- difficulty concentrating

The following are resources for spiritual growth and renewal. (See Prayer and Self-care Modules for more information.)

- daily devotions and prayer (See Appendix J, *21 Ways to Refresh Your Prayer Life.*)
- lectio divina (divine reading)
- visio divina (divine seeing)
- labyrinth
- imagery, visualization (See Appendix K, *Visualization.*)
- spiritual retreat
- theological reflection (See the Health, Healing and Wholeness Module.)
- spiritual direction
- reading
- walking
- spending time with a good friend
- laughter

Spiritual care is the gift you give out of who you are, making room for the other, making room for the Holy. Start where you are with your comfort level, tend to your own spiritual journey, and let God lead. God will bless whatever you offer!

Standards of Professional Performance for Faith Community Nursing

There is no specific standard related to spiritual care. However, "The primary focus of the FCN is the intentional care of the spirit" (ANA/HMA, 2012). The FCN integrates faith and health, tending to the spirit in all areas of practice with individuals, families, groups, and communities.

> **Critical Thinking**
>
> *What are the signs or symptoms of your personal need for spiritual care?*
>
> *How do you meet your own spiritual needs?*

Learning Activities

Prepare to Provide Spiritual Care

Instructions:
1. This assignment may be used as a pre-class activity to explore the concept of spirituality and spiritual care.
2. Assign participants to answer the questions below in a way that assesses their own thoughts and ideas about spirituality.
3. Suggest completing this assignment in a quiet place and to write out answers.

Questions:
1. What is your definition of spirituality?
2. Describe a spiritual experience you have had.
3. When do you feel most peaceful?
4. When do you feel most healthy?
5. What gives you fulfillment? Why?
6. How do you nurture your spiritual self?
7. Think back and describe your early childhood concepts of God. Describe your current concepts of God. Has there been a change or evolving of these concepts as you have journeyed through life? Explore that process.

Cup of Tea

Instructions:
1. On top of a table and underneath it, place plastic to catch the overflowing water during the drama.
2. Put a teapot of water, an empty bowl, and two cups on the table.
3. Ask for two volunteers to help you with a short drama. Give each volunteer a copy of the story "A Cup of Tea" from Appendix N.
4. Explain that you will be the narrator. Assign one volunteer to the role of master teacher to pour the tea. Assign the other person to the role of the university professor.
5. Ask both volunteers to raise their hands when their roles are mentioned in the first line of the story.
6. Ask the master teacher to pour the tea to overflowing and to say the "master teacher" lines at the appropriate time during your narration.
7. The professor will say the "professor" lines at the appropriate time and pour the water from the cup into a bowl at the end of the drama.
8. Ask the volunteers to take their places, and invite the group to watch and listen to a role-play. Read the story, "A Cup of Tea."

Question:
Guide the group discussion by leading participants through the questions and explanations found in Appendix N.

Case Study: Situation—Individual Living with Dementia

Instructions:
1. Review the case study below and then reflect upon the poem that follows.
2. Discuss the questions at the end of the case study.

Clara was in an advanced stage of dementia. She had been a volunteer in her faith community for many years. She always appeared pleasant, although she rarely talked. Clara had no children, and her husband died several years earlier. She lived at a skilled nursing facility and often sat in a reclining chair in the hallway, where she could watch the activity of the day.

The FCN visited regularly, holding Clara's hand, reading Scripture and saying prayers. One day, a few months before Clara died, the FCN found her more alert and talkative. The FCN asked Clara questions about her family and where she lived. Clara responded to some questions, but others were lost in the wanderings of her mind. Clara shared about her church and her love for the people she had served. After a time of conversation, the FCN introduced prayer and asked what Clara would want her to pray for. Clara was silent for a moment, appeared prayerful, and said, "For the remaining time that I have, that I might be in God's will." The FCN prayed with the sense of this being holy ground, and God was very near.

The FCN wrote this poem upon reflection on this visit.
> *Where are you? What are you thinking?*
> *Have you wandered off into your own little world?*
> *Or are you aware of the world we share?*
> *How can I reach you? How can I be reached by you?*
> *Lord, give me patience ... and the grace needed*
> *To not miss the joy of meeting your child!*

Questions:
1. Describe Clara's spiritual state in the midst of her illness. (She was spiritually well—faith intact, caring for others, aware of God's presence and care. Clara was a precious gift, unseen by the world, but not forgotten by God.
2. Describe the spiritual care the FCN provided. (Presence, active listening, silence, prayer, therapeutic touch, conversation, companionship.)

Case Studies: Assessing Spiritual Needs and Providing Interventions

Instructions:

1. Assign participants to small groups.

2. Read one or more of the case studies below and answer the discussion questions as they relate to that case.

Questions:

1. Reflect on how you would feel about making this visit.

2. What resources might you anticipate being useful during the visit?

3. How will you go about making an assessment on this visit? Consider FICA, HOPE, questions, or other methods.

4. What NANDA Nursing Diagnoses might you make? (See Appendix B, Sample Nursing Diagnoses and Interventions.)

CASE 1
Gregor

Gregor is 56 years old, married, and has three grown children. He is a member of the faith community and was more active when his children were young. He works full time. In the past year, he was diagnosed with prostate cancer and had surgery, chemotherapy, and radiation. Gregor continues to have scans periodically. He also continues to have difficulty with incontinence, which forces him to work mostly from home and limits his social activity. His wife attends worship regularly and has asked the FCN to visit, saying that she worries that Gregor is slipping into a depression.

CASE 2
Alicia

Alicia is a 74-year-old breast cancer survivor of 14 years. She was never married and lives alone in a townhome with many stairs. She was recently hospitalized with pneumonia, which led to a diagnosis of metastatic breast cancer to the lung. Alicia is concerned about many things—decisions about further treatment, possibly moving, fears about living alone when she is sick, and fears of the future. She is an active member of her faith community and has been a volunteer for some of the health and wellness activities. The FCN knows Alicia to be a kind and caring person who values her faith and privacy. Alicia has asked the FCN to visit.

CASE 3
Gloria

Gloria is 68 years old and married, has five grown children, and is an active member of the faith community. She and her husband are both retired and have particularly enjoyed going on mission trips and participating in small group Bible studies. Gloria recently had knee replacement surgery and her recovery has been slower than expected. This has limited her ability to participate in her regular activities and she has grown impatient and frustrated. Gloria's husband has asked the FCN to visit. Gloria agrees to the visit but states that she doesn't need one.

Offering Tangible Objects for Spiritual Care

Instructions:
1. Direct participants to Appendix F, *Tangible Objects of Spiritual Care.*
2. Ask participants to share personal experiencing with tangible objects such as prayer, holding crosses, care baskets and items from nature that have been useful in spiritual care.

Question:
What effect have you seen tangible objects have in spiritual care?

References

Required Textbook

American Nurses Association and Health Ministries Association (2012). *Scope and standards of practice: Faith community nursing* (2nd ed.). Silver Spring, MD: Nursesbooks.org.

References

Anandarajah, G. & Hight, E. (2001). Spirituality and medical practice: Using the HOPE questions as a practical tool for spiritual assessment. *American Family Physician, 63*(1), 81–89. Website: www.aafp.org/afp/2001/0101/p81.html#afp20010101p81-t4

Batcheller, J., Davis, J., & Yoder-Wise, P. S. (2013). Hope for the future: Intensifying spirituality in the workplace. *Nursing Administration Quarterly, 37*, 309–316.

Bauer, B. (2012). Unpublished lecture. Parish Nurse Ministry Program, Concordia College, Moorhead, MN.

BeFriender Ministry Coordinator Manual. (1997). BeFriender Ministry, St. Paul, MN: University of St. Thomas.

Burkhart, L. (2002). *Integration: A documentation system reporting whole person care.* Available at http://www.luc.edu/nursing/about/faculty/lisaburkhartphdrnmph.shtml

Carson, V. and Koenig, H. (2008). *Spiritual dimensions of nursing practice.* West Conshohocken, PA: Templeton Foundation Press.

Deffenbaugh, D. (2013). What is integrated health? *Church Health Reader, 3*(1), 8.

Dorn, K., Hook, J., Davis, D., Van Tongeren, D., & Worthington, Jr., E. (2014). Behavioral methods of assessing forgiveness. *The Journal of Positive Psychology, 9*(1), 75–80. doi: 10.1080/17439760.2013.844267

InterLutheran Coordinating Committee on Ministerial Health and Wellness of the ELCA and the LCMS. (1997). *Wholeness Wheel.*

Jewish Healing Program and the National Center for Jewish Healing. (2005). *Jewish Spiritual Companion for Medical Treatments: Resources for Patients, Family Members, Friends, Clergy and Health-Care Professionals.* Minneapolis, MN: Twin Cities Jewish Healing Program and the National Center for Jewish Healing.

Koenig, H. G., (2008). *Medicine, religion, and health: Where science and spirituality meet.* West Conshohocken, PA: Templeton Press.

MacKinlay, E. B. & Trevitt, C. (2007). Spiritual care and ageing in a secular society. *Medical Journal of Australia, 186,* S74–S76.

Martinson, R. (2001). Unpublished lecture. Luther Seminary, St. Paul, MN.

Mora-Ripoll R. (2011). Potential health benefits of simulated laughter: A narrative review of the literature and recommendations for future research. *Complementary Therapies in Medicine, 19*(3), 170–177.

O'Brien, M. E. (2011). *Spirituality in nursing: Standing on holy ground* (4th ed.) Sudbury, MA: Jones and Bartlett Learning.

Open doors, open minds, open hearts: A service of healing. (2005). Mental Health Education Project of Twin Cities Jewish Community and Jami Alanna Marks Tikkun Olam Fund.

Piderman, K. M. (2009). Unpublished lecture. Mayo Clinic, Rochester, MN

Schreiber, J. A., & Brockopp, D. Y, (2012). Twenty-five years later—what do we know about religion/spirituality and psychological well-being among breast cancer survivors? A systematic review. *Journal of Cancer Survivorship: Research and Practice 6*(1), 82–94.

Smucker, C. J. (2009). *Faith community nursing: Developing a quality practice.* Silver Spring, MD: American Nurses Association.

Solari-Twadell, P. A., & McDermott, M. A. (Eds.). (1999). *Parish nursing: Promoting whole person health within faith communities.* Thousand Oaks, CA: Sage Publications.

Solari-Twadell, P. A., & McDermott, M. A. (Eds.). (2006). *Parish nursing: Development, education, and administration.* St. Louis, MO: Elsevier Mosby.

Taylor, E. J. (2002). *Spiritual Care: Nursing theory, research, and practice.* Upper Saddle River, NJ: Prentice Hall.

Whiston, C. (1972). *Pray: A study of distinctive Christian praying.* Grand Rapids, MI: William B. Eerdmans Publishing.

Additional References

Balkin, R., Harris, N., Freeman, S., Huntington, S. (2014). The forgiveness reconciliation inventory: An instrument to process through issues off-forgiveness and conflict. *Measurement and Evaluation in Counseling and Development, 47*(1), 3–13. doi:10.1177/0748175613497037

Calhoun, A. (2005). *Spiritual disciplines handbook: Practices that transform us.* Downers Grove, IL: InterVarsity Press.

Carson, V. & Koenig, H. (2004). *Spiritual caregiving: Healthcare as a ministry.* Radnor, PA: Templeton Foundation Press.

Koenig, H. G., (2008). *Spirituality & health research: Methods, measurement, statistics and resources.* West Conshohocken, PA: Templeton Press.

Patterson, D. (2008). *Healing words for healing people: Prayers and peditations for parish Nurses and other health professionals.* Cleveland, OH: Pilgrim Press.

Patterson, D. (2010). *Balm in Gilead: Hymns of healing and wholeness.* St. Louis, MO: International Parish Nurse Resource Center.

Person, G. (2001). *Psalms for healing: Praying with those in need.* Minneapolis, MN: Augsburg Fortress.

Piderman, K. M. (2011). A pilot study of spirituality and inpatient rehabilitation outcomes in persons with spinal cord dysfunction and severe neurological illnesses. *Journal of Pastoral Care and Counseling, 65*, 1–13.

Rupp, J. (2000). *Out of the ordinary: Prayers, poems, and reflections for every season.* Notre Dame, IN: Ave Maria Press.

Online Resources

Model for Healthy Living: http://www.chreader.org

NANDA Nursing Diagnosis for 2012–2014:

http://faculty.mu.edu.sa/public/uploads/1380604673 .6151NANDA%202012.pdf

National Center for Jewish Healing: http://www.ncjh.org/ pubsorder.pdf

Prayer Shawls (patterns, prayers): http://www.shawlministry. com

Where to look in the Bible: http://clayyouth.tripod.com/ sitebuildercontent/sitebuilderfiles/wheretolook.pdf

Wholeness Wheel: https://www.porticobenefits.org/ PorticoBenefits/CallToLiveWell/FaithBasedWellBeing/ TheWholenessWheel.aspx and at www.wheatridge.org

Wrap-Up and Evaluation

Measuring Competency

This chart can be used to assess the individual outcomes in this module.

- A copy of this chart is attached to the Participant Module, so that each participant can complete this short evaluation.
- Have participants read each outcome and then place an X in the box that best matches their opinion about the objective being met.
- Encourage each participant to write a short reflection about this module in the space provided at the bottom of this chart.
- Use this data to make any necessary changes.

Outcome	Not Met	Somewhat Met	Met
1. Distinguish between spirituality and religion.			
2. Integrate faith and health to provide spiritual care to individuals, families, groups, and communities.			
3. Use a framework for spiritual assessment to discern spiritual needs.			
4. Identify resources for continuous personal spiritual growth and self-care.			
Reflection: *In one paragraph, write a reflection on this module.*			

Appendix A

Conceptual Models for Spiritual Care

1. **The Wholeness Wheel**

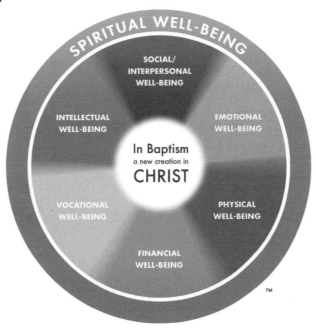

Portico Benefit Services' wholeness wheel emblems are trademarks of Portico Benefit Services. Used with permission.
(U.S. Patent and Trademark SN 86/238,903, 86/238,971, 86/252,356, 86/252,371, 86/252,365, 86/252,438, 86/257,977).

2. **The Model for Healthy Living from the Church Health Center**
   Available at http://www.chreader.org

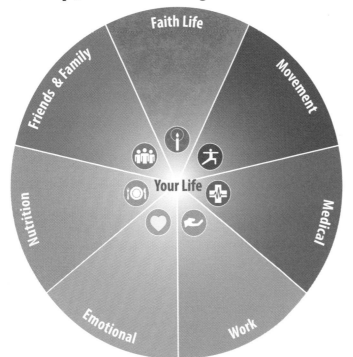

Faith Life
Building a relationship with God, your neighbors, and yourself.

Movement
Discovering ways to enjoy physical activity.

Medical
Partnering with your health care provider to manage your medical care.

Work
Appreciating your skills, talents, and gifts.

Emotional
Managing stress and understanding your feelings to better care for yourself.

Nutrition
Making smart food choices and developing healthy eating habits.

Family & Friends
Giving and receiving support through relationships.

3. **Philosophy of Parish Nursing**
   Parish nursing holds the spiritual dimension as central to its practice. It also encompasses the physical, psychological, and social dimensions of nursing practice (Solari-Twadell and McDermott, 1999).

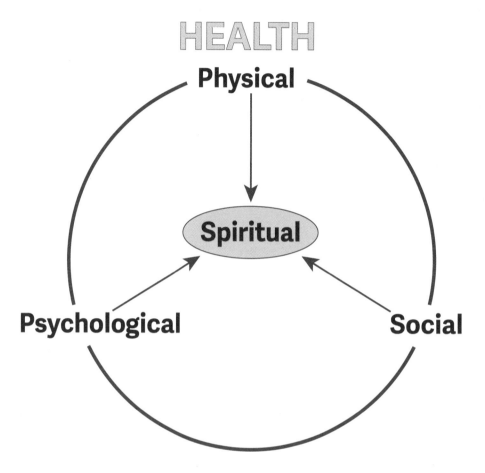

4. New Conceptual Model: Faith Community Nursing

A new conceptual model for faith community nursing visually presents the concept with the nurse/client (client as person, family, group, or community) relationship central.

The theoretical definition of faith community nursing is described as "... a method of health care delivery that is centered in a relationship between the nurse and client (client as person, family, group, or community). The relationship occurs in an iterative motion over time when the client seeks or is targeted for wholistic health care with the goal of optimal wholistic health functioning. Faith integrating is a continuous occurring attribute. Health promoting, disease managing, coordinating, empowering and accessing health care are other essential attributes. All essential attributes occur with intentionality in a faith community, home, health institution and other community settings with fluidity as part of a community, national, or global health initiative" (Ziebarth, 2014).

See Table 1 on page 24 for examples of how each essential attribute manifests in faith community nursing.

Established Conceptual Model
(Solari Twadell, et al, 1991)

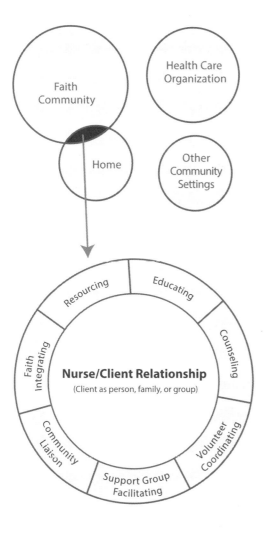

New Conceptual Model:
Faith Community Nursing (FCN)
A Method of Wholistic Health Care Delivery
(Ziebarth, 2014)

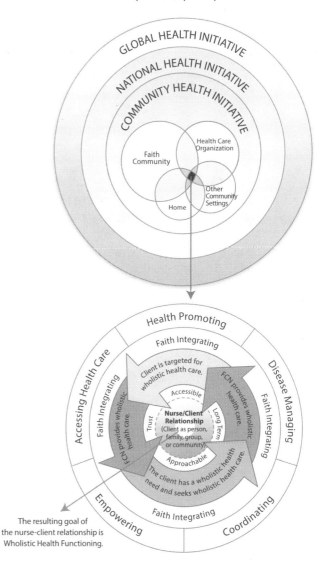

Ziebarth, D. (2014). Evolutionary conceptual analysis of faith community nursing. Journal of Religion and Health. DOI: 10.1007/s10943-014-9918-z

Table 1: Matrix

Essential Attributes	Faith Community Nursing Manifested
	Interventions from nurse to client (client as person, family, group or community)
Faith Integrating	• Intentional spiritual care and religious interventions: Presence, touch, spiritual and emotional support, prayer and meditation, spiritual growth facilitation, hope and forgiveness instillation, humor, faith related resources and referrals, showing compassion • Integration of faith traditions: Aligned religious readings, scriptures, songs, music, etc. • Cultural spiritual and religious activities: Communion, healing service, litany reading, etc. • Spiritual health assessment
Health Promoting and Disease Managing	• Management or surveillance • Disease focused programming • Disease counseling • Disease resources • Disease support services: Meals, transportation, calls, visits, cards, etc. • Advocacy • Primary, secondary and/or tertiary prevention activities • Referrals (multidisciplinary and interdisciplinary) • Symptom management • Care planning • Visits: Home, faith community, hospital, etc. • End of life planning • Assessment: Individual, family, faith community, community, etc. • Care giver support
Coordinating	• Recurring meetings: Health committee, social/community/global concerns, etc. • Identification of barriers and strategies • Ongoing activities: Volunteer training, support groups, CPR, community health events, screenings, education, articles, etc. • Survey development and results utilization • Referrals: Multidisciplinary and interdisciplinary • Health focused programming • Documentation: Coordinating the health record, data collection, reports, etc. • Care planning • Integrating health and faith • Health support: Meals, transportation, calls, visits, cards, etc. • Case managing

Essential Attributes	Faith Community Nursing Manifested
Empowering	• Capacity building • Supporting • Encouraging • Self-efficacy activities • Health counseling • Symptom management • Health promoting education • Health resourcing • Care planning • Education • Health support services: Meals, transportation, calls, visits, cards, etc. • Lifestyle change support • Care giver support

Accessing Health Care	• Health referrals:
	  Multidisciplinary and interdisciplinary
	• Practicing within a health care team
	• Providing health resources
	• Education and assistance:
	  How, when, where, and why to use the health care system
	• Health support services:
	  Meals, transportation, calls, visits, cards, babysitting, etc
	• Assistance:
	  Filling out forms, finding appropriate medical home, medical equipment, etc.
	• Advocating
	• Assessment:
	  Individual, family, faith community, community, etc.
	• Policy development
	• Research and literature reviews

Health Promoting	

Appendix B

Sample Nursing Diagnoses and Interventions

PARISH NURSING SERVICES
BRIEF CLIENT INTERACTION FORM—SPIRITUAL

Client's Name: _____

NURSING DIAGNOSIS[1]

Life Principles
- ☐ RFE Spiritual Well-Being
- ☐ Impaired Religiosity
- ☐ Decisional Conflict

Health Promotion
- ☐ Ineffective Health Maintenance

Activity/Rest
- ☐ Disturbed Sleep Pattern

Cognitive/Perceptual
- ☐ Disturbed Thought Process

Self-Perception
- ☐ Powerlessness
- ☐ Hopelessness
- ☐ Situational Low Self-Esteem
- ☐ Chronic Low Self-Esteem

Roles/Relationships
- ☐ Interrupted Family Processes
- ☐ Impaired Social Interaction

Comfort
- ☐ Chronic Pain
- ☐ Acute Pain
- ☐ Social Isolation

Coping/Stress Tolerance
- ☐ Anxiety
- ☐ Fear
- ☐ Ineffective Coping
- ☐ Compromised Family Coping
- ☐ Disabled Family Coping
- ☐ RFE: Family Coping

Safety/Protection
- ☐ Risk for Self-mutilation
- ☐ Risk for Injury

NURSING INTERVENTIONS[2]

Physiological Basic
- ☐ Pain Management
- ☐ Progressive Muscle Relaxation
- ☐ Sleep Enhancement
- ☐ Transport

Behavioral/Cognitive Therapy
- ☐ Bibliotherapy
- ☐ Music Therapy
- ☐ Mutual Goal Setting

Communication
- ☐ Acute Listening
- ☐ Complex Relationship Building
- ☐ Conflict Mediation
- ☐ Meditation
- ☐ Socialization Enhancement

Coping/Spiritual/Religion
- ☐ Anticipatory Guidance
- ☐ Body Image Enhancement
- ☐ Coping Enhancement
- ☐ Counseling
- ☐ Crisis Intervention
- ☐ Decision-Making Support
- ☐ Dying Care
- ☐ Emotional Support
- ☐ Forgiveness Facilitation
- ☐ Grief Work Facilitation
- ☐ Hope Instillation
- ☐ Humor
- ☐ Presence
- ☐ Recreational Therapy
- ☐ Religious Ritual Enhancement
- ☐ Role Enhancement
- ☐ Security Enhancement

Coping/Spiritual/Religion (cont.)
- ☐ Self-awareness Enhancement
- ☐ Spiritual Growth Facilitation
- ☐ Spiritual Support
- ☐ Support System Enhancement
- ☐ Touch
- ☐ Values Clarification

Psychological Comfort Promotion
- ☐ Anxiety Reduction
- ☐ Calming Technique
- ☐ Simple Guided Imagery
- ☐ Simple Relaxation Therapy

[1]Diagnosis labels reprinted with permission from NANDA.
[2]NIC labels reprinted with permission from Mosby.
Used with permission. Burkhart, L. (2002). Integration: A documentation system reporting whole person care. Available at http://www.luc.edu/media/lucedu/nursing/faculty/pdfs/Integration%20Manual.pdf

Appendix C

Scripture Resources for Spiritual Care

Where to look in the Bible for these emotions or life situations:

Afraid: Psalm 27, 56:3–4, 139:23–24; Isaiah 41:13; Romans 8:1827; 2 Corinthians 12:9

Alone or fearful: Exodus 14:13; Psalm 23:4, 27, 91; Proverbs 1:7; Luke 8:22–39; 2 Timothy 1:7; 1 Peter 4

Anxious: Psalm 107, 121; Philippians 4:6, Hebrew 12:4–11, 13:5; 1 Peter 5:6

Bereaved: Matthew 5:4; Luke 6:21; 1 Corinthians 15; 1 Thessalonians 4:13–5:28; Revelation 21, 22

Desiring peace: Psalm 46:10-11, 107, 119:165; Isaiah 26:3–4, 32:17–18; John 14:27; Romans 5:1–5, 8:18–30; Colossians 3:15; James 3:17–18

Discouraged: Isaiah 41:10; Psalm 23, 40, 42, 43, 107:19; Hebrews 12

Facing a crisis: Job 28:12–28; Proverbs 8; Isaiah 55; 2 Timothy 1:7; Hebrews 4:16

Needing comfort: Job 5:19; Psalm 25, 42:5, 103:11–13, 119:50–76; 121; 2 Corinthians 1:3–4

Sick or suffering: Psalm 6, 41, 42, 67; Isaiah 26; Matthew 26:39–42; Romans 8:18; 2 Timothy 2:2–13; James 5:11–15; 1 Peter 4:12, 13, 19

Needing forgiveness: Psalm 130:4; Luke 7:36–50, 15; Acts 13:38; Ephesians 2:1–10; Colossians 1:13–14; 1 John 1:8–9

Needing prayer: Psalm 4, 6, 25, 42, 51; 1 Kings 8:12–61; Matt 6:5–15; Luke 11, 18:1–14; John 17; 1 Thessalonians 5:16–18; 1 John 5:14, 15

Sad: Psalm 34, 71; Isaiah 40

Tired: Psalm 55:22, 73:26; Isaiah 40:31; Jonah 2:7; Matthew 11:28–30; 2 Corinthians 4:16

Troubled: Psalm 31, 38, 40; Romans 5:3–5, 8:18

Worried: Psalm 46; Matthew 6:25–34; Philippians 4:4–13; 1 Peter 5:6–7

Unable to sleep: Psalm 4, 46, 56, 130; Isaiah 26:3; Philippians 4:7

Selections from list at website:
http://clayyouth.tripod.com/sitebuildercontent/sitebuilderfiles/wheretolook.pdf

Other online Scripture sources:
Bible verses by topic: http://www.biblestudytools.com/topical-verses/
Bible search: http://www.biblegateway.com

Appendix D

Similarities Between a Home Visit and a Service of Worship

A Home Visit	A Service of Worship
Greeting and introduction	The gathering of the people
The grace to receive, small talk	Exchange of greetings, entrance rites The call to worship, praise
The purpose of the visit	Prayer and confession
A story unfolds	God's story as revealed through Scripture
Insights, information, new questions	The preached Word and Holy Communion
A resolution or response	Final closing prayers
Closing and farewell	Benediction, blessing

Adapted from BeFriender Ministry Training Manual IV.79. Used with permission from BeFriender Ministry—A Listening Presence. 1120 E. 80th Street, Suite 105, Bloomington, MN 55420. www. befrienderministry.org.

Appendix E

Spiritual Care During Crisis

Part 1: From Disorientation to Reorganization

1. **Status quo**—what we experience as normal.

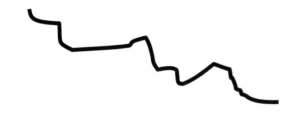

2. **Disorientation**—crisis tumbles us into a time of disorientation. Recovery is jagged with many ups and downs.

3. **Reorganization**—eventually reorientation and reorganization result in a return to status quo "normal" or a "new normal."

The angle of the disorientation (length and steepness) and the resulting new status quo or growth are impacted by the support and coping skills of the individual.

Four elements that help people cope with crisis:
- supportive community
- one caring person
- good information about the crisis
- sense of hope and anticipating positive future

Four elements that make crisis worse:
- sense of isolation
- "fix it" mentality
- shame—"buck up"
- bad or unhealthy information

Four spiritual care questions for recovery from crisis:
- Does the person feel supported? Does he or she have an accepting community?
- Does the person have helpful information about the crisis? Consider diagnosis, situation, what to expect with psychological experience of shock, denial, etc.
- Does the person have at least one individual who cares and listens with understanding and acceptance?
- Does the person have hope? Confidence that things will turn out for the best?

Source: Unpublished lecture by Roland Martinson, professor emeritus of children, youth and family ministry at Luther Seminary, St. Paul MN. Used with permission.

Part 2: A Story of Crisis: Highlighting Presence and Prayer

January 11, 2007

The call came to the church. "Janet's son was in the emergency room. He tried to kill himself."

"Which one? She has three boys."

"The youngest—Christopher."

Janet had been a member of my health ministry team and was a close friend. Grabbing a prayer shawl on the way out, I accompanied one of our pastors to the emergency room.

We found Janet alongside Christopher's bed in the emergency room. She was stroking his head—the part that wasn't covered with blood or bandages—and wondering out loud, "What were you thinking, Sweetie?" She hugged us and said her other boys were on their way and asked if we might be with her when she told them. Christopher's dad was also there, along with the hospital chaplain.

We stood by, watching, praying, and understanding that the situation did not look good.

When the boys arrived, we joined them in a small room off the waiting area. While we met there, the staff moved Christopher up to ICU. After telling the boys, we shared some prayers and gave Janet the prayer shawl. She clutched it to her heart.

Moving up to ICU, we watched as Janet and her boys reunited with Christopher. Janet took the prayer shawl and placed it over Christopher. We joined hands around Christopher's bed, touching him and each other, and said more prayers.

It struck me that in her mother wisdom, Janet was tucking her baby into God's care, into God's love.

The prayer shawl remained on Christopher. The staff understood its importance and did not remove it even when they needed to cool Christopher's body temperature.

More prayer shawls were brought for each family member. We spent more time just being there, listening, hugging, praying, weeping. Arrangements were made to donate Christopher's organs and a funeral. Janet kept Christopher's prayer shawl.

Janet Benz and her family established the Christopher Benz Foundation to provide education and awareness for the prevention of teenage suicide. Find more information at http://christopherbenzfoundation.org

Shared with permission by Annette Langdon, adjunct faculty for the Parish Nurse Ministry Program at Concordia College, Moorhead, MN.

Appendix F

Tangible Objects for Spiritual Care

Tangible objects, such as prayer shawls and holding crosses, can be symbolic of God's love and presence in times of grief or suffering. There are many stories of how people have experienced spiritual support through such items.

Tangible objects are items that people within the faith community can provide.

Prayer Shawls

A congregation may want to form a group for creating prayer shawls and presenting them to people in crisis, who are homebound, or who live with chronic conditions.

For more information on making and using prayer shawls, see http://www.shawlministry.com.

Holding Crosses

Members of the faith community who have woodworking skills can make holding crosses. These crosses are a comfortable size and design for holding in the hands as an aid to spiritual comfort and prayer. Holding crosses may also be purchased. See http://www.holdingcross.com.

Care Baskets

A care basket may be any basket holding a variety of items, such as candle, devotional reading, mug, packets of tea or soup, CareNotes (http://www.onecaringplace.com), artwork, prayer shawl, or holding cross.

A simple note may accompany the gift of a prayer shawl, holding cross, or care basket. Here is a sample note to use with a prayer shawl.

Prayer shawls have been used throughout the generations. Our ancient Israelite ancestors used prayer shawls to help them to pray and to remind them of God's constant presence.

This prayer shawl is for you to know that someone has been and continues to pray for you. And it is to encourage you to know that God is with you every step of the way, every day.

It is our prayer that you will use this shawl as a mantle of love. Wrap it around you as you go about your daily activities, when you go out, when you feel down, when you sleep, whenever you feel a need for love and support.

Always remember that the knitter wove prayers for God's love and healing into the shawl to create a covering of God's mysterious presence in the life of the recipient—you.

Loving hearts and hands make up the Knitting Ministry, sharing simple gifts for those who suffer in body, mind, and spirit. Our prayer is that this shawl might comfort you and remind you of God's healing presence with you.

Machine wash in cold water.
Tumble dry on low or delicate.

This prayer shawl was made for you by a member of the Prayer Shawl Ministry at (name and address of faith community).

Sample provided by Calvary Lutheran Church of Golden Valley, MN. www.calvary.org

Appendix G

Ritual of Thanksgiving
For a Dwelling That Has Blessed Us

by Annette Langdon

Invitation
Family and friends, gather to remember and give thanks for a home that has been a blessing.

Reading Psalm 121:8
The LORD will keep your going out and your coming in from this time forth and forevermore.

Hymn *Our Father, by Whose Name* (or other meaningful song)

Our Father, by whose name
All parenthood is known;
In love divine you claim
Each family as your own.
Bless mothers, fathers, guarding well,
With constant love as sentinel
The homes in which your people dwell.

O Christ, yourself a child
Within an earthly home,
With heart still undefiled
To full adulthood come;
Our children bless in ev'ry place
That they may all behold your face
And knowing you, may grow in grace.

O Holy Spirit, bind our hearts in unity
And teach us how to find
The love from self-set free;
In all our hearts such love increase
That every home, by this release,
May be the dwelling place of peace.

Reading Deuteronomy 4:9–10
But take care and watch yourselves closely, so as neither to forget the things that your eyes have seen nor to let them slip from your mind all the days of your life; make them known to your children and your children's children—how you once stood before the LORD your God at Horeb, when the LORD said to me, "Assemble the people for me and I will let them hear my words, so that they may learn to fear me as long as they live on the earth and may teach their children so."

Reading Psalm 90:1
Lord, you have been our dwelling place in all generations.

Reflection

Remembering God's special involvement in our lives gives us hope and encouragement for the future.

The procession of reflection from room to room may be led by the bearer of the candle, giving time for sharing memories and stories about the dwelling and its significance.

Conclude with prayers of thanksgiving in each room before moving on to the next.

The Lord's Prayer

Hymn *Now Thank We All Our God* (or other meaningful song)

Now thank we all our God
With hearts and hands and voices,
Who wondrous things has done,
In whom his world rejoices;
Who, from our mothers' arms,
Has blest us on our way
With countless gifts of love,
And still is ours today.

Oh, may this bounteous God
Through all our life be near us,
With ever joyful hearts
And blessed peace to cheer us,
And keep us in his grace,
And guide us when perplexed,
And free us from all harm
In this world and the next.

All praise and thanks to God
The Father now be given,
The Son, and him who reigns
With them in highest heaven,
The one eternal God,
Whom earth and heav'n adore;
For thus it was, is now,
And shall be evermore.

Blessing

May the Lord watch over our going out and our coming in, from this time forth and forever more. Amen.

Appendix H

Spiritual Assessment Acronyms: HOPE and FICA

Remembering the acronyms of HOPE or FICA can guide listening and help frame questions for discerning needs. While FCNs may assume some of the answers when interacting with members of their faith community, it is helpful to be aware of these assumptions and to keep open to a person's particular beliefs, values, and practices.

Select, adapt or find your own questions or ways to address the areas related to the acronyms. This does not have to be in one encounter, but rather gathered over time.

HOPE

H—Sources of Hope, meaning, strength, comfort, peace, love, and connection
- What are your sources of hope, strength, comfort, and peace?
- What do you hold onto during difficult times?
- What sustains you and keeps you going?

O—Organized Religion
- Do you consider yourself part of an organized religion or faith community?
- How important is this to you?
- What aspects are helpful? What's not so helpful?

P—Personal Spirituality and Practices
- Tell me about your personal spiritual beliefs.
- What kind of relationship do you have with God?
- What aspects of your spirituality or spiritual practices do you find most helpful to you personally? For instance, prayer, Scripture, meditation, attending worship services, listening to music, communing with nature. and so on.

E—Effects on care and end-of-life issues
- Has your current situation affected your relationship with God? Or affected your ability to do the things that usually help you spiritually?
- How might I be helpful in supporting you during this time?

Additional Questions

- What sustains you?
- What do you hope for?
- (For members) Do you consider yourself a part of the faith community?
- How would you like your beliefs addressed in our time together? (This may be through prayer, use of Scripture, devotionals, and so on.)

Adapted or reprinted with permission from Spirituality and Medical Practice: Using the HOPE Questions as a Practical Tool for Spiritual Assessment, January 1, 2001, Vol 63, No 1, American Family Physician Copyright © 2001 American Academy of Family Physicians. All Rights Reserved.

FICA

Clinician Questions	Patient Responses
F - Faith and Belief	
Do you consider yourself spiritual or religious?	
Do you have spiritual beliefs that help you cope with stress?	
If the patient answers "No," the health care provider might ask,	
What gives your life meaning?	
Sometimes patients respond with answers such as family, career, or nature.	
I - Importance	
What importance does your faith or belief have in your life?	
Have your beliefs influenced how you take care of yourself in this illness?	
What role do your beliefs play in regaining your health?	
C - Community	
Are you part of a spiritual or religious community?	
Is this of support to you and how?	
Is there a group of people you really love or who are important to you?	
Communities such as churches, temples, and mosques, or a group of like-minded friends can serve as strong support systems for some patients.	
A - Address in Care	
How would you like me, your healthcare provider, to address these issues in your healthcare?	

The FICA Spiritual History Tool was developed by Christina Puchalski (1996; consultgerirn.org/uploads/File/trythis/ try_this_sp5.pdf). Reprinted with permission.

Appendix I

Questions for Spiritual Assessment

Children & Youth

Children have trouble understanding God, especially when bad things happen. Asking questions like these can help the adults in their lives understand what children and youth are thinking. They also can assist the child in dealing with feelings.

Preschool Age:
- Who is God?
- How does God help you?
- When do you feel close to God?
- What helps you when you are scared?
- What does God think about you (or your family member's) illness?
- What do you think caused your sickness or trouble?
- Do you think God can help you get better?

School Age:
- Do you think about God?
- What does God mean to you?
- What does God do for you?
- Who do you turn to when you are in trouble?
- Do you pray? Does it help?
- How does God answer your prayers?
- What things at church make you feel better?

Adolescent:
- Is God important to you?
- What is your source of strength and hope?
- When have you felt that you really needed God?
- Is prayer helpful to you?
- How has God answered your prayers?
- Do you ever wonder how God is involved in certain situations?
- How does your relationship with God affect your daily life?
- How do troubled times affect your relationship with God or church?

Adults

Spirituality:
- What gives you "life," energy, a reason to get up?
- What gives you meaning?
- What gives you hope? Or, where do you find hope these days?
- What is the "fire within"?
- What do you look forward to? What are your goals? Your dreams? Your plans?

- If you were to die suddenly, is there anything that would seem unfinished?
- How have you been gifted by life? For what and to whom are you grateful?
- What have you contributed to life, to others, to society? What are your gifts and talents? Accomplishments?
- What fears to do you have? What concerns?
- Do you have any regrets? Any guilt?

Faith:
- What do you believe about God?
- What is God like for you?
- What is God like for you in this illness?
- What are your memories of God from your childhood?
- Was there anyone in your life who helped you in your relationship with God? Is there now?
- Do you have any fears about God?
- What do you believe happens after death? What will happen to you?

Worship:
- What is your religious background?
- Were you raised in a church?
- Is there anything you miss about church now that you are sick?
- Do you pray? What is your prayer like? Is it helpful?
- Would you like me to pray with you?
- Are there any prayers, songs, scripture readings, or rituals that are meaningful?
- Is there anything you would like in terms of worship, ritual or prayer when you can't speak? When you die?

From unpublished lecture by Chaplain Katherine M. Piderman, Ph.D., Mayo Clinic, Rochester, MN.

Additional Questions for Spiritual Care

- Tell me more.
- Tell me more about ...
- What do you find yourself thinking about or wondering about?
- What would you like me to share with (pastor, members, others)? What would you like them to know about your situation?
- What relationships are important to you at this time?
- Who is supportive of you? With whom can you share openly and honestly?
- If discord is noted in a relationship: How would you like this relationship to be? How might you move toward this?
- What gets in the way for you in relating to ...?

Appendix J

21 Ways to Refresh Your Prayer Life

by Betsy Lee, Prayer Ventures www.prayerventures.org

1. Sing a psalm. Many of the psalms were originally composed on David's lute. Make up your own melody and sing or hum the words.

2. Take a prayer walk around a lake, in a park, or through the neighborhood. Imagine Jesus walking beside you like a friend. Feel free to share your heart. He will listen.

3. Use a picture calendar for a devotional focal point. You might enjoy ocean scenes or gardens or mountainscapes. Imagine yourself in the scene; commune with God there.

4. Kneel as you pray. It will increase your humility and attitude of reverence and worship.

5. Dance to the Lord as David did (2 Samuel 6:14). Make up your own steps while listening to praise music. Clap your hands or lift them up as you sway to the music. Release your whole body to be an instrument of worship!

6. Pray while lying down outstretched on the floor.

7. Be completely silent. Silence is restful, and it allows us to rest in God's love. Empty your mind of preoccupations and let God fill you up with himself.

8. Rest your hands on your lap, palms up, ready to receive what God has to give in prayer.

9. Light a candle. Focus on the flame. Let its quiet beauty still your mind. Draw close to God and he will draw close to you.

10. Personalize Scripture. For example, hear God speak these words personally to you: "I will exult over you, (insert your name), with joy, I will be quiet in my love, I will rejoice over you with shouts of joy" (Zephaniah 3:17). Drink the words in deeply. Or you could pray this for a friend: "Lord, exult over Jane with joy, be quiet in your love, rejoice over her with shouts of joy!" Imagine your friend drinking these words in deeply.

11. Type out a verse of Scripture and tape it to the steering wheel of your car. When your eyes glance down at it while waiting at a red light, ponder it and let God speak to you through those words. Let God's Word nourish your spirit.

12. Pray while engaging in a relaxing activity, such as pushing your preschooler in the backyard on a swing or jogging or gardening. This will slow your praying down to a more leisurely pace.

13. Use the outdoors to inspire your prayers. For example, as you drive down the highway, gaze at the sky and recall this verse, "For great is your love, higher that the heavens; your faithfulness reaches to the skies" (Psalm 108:4, NIV). Thank God for his vast, immeasurable faithfulness to you.

14. Journal as you pray. If a particular Scripture verse seems to strike a chord in your heart and it seems that God is speaking those words directly to you, he probably is. Jot the verse down, reflect on it, let it unfold in your thinking over weeks, even months. Little by little, the full intent of what God is saying will be revealed.

15. Use concrete objects to focus your prayers. For example, if you need to give God a burden or heartache, hold a small wooden cross in your hand and let the pain literally be transferred from you to Jesus. Scripture invites us to do this: "Cast all your anxiety upon him, because he cares for you" (1 Peter 5:7, NIV). If you need to let someone go in your life, hold a miniature basket in your hand and imagine putting that person in the basket as Moses' mother put her son in a basket and let him go, trusting him to God.

16. Use life-size objects, too. For example, if God is calling you to take a step of faith, think of your ottoman in the living room as an altar; place your shoes on the ottoman to signify your willingness to be fully yielded to where he is asking you to go.

17. Organize your prayer life by focusing on different subjects every day of the week. You could pray for family members on Monday, your church on Tuesday, missionaries on Thursday, and so on. Be sure to reserve Wednesday just for praise—no petitions. Nothing overcomes a midweek slump like a surge of worship and praise!

18. Pray thematically. Use the theme from a single verse to guide your prayers: "I am the light of the world" (John 8:12). Pray that Jesus would infuse the lives of those you love with light; ask for his light to illumine a confusing situation you are wrestling with; imagine the light of his presence bathing a dark place in the world.

19. Step into a scene of Scripture. Experience through your senses the actual sights, sounds, and smells of the setting of a gospel story. Imagine yourself in the story face-to-face with Jesus. Let him touch the leprosy in you, heal your blindness, call you back to life like Lazarus.

20. Draw pictures in the margins of your Bible or in a notebook as you pray. If you are a visual person, this is a powerful way to process prayer and let it do its deep work.

21. Listen. Listen. Listen. God speaks in many ways: through pictures, dreams, impressions, words of Scripture, circumstances, other people.

Appendix K

Visualization

Many people find it helpful to use their imagination to create a mental "vacation" or a "private place" where they can go at any time to feel peaceful and relaxed.

1. Sit or lie down in a comfortable position. Try not to cross your legs. Leave your arms relaxed at your sides or in your lap.
2. Close your eyes.
3. Take a couple deep, relaxation breaths.
4. Imagine yourself in a place that is comfortable, safe, relaxing, and beautiful for you. It can be a place you have been or an imaginary place.
    -   an ocean beach
    -   a forest
    -   a garden etc.
5. Now, fill in the details:
    -   What do you *see* around you? In your mind look around you, create each detail—the colors of the leaves, the sun sparkling on the water, etc.
    -   What *sounds* do you hear? Listen to the waves lapping against the shore, the birds chirping, and so on.
    -   What do you *feel*? Feel the warmth of the sun on your skin and between your toes, etc.
    -   What do you *smell*? Salt water? Flowers?
    -   Is anyone with you? Are you alone?
    -   Fill in any other details.
6. Build this image in your mind, and rest here. When you feel at peace and relaxed, slowly leave your special place and return your mind to the present.
7. Take a couple deep relaxation breaths.
8. Slowly open your eyes.

The place you create is yours alone, and you can return there whenever you need peace and relaxation.

Hint: Some find it helpful to create a transition to and from a relaxation place. For example, you could begin and end your visualization by walking down a hallway or a path to, then from, your place.

Quick Stress Reducer: You can also use visualization as a tool to help you prepare for a stressful situation. Preview the event in your mind. Imagine yourself doing the task perfectly. For example, if you are anxious about a speech, imagine yourself in front of the audience calm and confident. Hear yourself speaking with a strong and steady voice.

Used with permission from Trinity Unity Point Health and Trinity Parish Nurse Program.

Appendix L

Prayers for Spiritual Care

Prayers for Strength and Courage (http://edwinagateley.com/)
"The LORD is my light and salvation; whom shall I fear? The LORD is the strength of my life; of whom shall I be afraid?" (Psalm 27:1, KJV)

" ... those who wait on the LORD shall renew their strength; They shall mount up with wings like eagles, they shall run and not be weary, they shall walk and not be faint." (Isaiah 40:31)

Christ be with_____and her/his family, be within _____ and her/his family, be behind _____ and her/his family, be before _____ and her/his family, be beside _____ and her/his family, be beneath _____ and her/his family, be above _____ and her/his family. Let them know your peace that passes all human understanding. Give them strength and courage on this journey. Bless and keep them in loving arms.
(Inspired by the Breastplate of St. Patrick)

Prayers for Healing, Hope and Peace
Lord, we hold (name) and her (his) family lovingly, trustingly before you. Please surround them with your healing power. Let their hearts be hushed and quieted knowing that you have them in your healing arms.

"Be still and know that I am God." (Psalm 46:10)

Centering Prayer
"Let the words of my mouth and the meditation of my heart be acceptable in your sight, O LORD, my strength and my redeemer." (Psalm 19:14, KJV)

All will be well, and all will be well
And all manner of things will be well.
        —Julian of Norwich, c. 1416

Care for Caregivers
My soul thirsts for the living God (Psalm 42:1–3)
Our eyes look to God (Psalm 123)
Those who wait on the Lord will renew their strength (Isaiah 40:27–31)
I will give you rest (Matthew 11:28–30)
We have treasure in clay jars (2 Corinthians 4:7–12)
God's power made perfect in weakness (2 Corinthians 12:7–10)

O Lord, we sometimes feel that we are at our limits of power to help. We struggle to know what to do to be helpful. We place into your hands ourselves that care so deeply for (name) and (his or her) family. We thank you for all you have done and helped us to do. We ask you to lend your strength and courage to all those that are providing care support. Now shelter us in your peace, which surpasses our understanding. Amen.

Adapted from Evangelical Lutheran Worship, Pastoral Care *(Augsburg Fortress).*
Prayers and resources offered by Mary Nordtvedt, FCN, Augustana Lutheran Church, West St. Paul, MN. http://www. augustana.com

Appendix M

Daily Texts

The Daily Texts are Bible verses selected annually for each day of the year by the Moravian Church and shared worldwide since 1731. The *Daily Texts* booklet adds prayers to the Bible texts and is available through Mount Carmel Ministries, Alexandria, Minnesota. www.MountCarmel Ministries.com

The following process of using the Daily Texts is shared by retired Pastor Dale Vitalis of Moorhead, Minnesota, and used with permission.

There are many ways to feast on God's Word. I think some of these thoughts may lead you to find the manna for your journey.

When I am alone and using the Daily Texts, it is helpful for me to speak these verses aloud. Then I write down my thoughts. I have learned that when I write, I tap the treasure of my subconscious mind. I think of this as a way that Christ is *at work in you, enabling you both to will and to work for his good pleasure* (Philippians 2:13).

When we write we experience part of the way in which we speak the truth in love, ... *grow up in every way into him who is the head, into Christ* (Ephesians 4:15).

It is a bonus to be able to share our thoughts with someone else and to enter into a time of prayer, but it is not essential to the process. After all, we are with the Spirit who intercedes on our behalf and with Jesus, the author and perfecter of our faith. So we are never alone in our quiet time.

Here are some specific steps to expand your use of the Daily Texts that I have learned through my own habitual practice and experience.

Ways to Pray the Daily Texts
- Read the texts beginning with the Old Testament verse. Read it twice, once out loud.
- Read the New Testament verse. Read it twice, once out loud.
- Identify the words or themes that are similar or reflect one another in the verses.
- Underline or circle any of these words, or write down the theme that corresponds to the other text.
- Look at the action verbs in the verses. Who is initiating the action?
- Shut your eyes and reflect on these verses. Be still before the Lord. Talk to your Lord about what you are seeing in the verses. Read them again, if you like.
- Write down or draw any images as a question or a thought of what these verses are giving you as a message from God today.
- Pray for whatever comes to you for this day as you lift up your voice to God.

Appendix N

A Cup of Tea

1. On top of a table and underneath it, place plastic to catch the overflowing water during the drama.
2. Put a teapot of water, an empty bowl, and two cups on the table.
3. Ask for two volunteers who will help you with a short drama. Give each volunteer a copy of the story "A Cup of Tea" (below).
4. Explain that you will be the narrator. Assign one volunteer to the role of master teacher who will pour the tea. Assign the other person to the role of the university professor.
5. Ask both volunteers to raise their hands when their roles are mentioned in the first line of the story.
6. Ask the master teacher to pour the tea to overflowing and to say the "master teacher" lines at the appropriate time during your narration.
7. The professor will say the "professor" lines at the appropriate time and pour the water from the cup into a bowl at the end of the drama.
8. Ask the volunteers to take their places, and invite the group to watch and listen to a role-play. Read the following narration.

    Narrator: There is a story about a university professor (volunteer raises hand) who came to a master teacher (volunteer raises hand) to learn about human psychology. The master teacher began explaining his philosophy but the professor kept interrupting, saying:

    Professor: "Oh yes, we teach that, too. Ah, I've heard that before."

    Narrator: Finally, the master teacher stopped talking and poured his visitor a cup of tea. Once the cup was full, though, he kept pouring until the tea overflowed onto the table. The professor exclaimed:

    Professor: "Stop! No more can go into the cup."

    Narrator: The master teacher responded:

    Master Teacher: "Like this cup, you are full of your own opinions and speculations. How can I teach you about the subject unless you first empty your cup?"

    Narrator: The professor paused and then slowly poured most of the water from the cup into the empty bowl at his side.

9. Thank the volunteers for participating and ask them to return to their seats.

Guide the group discussion by leading participants through these questions and explanations.

How did you feel about what you saw in this short drama?

Explain that the message for BeFrienders (and FCNs) is that the master teacher in the story is those whom they befriend (visit). A BeFriender (FCN) is the student or listener. However, if we come to listen to the story with our cups full, we can't hear the story.

What might be in your cup that could prevent you from really hearing the story?

To help participants reflect on this question suggest that possibilities could stem from their judgments, personal agendas, desire to "fix" things, expectations, assumptions, resistance, and leftover emotions from previous experiences. Allow some time for discussion and silent reflection.

What impact might good intentions or positive feelings have on listening?

Explain that things like optimism, excitement, or care for the other may also prevent us from really hearing.

Are the things in your cup good or bad?

Explain that it is neither good nor bad. It simply is. Anything in one's cup can be helpful to another at some times and not helpful at others.

What is the purpose of knowing what is in your cup?

Let participants talk this through for a minute or two. Be sure to cover the following points if they are not brought forward.

- Being aware of the contents enables you to have the possibility of choice. You may either set it aside and leave it there, or use it at the appropriate time.
- If you don't know what is in your cup, what is in it will have an effect on your ministry.
- If you are aware, you can empty your cup and be fully present to hear the other person's story.

At the end of the drama, was the cup completely emptied by the professor?

No. At times we have something in our cup but there is still space to openly receive what we hear. It is also important to note that what is emptied from our cup doesn't disappear. It is set aside like the tea poured into the bowl.

What are some things you can do to help empty your cup?

Suggest the following if they are not mentioned.

- journal
- self-talk
- talk with a friend
- pray
- exercise
- experience nature

What if you can't empty your cup or it becomes full during a visit?

Point out that while an empty cup is our goal, one that is partially full can still receive. However, if it is so full that no more will go in, it is appropriate to tactfully bring the visit to a close or postpone a visit.

Used with permission from BeFriender Ministry—
A Listening Presence
120 E 80th St, Suite 105
Bloomington, MN 55420
www.befrienderministry.org

Unit I: Spirituality
Prayer

Prayer

Introduction

Learning Outcomes

Upon completion of this module, the participant will be able to:

1. Use prayer as an intervention for individuals and groups in the practice of faith community nursing.
2. Explore various theological concepts about prayer and healing.
3. Use pertinent scriptural resources for prayer sessions related to physical and spiritual healing.
4. Examine prayer practices that can promote personal spiritual growth.

Description

This module focuses upon expanding the knowledge, resources, and prayer leadership skills of the faith community nurse (FCN). Prayer is a central component of the expression of all faith traditions and key to the integration of spirituality and health. Prayer practices are important for one's personal faith development as a spiritual leader, as well as for the support of individuals and groups within a faith community.

Hours: 2

Research

Relying upon reports from the world's diverse religious communities, Dossey (1993) provided examples of instances when prayer seemed to induce physical healing. Making the connection between physical health and spirituality, he examined prayer from a scientific point of view. A number of more recent studies that clarify the link between prayer and healing are documented by Koenig et al., (2012). The nurse's own personal and professional experience, which draw the individual toward the profession of faith community nursing, may embrace prayer as a powerful nursing intervention that helps facilitate desired outcomes, such as reduced spiritual distress, reduced risk for loneliness, or grief work facilitation. Kim-Godwin's (2013) review of research on prayer for health and in nursing practice offers evidence-based suggestions for prayer with and for patients in clinical settings.

Faith Tradition

Most religions are characterized by the practice of praying even though the usual practices are varied and reflect cultural differences. Prayer is an essential discipline in the Judeo-Christian faiths, and Christians are commanded to include prayer in their everyday lives. Both private and corporate prayers are encouraged. Prayer can be liturgical, as is often seen within Catholic, Lutheran, and Episcopal churches. Non-liturgical informal prayer is more common within evangelical faith communities, and charismatic prayer may include song and dance and is often seen within gospel traditions.

Key Terms

Centering prayer: praying while reading and reflecting on scripture

Lectio divina: slow, contemplative praying while meditating on the scriptures

Meditation: process of focusing and calming your mind

Prayer: a vehicle for communication with God (Judeo-Christian tradition)

Reflection

The Inescapable God
To the leader. Of David. A Psalm.

"O Lord, you have searched me and known me.
You know when I sit down and when I rise up;
you discern my thoughts from far away.
You search out my path and my lying down,
and are acquainted with all my ways.
Even before a word is on my tongue,
O Lord, you know it completely.
You hem me in, behind and before,
and lay your hand upon me.
Such knowledge is too wonderful for me;
it is so high that I cannot attain it.
Where can I go from your spirit?
Or where can I flee from your presence?
If I ascend to heaven, you are there;
if I make my bed in Sheol, you are there.
If I take the wings of the morning
and settle at the farthest limits of the sea,
even there your hand shall lead me,
and your right hand shall hold me fast.
If I say, 'Surely the darkness shall cover me,
and the light around me become night,'
even the darkness is not dark to you;
the night is as bright as the day,
for darkness is as light to you.
For it was you who formed my inward parts;
you knit me together in my mother's womb.
I praise you, for I am fearfully and wonderfully made.
Wonderful are your works;
that I know very well.
My frame was not hidden from you,
when I was being made in secret,
intricately woven in the depths of the earth.
Your eyes beheld my unformed substance.
In your book were written
all the days that were formed for me,
when none of them as yet existed.
How weighty to me are your thoughts, O God!
How vast is the sum of them!
I try to count them—they are more than the sand;
I come to the end—I am still with you. ...
Search me, O God, and know my heart;
test me and know my thoughts.
See if there is any wicked way in me,
and lead me in the way everlasting."
—Psalm 139: 1-18; 23-24

Prayer
Content Outline

KEY TERM
Prayer *is a vehicle for communication with God.*

OUTCOME 1

Use prayer as an intervention for individuals and groups in the practice of faith community nursing.

In the Judeo-Christian tradition, prayer is a vehicle for communication with God. Prayer is lifting the mind and heart to God. This ancient definition, generally attributed to St. Augustine, allows for a wide range of prayer forms. Prayer and meditation facilitate time for centering and focusing on one's spiritual wellness. Prayer helps people to alleviate anxiety, lift the spirit, and express gratitude.

The Judeo-Christian tradition provides illustrations of various types of prayer.
- prayer of praise and adoration of God
- prayer of penitence, asking forgiveness of sin
- prayer of petition, asking for answer to a specific request
- prayer of thanksgiving, expressing gratitude to God
- prayer of intercession, praying on behalf of another
- prayer of blessing, asking a special blessing on another
- prayer of meditation, pondering the nature of God

Often several types of prayers such as thanksgiving, intercession, and praise, may be combined into one prayer. These prayers can be either liturgical (scripted prayers for corporate worship) or personal prayers.

Other faith traditions also value prayer.
Jewish Prayer
In the Jewish tradition, prayer means to stand in self-judgment (Weinberg, 2009). "Prayer has the ability to lift human beings upward toward God and to bring God closer to human beings" (p. 86). The Jews have special prayers for each situation in their lives. The prayers pronounced on ecclesiastical holidays differ from the ones for average days. Generally, modern Jews say the special prayers only on Saturdays and on special occasions such as Hanukkah or Pesach. All forms of Judaism use established prayers.

- The *Shema* "is the most significant prayer relating to Jewish identification—be it an individual or entire community" (p. 81). This prayer is about hope, courage and commitment to the faith.
- The *Mi she-Berakh* is the prayer of healing and represents the "role that health plays in the everyday lives of Jews" (p. 84).
- The *Kaddish*, the prayer of mourning, is used by family members daily for 11 months after the death of a loved one.

Muslim prayer (*Salat* or *Namaz*), in the sense of worship, is the second pillar of Islam. Adherents to the Islamic faith tradition believe that prayer is obligatory and must be done five times a day. Every time of day begins with prayer; the first one is pronounced during dawn and the last one is pronounced at sunset.

- The five times are dawn (*al-fajr*), immediately after noon (*al-zuhr*), midafternoon (*al-'asr*), sunset (*al-maghrib*), and early night (*al-'isha*).
- Prayer involves uniting body, mind, and soul in worship.
- Islam teaches that in prayer, each person is in direct contact with Allah.
- Muslims may pray anywhere, but praying together in a mosque helps believers realize that all are equal in the sight of Allah.
- Ritual washing, called *wudhu*, is required before prayer (http://www.bbc.co.uk/religion/religions/islam/practices/salat.shtml).

Hinduism has no single founder or sacred text, though most Hindus revere the *Veda* texts and draw on *dharma* as a system of morality.

- Most Hindus believe in a Supreme God. Because God is unlimited, a multitude of deities emanate from God.
- Most worship and prayer is individual rather than corporate.
- Prayer involves using a mantra (http://www.bbc.co.uk/religion/religions/hinduism/worship/worship.shtml).

Exceeded in numbers only by Christianity, Islam and Hinduism, **Buddhism** is the fourth largest religion in the world.

- Rather than worshiping gods or deities, Buddhists seek a path to Enlightenment about the true nature of life through morality, meditation, and wisdom.
- Though Buddhism does not teach about a supreme creator God, prayer and meditation are central to its practice.
- Prayer aids include mantras (a word, syllable or phrase repeated), which are thought to have profound spiritual effect, and prayer wheels and flags that may be used as a method of repeating the mantra (http://www.bbc.co.uk/religion/religions/buddhism/customs/worship_1.shtml).

Prayer and the Nurse-Client Relationship

The FCN should undertake **assessment** to ascertain whether or not individuals would like to have prayer and what their experience and understanding of prayer has been.

- It will be important to discover whether or not they are familiar with praying individually or in groups.
- It is desirable to determine how they prefer to reference God (Heavenly Father, Creator, Lord, Jesus).
- It will also be essential to discern what specific needs and concerns they would like to bring to God.
- Developing a therapeutic nurse-client relationship is key to assessing and discerning individual prayer preferences.

Established prayers for personal and communal praying are common in many faith traditions. Numerous books are available that contain prayers for every occasion. There are many famous prayers that the FCN can use when leading prayer sessions, including these examples.

The Prayer of St. Francis

Lord, make me an instrument of thy peace;
where there is hatred, let me sow love;
where there is injury, pardon;
where there is doubt, faith;
where there is despair, hope;
where there is darkness, light;
and where there is sadness, joy.
O Divine Master,
grant that I may not so much seek to be
consoled as to console;
to be understood, as to understand;
to be loved, as to love;
for it is in giving that we receive,
it is in pardoning that we are pardoned,
and it is in dying that we are born to eternal life.
Amen.

The Serenity Prayer

Lord, grant me the serenity to accept
the things I cannot change,
The courage to change the things I can,
And the wisdom to know the difference.

Personalized prayers can be helpful. A parish nurse in the United Kingdom (UK) was unused to praying with her hospitalized patients, since this is not allowed in state hospitals in the UK. At first she felt awkward and embarrassed about doing it. Then she had an idea: perhaps she could offer to write a personalized prayer for a patient and bring it back at a later date. Being quite artistic, she embellished cards with artwork from software and made two copies: one for herself and one for the patient. In this way the patients would know what the nurse was praying for, and could also use the prayer whenever they felt the need. An activity like this may be some individuals' first introduction to praying, even though in faith community nursing as opposed to secular nursing, prayer often is an expectation.

Praying with children should be given special consideration. Helpful resources for this may be found in Online Resources at the end of this module.

- Young children learn spiritual practices by imitating what they see adults around them doing. Let children see you praying even before they understand all the words.
- Look for ways to include children in the prayer life of the faith community, whether alongside adults or in a children's program.
- Change prayers with the changing age of children. Young children may be more concerned about praying for their sick pet to get well than anything else. Accept the prayers children offer without judgment. As they grow into more abstract thinking, encourage more reflective prayers.
- Give children words for prayer. Use established prayers in the faith tradition, such as the Lord's Prayer in Christian churches, or lead children through prayer by asking them to repeat after you or finish sentences that you begin.
- Encourage habits of prayer by including prayer in interactions with groups of children or assuring individual children you are praying about concerns they express.
- Respect personalities. Don't put a shy child on the spot by expecting everyone to pray aloud.

Praying in groups can be a very positive way to connect family, friends, and colleagues. It is important to ask individuals what they would like to have included in the prayer. FCNs may have varying comfort levels with praying out loud depending upon his or her faith tradition. If this is the case, the FCN may need to gain experience before being fully comfortable with praying out loud.

Group prayer also raises issues of confidentiality. A simple policy for observing professional guidelines when sharing news for prayer in the context of worship or small groups is essential. Such a policy needs to be agreed to by all involved and placed in a prominent position in the building. (See sample confidentiality policy in Appendix A.)

Critical Thinking

How does your ability to offer prayer for or with someone affect your practice as an FCN?

When encouraging someone from a different faith to pray, what factors does the FCN need to consider?

OUTCOME 2
Explore various theological concepts about prayer and healing.

Concepts Implicit in Prayer for Healing

Here are some questions the FCN can explore for a deeper understanding of prayer for healing.

What is the nature of God?
Words that express what we believe about God may be useful. For Christians the ultimate answer to this question lies in the ministry, nature and action of Jesus. Through Christ's suffering, death and resurrection, God reached out in a ministry of love, healing and reconciliation. God offers to everyone the gift of salvation and hope for a future lived in a recreated and redeemed world (John 3:16).

What is the importance of finding meaning in one's life?
In Christianity and Judaism each person is unique, special and created by God for a relationship with Him. We are called to love

God and love our neighbor. Jesus called people to follow him and to make disciples of all nations (Matthew 28:19–20). Paul called Christians to share in the ministry of reconciliation (2 Corinthians 5:18–19). Prayer may be the only way some people can engage in this relationship, but whatever our gifts and physical or mental abilities, finding this kind of meaning in one's life gives a sense of purpose and peace.

What is the role of touch in healing?
Look at the way touch was involved in the various healing stories in the Bible. Consider these examples: 2 Kings 4:32–37; Matthew 8:1–3, 14–15, 20:29–34; Mark 5:22–34; Acts 9:17–19, 28:7–9; James 5:14.

How can those who are suffering from illness care for others?
The story of St. Cuthbert and St. Aidan, early Celtic saints in the Christian history of England, is inspirational. Even when they were too ill to walk, they were carried around the countryside by their contemporaries, and they prayed for healing for those around them.

What role can the faith community play for those who are sick?
Think not only about the role of the faith community for those who are part of it, but also for those who are not (James 5:14–15).

The FCN must focus on the intentional care of the spirit as well as on the promotion of wholistic health and prevention or minimization of illness within the context of the faith community. The **FCN's personal prayers** for strength, courage, wisdom, and insight can have a positive impact on the care provided to individuals and families in difficult situations. The FCN may want to consider this prayer:

> *Loving and tender God, touch my heart with hope, touch my mind with clarity, touch my soul with peace, and touch my body with the warmth of your healing presence.*
>
> *Grant me courage to face the future, insight to understand life's trials, wisdom to discern how I can touch the lives of others, and comfort of people who care about me as I reach for your loving hands. In your holy name, amen* (Patterson, 2008, p. 77. Used by permission.).

Critical Thinking

How does an understanding of various theological concepts of prayer and healing enhance the practice of an FCN?

How important is it for the FCN to pray with individuals, families, groups, and others in the broader community?

OUTCOME 3

Use pertinent scriptural resources for prayer sessions related to physical and spiritual healing.

Physical healing is one of the most common themes within the Judeo-Christian Scriptures.
- Jesus healed and forgave sins. This happens throughout the Gospels (Matthew, Mark, Luke, and John).
- The apostles continued to heal. See, for example, Peter's healing of a lame beggar in Acts 3 and the apostles' healing many in Acts 5:12–16.

- A number of Old Testament figures had the power to heal. For example, see the story of Elisha healing Naaman of leprosy (2 Kings 5:1–14), Elijah raising a widow's son from death (1 Kings 17:17–24), or Abraham healing Abimelech and his family (Genesis 20).

Spiritual healing is a prominent theme in faith community nurse ministry, with many prayers found throughout the Scriptures. The book of Psalms, for example, has a number of beautiful psalms suitable for use in healing prayers, or for meditation.
- Psalm 1— ... they are like trees planted by streams of water ...
- Psalm 18— I love you, O LORD, my strength ...
- Psalm 19—The heavens are telling the glory of God ...
- Psalm 20—The LORD answer you in the day of trouble!
- Psalm 22—My God, my God, why have you forsaken me?
- Psalm 23—The LORD is my shepherd ...
- Psalm 24—The earth is the LORD'S, and all that is in it ...
- Psalm 46—God is our refuge and strength ...
- Psalm 91—You who live in the shelter of the Most High ...
- Psalm 121—I lift my eyes to the hills ...

A number of passages speak specifically about prayer, including these.
- Psalm 46:10—Be still, and know that I am God!
- Romans 8:26—The Holy Spirit intercedes for us.
- Matthew 6:6—Go into your room and shut the door ...
- Matthew 6:7—Do not heap up empty phrases ...
- Matthew 6:9—Pray then in this way: Our Father in heaven ...

Critical Thinking
What prayer resources are available for physical and spiritual healing in your faith tradition?

What kind of prayer would be helpful for someone who is terminally ill?

OUTCOME 4

Examine prayer practices that can promote personal spiritual growth.

Personal prayer practices may include the following.

Meditation involves focusing and calming your mind.
1. Seek out a quiet place. Find a comfortable, upright position in which you are relaxed but alert, with your eyes lightly closed. Remain as still as possible.
2. Silently, begin to say interiorly a single word or phrase selected from the context of Christian faith (*Maranatha* is frequently recommended). Listen to it as you say it gently but continuously with faith and love. Do not think or imagine anything, spiritual or otherwise. If thoughts and images come and your attention strays, as soon as you become aware of this, return to saying your word.
3. Meditate each morning and evening for between 20 and 30 minutes (Finley, 2005).

Lectio divina, praying while meditating on the Scriptures has been the most traditional springboard to contemplative prayer. Taking a variety of forms, it is sometimes called sacred reading.

KEY TERM
Meditation *is the process of focusing and calming your mind.*

KEY TERM
Lectio divina *is slow, contemplative praying while meditating on the scriptures.*

KEY TERM

Centering prayer *is praying while reading and reflecting on scripture.*

One form uses these steps.

1. Relax. Settle in. Be aware that God is here, now, loving you.
2. Read a short passage of Scripture as though God were speaking directly to you in it.
3. Choose a phrase from the passage that strikes you and repeat it slowly and prayerfully.
4. When your heart is full, express to God the needs and sentiments awakened by your meditation. When you're done, read another passage and repeat steps 3 and 4.
5. If, at any time, you feel moved to simply be present to God in loving silence, put the Scripture aside and rest in God (Keating, 2009).

Centering prayer involves taking time to read and reflect on Scripture.

1. Choose a sacred word as the symbol of your intention to consent to God's presence and action within.
2. Sitting comfortably and with eyes closed, settle briefly, and silently introduce the sacred word as the symbol of your consent to God's presence and action within.
3. When you become aware of thoughts, return ever-so-gently to the sacred word.
4. At the end of the prayer period, remain in silence with eyes closed for a couple of minutes (Keating, 2009).

Other prayer practices include:
- praying the rosary
- walking a labyrinth
- prayer-walking
- singing hymns
- breath prayer
- journaling as prayer
- working with a spiritual director
- finding a prayer partner
- attending a prayer group
- participating in a prayer chain
- bringing prayer requests to others, such as religious orders who practice perpetual adoration
- praying together with others in worship services

Standards of Professional Performance for Faith Community Nursing

Prayer is an important competency for faith community nurses whose specialty practice focuses on intentional care of the spirit. However, there is no specific professional standard that relates to prayer.

Learning Activities

Prayer Roles and Practices

Instructions:
1. Discuss the various roles of prayer in a faith community, including the concepts of invocation, blessing, supplication, dedication, and intercession.

2. Discuss various prayer practices that occur in a variety of faith traditions, from private prayer, to prayer partners, to prayer groups, to congregational prayer.

Question:
What new practice of prayer are you interested in exploring?

A Prayer for Healing

Instructions:
1. Read this prayer aloud together as a group.
   Loving and tender God, touch my heart with hope, touch my mind with clarity, touch my soul with peace, and touch my body with the warmth of your healing presence.

   Grant me courage to face the future, insight to understand life's trials, wisdom to discern how I can touch the lives of others, and the comfort of people who care about me as I reach for your loving hands. In your holy name, amen (Patterson, 2008, p. 77. Used by permission.).

2. As a large group or in small groups, ask participants to identify theological concepts implicit in this prayer.

Question:
How would you explain your personal view of the role of prayer in healing?

Prayer Needs

Instructions:
1. Pair participants.

2. Ask one participant to tell the other about a personal prayer request. The second will then prepare a short prayer or read a prayer that meets the need of the first.

3. Have participants switch roles.

Question:
How do you feel when you hear others praying for you? How do you feel when you have the opportunity to pray for someone else?

Prayer Resources

Instructions:
1. Ask participants to form small groups.
2. Discuss prayer resources that can be used for physical and spiritual healing. If Internet access is available, encourage participants to explore online resources listed at the end of the module.
3. Ask groups to share their resources with the larger group.

Question:
What resources for prayer have you found most meaningful to you personally?

Advance Resources

Instructions:
As a pre-class assignment, ask participants to make a resource list of CD or downloadable music that helps them pray and bring it to share with others. In addition, they could research and include the liturgies or source books for prayer they have found to be particularly useful or resources published by their own denominations. In this way, each participant can benefit from the experience of others and collect a personal library of resources.

References

Required Textbook

American Nurses Association and Health Ministries Association. (2012). *Faith community nursing: Scope and standards of practice* (2nd ed.). Silver Spring, MD: Nursesbooks.org.

References

Buttrick, G. A. (1947). *Prayer.* Nashville, TN: Abingdon.

Dossey, B. M. & Keegan, L. (Eds.) (2012). *Holistic nursing: A handbook for practice.* Burlington, MA: Jones and Bartlett Learning.

Dossey, L. (1993). *Healing words: The power of prayer and the practice of medicine.* San Francisco, CA: Harper Collins.

Dysinger, L. *How to practice lectio divina.* Retrieved June 29, 2014 from http://www.beliefnet.com/Faiths/Catholic/2000/08/How-To-Practice-Lectio-Divina.aspx

Finley, J. (2005). *Christian Meditation: Experiencing the presence of God.* San Francisco, CA: HarperOne.

Foster, R. J. (1992). *Prayer: Finding the heart's true home.* San Francisco, CA: HarperOne.

Hallesby, O. (1931). *Prayer.* Minneapolis: Augsburg Fortress.

Keating, T. (2009). *Intimacy with God: An introduction to centering prayer.* Colorado Springs, CO: Crossroads Publishing Company.

Kim-Godwin, Y. (2013). Prayer in clinical practice: What does evidence support? *Journal of Christian Nursing, 30*(4), 208–217.

Koenig, H. G., (2008). *Medicine, religion, and health: Where science and spirituality meet.* West Conshohocken, PA: Templeton Press.

Koenig, H .G., King, D. E., and Carson, V. B., (2012). *Handbook of religion and health* (2nd ed.). New York: Oxford University Press.

O'Brien, M. E. (2003). *Prayer in nursing: The spirituality of compassionate caregiving.* Sudbury, MA: Jones and Bartlett Learning.

Patterson, D. (2008). *Healing words for healing people: Prayers and meditations for parish nurses and other health professionals.* Cleveland, OH: Pilgrim Press.

Rupp, J. (2007). *Prayer.* New York: Orbis.

Weinberg, L. (2009). A model of Jewish congregational nursing. In Smucker, L., *Faith community nursing.* Silver Spring, MD: Nursesbooks.org.

Westberg, G. (1955). *Nurse, pastor, and patient: A hospital chaplain talks with nurses.* Rock Island, IL: Augustana Press.

Yancey, P. (2006). *Prayer: Does it make any difference?* Grand Rapids, MI: Zondervan.

Additional References

Beech, V. (2010). *My God book.* Bletchley, England: UK Scripture Union Press.

Krause, N., Hayward, R. D. (2013). Prayer beliefs and change in life satisfaction over time. *Journal of Religion and Health, 52,* 674–694.

Patterson, D. (2010). *Balm in Gilead: Hymns of healing and wholeness.* St. Louis, MO: International Parish Nurse Resource Center.

Patterson, D. (2011). *Prayers for the soul: Comfort for parish nurses and the people they serve.* St. Louis, MO: International Parish Nurse Resource Center.

Roberts, L., Ahmed, I., & Davison, A. (2009). Intercessory prayer for the alleviation of ill health. *Cochrane Database of Systematic Reviews 2.* Art. No.: CD000368. doi: 10.1002/14651858.CD000368.pub3.

Online Resources:

Prayers from different faiths can be found at i-church.org: http://www.i-church.org/gatehouse/index.php?page=16

Prayers from the Muslim tradition are explained here: http://www.bbc.co.uk/religion/religions/islam/practices/salat.shtml

Prayers from the Hindu tradition here: http://www.bbc.co.uk/religion/religions/hinduism/worship/worship.shtml

Prayers from the Buddhist tradition here: http://www.bbc.co.uk/religion/religions/buddhism/customs/worship_1.shtml

Prayers from the Jewish tradition here: http://www.bbc.co.uk/religion/religions/judaism/worship/prayer_1.shtml

Christian Meditation Links:

Center for Action and Contemplation: http://www.cac.org

Christian Meditation Center: http://christianmeditationcenter.org

Christian Meditation Downloads: http://www.thechristianmeditator.com/christian-meditation-products/meditation-affirmation-bundles/

Contemplative Outreach: http://www.contemplativeoutreach.org

Contemplative Way: http:www.contemplativeway.org

Loyola Press: Praying with Children: Tips to Remember, http://www.loyolapress.com/tips-for-praying-with-children.htm

Pediatric Chaplaincy Network: http://www.paediatric-chaplaincy-network.org/media

Shalem Institute: http://www.shalem.org

Taize: http://www.taize.fr/en

Wisdom Ways: http://wisdomwayscenter.org/christianmeditation.html

World Community for Christian Meditation: http://wccm.org

Quiet Musical Resources:

Perfect Peace. Westminster Abbey Choir, Sony classical productions: http://www.gemm.com/store/CHILTERNS/item/WESTMINSTER-ABBEY-CHOIR-PERFECT-PEACE-CD/757837664

Spirit Wings by Room 217 recordings: http://www.cdbaby.com/cd/room2172

Taize music recordings: http://www.exultet.net/eshop/media/music_samples/M000638-02s.mp3

The Sounds of Shenandoah: www.orangetreeproductions.com

Wrap-Up and Evaluation

Measuring Competency

This chart can be used to assess the individual outcomes in this module.

- A copy of this chart is attached to the Participant Module, so that each participant can complete this short evaluation.
- Have participants read each outcome and then place an X in the box that best matches their opinion about the objective being met.
- Encourage each participant to write a short reflection about this module in the space provided at the bottom of this chart.
- Use this data to make any necessary changes.

Outcome	Not Met	Somewhat Met	Met
1. Use prayer as an intervention for individuals and groups in the practice of faith community nursing.			
2. Explore various theological concepts about prayer and healing.			
3. Use pertinent scriptural resources for prayer sessions related to physical and spiritual healing.			
4. Examine prayer practices that can promote personal spiritual growth.			
Reflection: *In one paragraph, write a reflection on this module.*			

Appendix A

Good Practices in Confidentiality for Church Prayer Groups and Services

"A gossip betrays a confidence,
but a trustworthy person keeps a secret."
—Proverbs 11:13 (NIV)

Parish Nurses have developed these guidelines to safeguard and protect the privacy and identity of the individual, family group, congregation and the wider community when the church is engaging in prayer for them.

Aim: To promote wholeness, trust and healing.

1. Prayer requests should be anonymous unless the consent of the person/family being prayed for has been gained.

2. If consent to share information has been given then the person receiving that consent should clarify
   - what information is permitted
   - what is to be prayed for
   - with whom it may be shared
   - when it may be shared
   - where it may be shared

3. Prayer will be offered with the information as given.

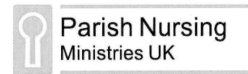

www.parishnursing.org.uk. Used by permission.

Unit I: Spirituality

Self-Care
for the Faith Community Nurse

Self-Care for the Faith Community Nurse

Introduction

Learning Outcomes

Upon completion of this module, the participant will be able to:

1. Develop a deeper intimacy and personal connection with God through care of one's own body, mind, and spirit.
2. Discern the will of God.
3. Engage in the practice of Sabbath, keeping it integral for care of mind, body, and spirit.

Description

This module explores the necessity of caring for one's own body, mind, and spirit. This is important because it is what we are called to do. In order to be wholly present and able to fulfill the role of a faith community nurse (FCN), one must take full responsibility for one's well-being. In addition to being called by God to maintain our well-being, we are at the same time role modeling this concept. It is through mindful and deliberate care of one's whole self that this is achieved. The concept of the ongoing development and maturation of a strong faith in God and how this is linked to self-care will be explored. The theory of developing a deep spiritual connection and discerning the will of God is used as the basis of self-care. Attending to personal care through application of Sabbath-keeping practices and traditions is also presented.

Hours: 2.5

Research

In keeping with Rosemary Rizzo Parse's theory of human becoming, each person is the expert for himself or herself. Each person knows what is best for himself or herself, and no one else can dictate what he or she should do or the decisions he or she should make for personal health care. Therefore, each FCN needs to discover a definition of health and what personal optimum health would be. The way to discover this is to spend time each day meditating and praying. In this way you will discover what your definition is according to the will of God. Research suggests that self-care is vital for the treatment and prevention of burnout and compassion fatigue (Babbel, 2012). Many studies have been done linking faith and health and the benefits of a strong faith to maintain a sense of well-being (Johnstone et al., 2012).

Faith Tradition

Self-care is essential and central to Jewish thought and belief, especially for individuals who are in charge of the care of another. It is believed that each person has the strength within to persevere and is admired and applauded when one not only perseveres on his or her own but calls upon God for strength. Reaching out to others personally or professionally when needed is also respected. "Do not worry about tomorrow's troubles for you may not know what the day will bring. Tomorrow may come and you will be no more and so you will have worried about a world that is not yours" (Talmud Balvi, Tractate Yevamot 63b).

Key Terms

Self-care: deliberate expenditure of energy and time to perform those activities required for well-being and good health, including rest and relaxation

Boundaries: personal property lines that define who you are, and who you are not, and influence all areas of your life (Cloud and Townsend, 1992)

Compassion fatigue: the gradual decline of compassion over time that results when nurses or other health professionals are exposed to events that have traumatized their clients

Discern: to separate; to distinguish; to determine; to sort out

Discernment of God's will: seeking to do God's will, not your will

Sabbath: Hebrew meaning of the word *Sabbath* (Shabbat) is "cessation of work" or "rest"

Reflection

"For surely I know the plans I have for you, says the LORD, plans for your welfare and not for harm, to give you a future with hope."
—Jeremiah 29:11

"For everything there is a season, and a time for every matter under heaven: a time to be born, and a time to die; a time to plant, and a time to pluck up what is planted; a time to kill, and a time to heal; a time to break down, and a time to build up."
—Ecclesiastes 3:1–3

"The thief comes only to steal and kill and destroy. I came that they may have life, and have it abundantly."
—John 10:10

"Remember the sabbath day, and keep it holy."
—Exodus 20:8

"Then he said to them, 'The sabbath was made for humankind and not humankind for the sabbath.'"
—Mark 2:27

"I can do all things through him who strengthens me."
—Philippians 4:13

Self-Care for the Faith Community Nurse

Content Outline

OUTCOME 1

Develop a deeper intimacy and personal connection with God through care of one's own body, mind, and spirit.

Scriptural Basis for Self-Care

As people of God, we are called to practice **self-care**, the deliberate expenditure of energy and time to perform those activities required for well-being and good health, including rest and relaxation and being interactive with God. By being still and offering up *all*, we empty ourselves and make room for the grace of God to fill us and the Spirit of God to move within us.

Discuss the following Scriptures as a basis for developing intimacy and a personal connection with God.

- "The thief comes only to steal and kill and destroy. I came that they may have life, and have it abundantly" (John 10:10).
- "Do not be conformed to this world, but be transformed by the renewing of your minds, so that you may discern what is the will of God—what is good and acceptable and perfect" (Romans 12:2).
- "And all of us, with unveiled faces, seeing the glory of the Lord as though reflected in a mirror, are being transformed into the same image from one degree of glory to another; for this comes from the Lord, the Spirit" (2 Corinthians 3:18).

Suggested Daily Routine for Self-Care of Body, Mind and Spirit

Body

Exercise daily or as many days as time allows.

- A 20-minute walk is a good start. Gradually increase.
- Outdoors is best, weather permitting. Be sure to connect with nature as you walk.

Eat a balanced diet. Give your body the proper nutrition and it will serve you well.

- Choose a wise food plan (such as the Daniel Plan, Mediterranean, Paleo, South Beach or Weight Watchers).
- Before making choices, ask a nutritionist or health care provider whether or not this is a good choice for your body and one that will nourish you.

Many studies show the ill effects of gluten, sugar, processed foods and dairy. A complex range of diseases may result from consumption of wheat, including ulcerative colitis, celiac disease, and irritable bowel syndrome to an assortment of neurological disorders, diabetes, heart disease, fibromyalgia, arthritis, and curious rashes (Davis, 2012; Hyman; 2012, Brown and Roy, 2010; Eswaran, et. al, 2013; Merrin, et. al, 2014).

- Practice moderation. All things are God-given, but we must practice moderation.
- Stop eating as soon as you are full no matter how much is left on your plate. If you want one more bite, resist it and offer the sacrifice for the good of something you want or need. This is a form of fasting.
- Take a quality multivitamin and mineral supplementation. All vitamins are *not* alike. Many of the cheaper brands are not absorbed, so you are not getting any of the benefits. Many good mineral supplements are available, such as concentrated vegetable and fruit powders.
- Use caution when taking additional dietary supplements and megadoses of vitamins.
- Our goal should be a healthy, balanced diet, but most of us do *not* get everything we need from our diet.
- When you give your body the proper nutrients that it needs, your hunger is greatly diminished, and you feel more satisfied more often.
- Maintain a healthy weight and Body Mass Index (BMI) following these recommendations:
  - Underweight = <18.5 BMI
  - Normal weight = 18.5–24.9
  - Overweight = 25–29.9
  - Obese = BMI of 30 or greater

Get adequate sleep. Chronic sleep restriction is increasingly pervasive in the community.
- Studies about short sleep duration have shown that this restricted sleep can be associated with increased sleepiness, poor performance, and increased health risks or mortality (Laugsand et al., 2013).
- Lack of sleep may compromise alertness and performance.
- However, because it becomes a chronic condition, sleep loss may be unrecognized by the sufferers, who accept it as their norm.
- Some clues to an overly sleep-restricted life include the need for stimulants like coffee to wake up or get going each morning, difficulty remaining focused and productive when sitting for a while, negative mood, or poor memory.

- Short sleep duration is linked with:
  - increased risk of driving while drowsy
  - increase in BMI; greater likelihood of obesity due to an increased appetite caused by sleep deprivation
  - increased risk of diabetes and heart problems
  - increased risk for depression and substance abuse
  - decreased ability to pay attention, react to signals or remember new information

HELPFUL RESOURCE

Appendix A features the Church Health Center's Model for Healthy Living.

Sleep hygiene comes from a variety of practices necessary to have normal, quality nighttime sleep and full daytime alertness.

- The most important measure of sleep hygiene is to maintain a regular wake and sleep pattern seven days a week.
- It is also important to spend an appropriate amount of time in bed—not too little, or too much. This may vary by individual; for example, if you have a problem with daytime sleepiness, you should spend a minimum of eight hours in bed. If you have difficulty sleeping at night, you should limit yourself to seven hours in bed in order to keep the sleep pattern consolidated.

Sleep hygiene practices include:

- **Avoid stimulants such as caffeine, nicotine, and alcohol too close to bedtime.** While alcohol is well known to speed the onset of sleep, it disrupts sleep in the second half of the night as the body begins to metabolize the alcohol, causing arousal. Remember, chocolate has caffeine.
- **Exercise can promote good sleep.** Vigorous exercise should be done in the morning or late afternoon. A relaxing exercise, like yoga, can be done before bed to help initiate a restful night's sleep.
- **Avoid large meals before bedtime.** Stay away from large meals close to bedtime. Also, dietary changes can cause sleep problems. If you are struggling with a sleep problem, it's not a good time to start experimenting with spicy dishes.
- **Establish a regular relaxing bedtime routine.** Try to avoid using the computer or other electronic devices before trying to go to sleep.
- **Associate your bedroom with sleep.** Avoid using your bedroom to watch TV, listen to the radio, or access mobile devices.

Remember, your body is the temple of the Holy Spirit. It is our spiritual responsibility to be good stewards of our bodies. Here are some helpful tools to identify the stress areas of your life. Keep in mind that what affects the body also affects the spirit, and what affects the spirit affects the body.

Model for Healthy Living. This model was developed by the Church Health Center based on the beliefs that God created us body and spirit, and that we have a responsibility to be good stewards of our health and help others do the same. Living healthy lives doesn't just mean that you see the doctor regularly. Rather, healthy living means that all aspects of your life are in balance.

Your faith, work, nutrition, movement, family and friends, emotions, and medical health all contribute to a life filled with more joy, more love, and more connection with God. The Model for Healthy Living (Appendix A) visually illustrates how these seven key dimensions of our body and spirit experience overlap at the core of our lives.

Once you have identified areas of less satisfaction, look for ways where you can increase those areas to achieve a more balanced life.

Holmes and Rahe Stress Scale. This scale consists of 43 stressful life events that can contribute to illness. To measure stress according to the Holmes and Rahe Stress Scale, the number of "Life Change Units" that apply to events in the past year of an individual's life are added and the final score will give a rough estimate of how stress affects health. (See Appendix B accessed at http://shar.es/DKhRz April 29, 2014.)

Mind

Connect with someone at least on a daily basis if not more frequently.

- Laugh with someone.
- Share with someone.
- Be of service to someone.
- Practice compassion and forgiveness on a regular basis.
- Remember to take the ego out of any situation.

Set boundaries. Mental, emotional, physical and spiritual boundaries are unlike physical property boundaries that are easy to see. However, they are just as important and harder to define. Boundaries are personal property lines that define who you are, and who you are not, and influence all areas of your life (Cloud and Townsend, 1992).

- A variety of things, including **past hurts, poor models, and misunderstood teachings**, result in weak boundaries or in no boundaries at all.
- Boundaries define what is me and what is not me. A boundary shows where each individual ends and someone else begins, leading each person to a sense of ownership and responsibility.
- Boundaries also protect us from the bad.
- Defining personal boundaries is biblically based. The reality God has established is an orderly one based on laws and principles that are seen in the Bible and are very real. The **Laws of Boundaries** (Cloud and Townsend, 2007) include:
  - **Law of Sowing and Reaping.** This is a basic law of cause and effect and of life. God tells us in Galatians 6:7–8 that we will reap what we sow. This is not a punishment, but the way things are in reality.
  - **Law of Responsibility.** This includes loving others as stated in John 15:12 and Galatians 5:13–14. We are responsible for ourselves and to love one another, but not *be* one another.

Critical Thinking
What physical, mental, spiritual, and behavior symptoms do you experience when one area of your life becomes unbalanced?

HELPFUL RESOURCE
Appendix B features the Holmes and Rahe Stress Scale, a tool for both self-care and ministry.

KEY TERM
Boundaries *are personal property lines that define who you are, and who you are not, and influence all areas of your life.*

*The **Serenity Prayer** is a boundary prayer:*

God, grant me the serenity to accept the things I cannot change, the courage to change the things I can, and the wisdom to know the difference.

COMMON BOUNDARY MYTHS

Myth#1 *If I set boundaries I'm being selfish.*

Myth #2 *Boundaries are a sign of disobedience.*

Myth #3 *If I begin setting boundaries, I will be hurt by others.*

Myth #4 *If I set boundaries I will hurt others.*

Myth #5 *Boundaries mean that I am angry.*

Myth #6 *When others set boundaries, it injures me.*

Myth #7 *Boundaries cause feelings of guilt.*

Myth #8 *Boundaries are permanent and I am afraid of burning my bridges.*

Taken from Boundaries: When to Say Yes, How to Say No to Take Control of Your Life *by Henry Cloud and John Townsend, Copyright © 1992 by Henry Cloud and John Townsend. Use by permission of Zondervan. www.zondervan.com*

- **Law of Power.** Your boundaries define what you do and do not have power over. God will do what you are unable to do (1 John 1:9; James 4:7–10; Matthew 5:3, 6).
- **The Law of Respect.** We fear that others will not respect our boundaries; when we accept others' freedom of choice, we feel better about our own (Matthew 7:12).

Establish work-life balance. Work-life balance is something that many desire but few successfully achieve without a serious attitude adjustment. In an age when we are always connected to our work through mobile devices, it can be difficult to have a fulfilling personal life. When our work is also our ministry, it can be even more difficult. Incorporating the following strategies will help improve work-life balance.

- **Recognize the role of work.** Adopting the right mindset allows you to celebrate and enjoy the fruit of your labor.
- **Tap into your support system.** Be sure to carve out family time, exercise time, and laughter time.
- **Maintain one calendar for work and family.** This will help you define the work day and establish a cut-off time to be with family.
- **Be present, consistent and accountable.** Being present requires you to be attentive at home, at work, and during free time. The quality of being present makes a significant and positive impact on your surroundings.
- **Learn to breathe.** Slow down, relax, and breathe; this will give you the opportunity to regroup and assess where you are.

Take a break when needed to prevent compassion fatigue, the gradual decline of compassion over time that results when nurses or other health professionals are exposed to events that have traumatized their clients. Health professionals who help traumatized clients may develop symptoms as an indirect response to their clients' suffering. This phenomenon is called compassion fatigue.

- The helpers' symptoms, frequently unnoticed, may range from psychological issues, such as anxiety and sleep disturbances, to feeling powerless.
- However, professional caregivers may also experience physical symptoms such as nausea, headaches, dizziness, fainting spells, and impaired hearing.
- All are important warning signals that need to be addressed or otherwise might lead to health issues or burnout.
- Giving oneself permission to take a break for a short time and taking care of oneself may not only help the FCN but may also provide a role model of self-care for his or her clients.
- Studies have also shown that self-care strategies such as balancing work and private life, relaxation techniques, and vacation time have been useful in preventing compassion fatigue (Babbel, 2012).

Seek professional counseling for difficult situations.
- Seek a counselor, preferably one of your faith tradition.
- Seek a counselor who does boundary work.
- Seek out healing ministries.
- Seek a spiritual leader of your faith community to pray healing over you.

If you want to live your life, and live it well, don't take anything personally!

Spirit

Upon awakening, get out of bed, and mentally and physically prepare for spending quiet time with God. Go to a designated spot in your home which is sacred and special to you. Create a prayer place.

- **Read the Bible** or other sacred text.
- **Pray prayers** that are meaningful to you.
- **Meditate.** There are many forms of meditation. One way to meditate is to sit upright, eyes closed and hands on your thighs. Begin breathing and concentrate on your breath. Before beginning to meditate, it is helpful to choose a mantra of the Holy Name of God in whatever form resonates with you. After focusing on your breath, begin saying your mantra repeatedly. As thoughts pass through your mind, acknowledge them, honor them and offer them up to God, one by one. Do this for each passing thought. You will know when you are finished.
- **Journal your experience** or simply what you are feeling at this time.

Until the daily routine of self-care of body, mind, and spirit becomes a habit, it will be difficult to carve out the time for it. Remember to bring all of the concerns and issues around time to God. Your schedule will be rearranged as you align yourself with the will of God.

- quiet time for personal reflection and prayer
- time dedicated to exercise
- time to prepare or select nutritious meals
- time to spend with family, friends and others who are significant in our lives
- time for worship with our faith communities
- time for study, learning or intellectual pursuits
- time for work

KEY TERM

Compassion fatigue *is the gradual decline of compassion over time.*

Critical Thinking

In what ways might poor boundaries contribute to compassion fatigue?

PERSONAL RELAXATION RECORDINGS

Many people find it helpful to listen to music or readings while doing relaxation exercises. You can create your own playlist of favorite music you already own to use specifically when you are relaxing. If your music is on CDs, a computer application such as iTunes will help you transfer the tracks you choose to a smart phone or an iPod for listening. You also could record a favorite reading or something you have written to help you relax, such as a description of the relaxing place you imagine. This is especially helpful for visualization.

- *Try to minimize distraction and outside noise while you are recording.*
- *Speak slowly and allow long pauses between each step of the instructions. Remember, when you listen to the recording later, you will need time to act on each instruction.*
- *Try adding special quotations, verses or songs that are comforting to you.*
- *Don't be afraid to ask someone with stronger computer skills to help you if needed.*

- time for being in service to others
- time for rest
- time for play
- there is a time for everything under heaven (Ecclesiastes 3:1–3)

OUTCOME 2
Discern the will of God.

"I appeal to you therefore, brothers and sisters, by the mercies of God, to present your bodies as a living sacrifice, holy and acceptable to God, which is your spiritual worship. Do not be conformed to this world, but be transformed by the renewing of your minds, so that you may discern what is the will of God—what is good and acceptable and perfect" (Romans 12:1–2).

Seeking God's Will

To **discern** is to separate, distinguish, determine, or sort out. The **discernment of God's will** is seeking to do God's will, not your will.

What one listens for and distinguishes is the will of God from his or her own will. Questions to ask yourself would be: "What does God desire for *me* in this situation?" and "What is God's will for me?"

Discernment is the *ear for God*. Just as a musician has an *ear for music*, in the same way, the discerner uses his or her ear of discernment to notice the voice of God speaking through life experiences.

People of faith can agree to the idea or concept of discernment. It makes sense. The challenge comes in the lived experience. The discerner realizes that he or she has many choices or options. So the discerning choice is generally not a readily clear one.

Exploring the Discernment Process

Some **discernment assumptions** or beliefs about God can aid the process of discovering God's will.
- God is loving and created me out of love; I am important, but not necessary.
- God desires me to fulfill my purpose; he knows what my purpose is and wants me to discover it.
- God works collaboratively with me in helping me uncover my purpose, gifts, and mission.

Building on these assumptions is the question, **How is God communicating with me?** God is always already communicating with me in the everyday events and people in my life. God may speak in the following ways.

In most instances God speaks with a **voiceless voice**. We experience God communicating to us through our own experiences.

Critical Thinking

What types of activities best nourish your spirit? What interferes with caring for yourself in these ways?

KEY TERM

To discern *is to separate, to distinguish, to determine, to sort out.*

We get a *felt sense*, an *intuition*, or an *inclination* that this is the will of God. Therefore, discernment is an act of faith.

Discernment is listening, acknowledging, and **balancing your interior life** (perceptions, interpretations, affect and desires) with the external world. It is the intersection and interplay of God within and through you, the faith community, and events and situations.

In any one of these areas, there is a lot going on. If you doubt that, just try sitting quietly for two minutes and observe the number of ideas and feelings that come into your awareness. The main elements related to discernment in each of these areas are listed below.

Yourself
Look within yourself and strive for personal awareness by taking inventory of the following things.
- open inner disposition, readiness, attentiveness
- interior freedom—free from your learned reaction and free for growth and new opportunities
- gratitude and appreciation—where do I appreciate what is?
- blocking and resisting—notice when you get defensive and resistant
- intuition—pay attention to that sixth sense about things
- triggers and hot buttons
- personality differences
- defense mechanisms
- unrestricted readiness
- willingness to act
- willingness to be of service
- willingness to do God's will
- willingness to serve the common good
- willingness to embrace self-sacrifice

Faith Community
Identify wise truth-speakers to balance your self-perception. Ask for feedback and for another viewpoint. Listen in humility.

Events and Situations
View events and situations through the eyes of discernment.
- Events and situations are part of a continuous narrative through which God communicates with you.
- Realize that you participate in a story greater than your own making.
- View events and situations with an open mind and humble heart; events can speak to you about reoccurring patterns.
- Ask:
    - What is really happening here?
    - God, what are you trying to teach me?
    - Is this a roadblock or a dead end?
    - Is this temporary or permanent?
    - Is it consistent or occasional?
    - Is it particular or pervasive?

KEY TERM
The **discernment of God's will** *is seeking to do God's will, not your will.*

Starting at age 30, Florence Nightingale meditated three times a day for 15 minutes to find out what the will of God was for her in her life (Ascension Health, 2007).

Critical Thinking
Describe a time when you felt you clearly discerned God's will? What factors contributed to your confidence?

Sometimes you will experience **confirming signs** when you act in accordance with God's will, such as:
- consolation or deep peace about the choice you made
- a sense of "*feels right and flows*"

Daily Discernment Practices

Daily discernment is taking time to listen and attune yourself to God speaking in and through you and the events of your day. Daily discernment means taking a little time each day to be attentive and listen. It means stepping back to create a space to observe yourself, your situation, and how you are relating to the present moment to better understand God's will and direction for your life. Spending time with God may take many forms.

Lectio Divina
Lectio divina is a Latin phrase meaning a "holy reading" or a "divine reading." The point is to take your time and read slowly, interacting with what you are reading. This method will work with any wisdom literature, sacred writings, or thought-provoking writings.
- Select a small section from any sacred or inspirational writing.
- Read the section *slowly* and *out loud* three times, pausing between the readings.
- After the first time, notice what strikes you or stands out to you.
- After the second time, ask yourself, what does this mean to me?
- After the third time, ask, what is my response?
- Go back to this reflection throughout the day.

Life Examination
To examine life during a stressful or anxiety-filled situation:
- Ask what Jesus or a holy and wise person would do?
- Try mental moviemaking. Once you see in your mind's eye what the wise person does, it will be easier for you to picture yourself doing it.
- Have an attitude of openness.

Release
Let go of your:
- past and current painful experience
- present tension and anxiety
- future fear and uncertainty

Invite God In
- Seek to know and prefer the will of God to your own will.
- Pray short prayers: "If in all your life the only prayer you ever say is 'Thank You,' that would be enough" (Meister Eckhart).

Offer Time Wisely
- Time is life (not money).
- Our use of time is the real measure of who we are and what we value.

- What is the lasting gift you gave to others today?

By Yourself
- Create space for silence.
- Leave the car radio off on your drive to or from work.
- Watch 30 minutes less television each day.
- Either before or at the end of the day pray over your calendar.
- Spend a few moments praying over each meeting and appointment, placing the meeting in the hands of God.
- Notice where you feel grateful and where you need help.

With Others
- Seek feedback and feed-forward.
- Seek two or three wise truth-speakers.
- Ask for their honest feedback.
- Listen with humility to their response.
- Weigh their feedback with your thinking before acting.

Remember we are here to **serve**, as Jesus Christ modeled for us. When we focus on others and how we can serve according to God's will, we will prevent compassion fatigue, burnout, and imbalances in our ministries.

OUTCOME 3

Engage in the practice of Sabbath, keeping it integral for care of body, mind, and spirit.

Complete this sentence: The Sabbath is_____.
   Hebrew meaning of the word **Sabbath** (Shabbat) is "cessation of work" or "rest."
   Caring for the domains of body, mind, and spirit includes identifying the stressors that might impact each domain and interfere with the practice of Sabbath.
- Body: tension, back pain, elevated blood pressure, headaches, joint pain, decreased exercise
- Mind: worries, expectations, shouldering, depression, mood swings, low self-esteem
- Spirit: lack of meaning, no time for God or prayer, emptiness

Suggestions for How to Practice the Sabbath
Preparation
- Shop for food and other needed items.
- Prepare the food.
- Clean the space so it is comfortable.
- Prepare needed laundry or other items.

Celebration
Practice the Sabbath by doing something special and enjoyable.
- Plan a beginning.
- Plan an ending.

Critical Thinking

How is Sabbath a deeper concept than merely a "day off"?

- Use candles.
- Include prayer.
- Include readings.
- Include music or song.

Rituals
- Conduct worship.
- Invite family and friends.
- Disconnect the phone, television, computer, and all mobile devices.
- Play games, walk, read, paint, garden.
- Participate in other leisure activities.
- Forget the "to do list."
- Be mindful of self-care.

Beauty
- Enjoy nature.
- Use the five senses.
- Listen to special music.
- Enjoy aromas.
- Participate in art.
- Enjoy elegant fabrics (velvet, chenille, cashmere, silk) and fine table settings.
- Eat special foods and drink healthy beverages.

Attitude
- Gratitude
- Mindfulness
- Reflection

Self-Care that Reflects Sabbath

Based on previous reflection and journaling, develop a **personal plan of self-care that keeps the Sabbath.**
- Conduct a spiritual assessment from the Learning Activities. Complete the following sentence: "A spiritual assessment is important in a personal plan of care because ... "
- Identify Sabbath rituals to incorporate into your personal plan of self-care.

Standards of Professional Performance for Faith Community Nursing

Standard 14. Professional Practice Evaluation

The faith community nurse evaluates his or her own nursing practice in relation to professional practice standards and guidelines, relevant statutes, rules, and regulations.

COMPETENCIES

The faith community nurse's practice reflects the application of knowledge of current practice standards, guidelines, statutes, rules, and regulations.

The faith community nurse:

- Engages in self-evaluation of practice regularly, identifying areas of strength as well as areas in which professional development would be beneficial.
- Obtains informal feedback regarding her or his own spiritual care and nursing practice from healthcare consumers, peers, spiritual leaders, health committee members, faith community volunteers, professional colleagues, and others.

Learning Activities

Reflection Exercise

Instructions:
1. Create a calm, quiet environment. (If you are using this exercise in a retreat setting and weather permits, this is a great outdoor activity.)
2. Use soft instrumental music or nature sounds CD because it makes a nice background for this exercise. Rhythmic Medicine Series (http://www.rhythmicmedicine.com) works well and is a great resource for participants.
3. Have the participants think about the impact that a few small changes could make in both the quality of their lives and the examples they can set for others.
4. Have the participants consider their current states; then write out their desired future states.
5. Instruct the participants to turn their thoughts inward for the next 15 minutes to reflect on the questions below.

Questions:
1. How do you currently prepare for the Sabbath in your household?
2. How might you prepare for the Sabbath in the future?
3. What are one or two things that would be helpful to get done before the Sabbath?
4. What enjoyable things are you unable to do during the week that you could do during Sabbath?
5. What do you need to take a rest from during the Sabbath?
6. What is your attitude toward rest?
7. What is your behavior regarding rest?
8. What type of role model are you in regard to self-care for the faith community and ministry team you serve?
9. Are you willing to do for yourself what you so freely do for others?

Case Study

Instructions:
Review the following case study and apply what you have learned about self-care. Also think about how keeping the Sabbath may be used to both model self-care and help others establish self-care routines.

You have a faith community nurse colleague, Mary, who has become the primary caregiver for both her elderly sister and mother. Both the sister and mother have several chronic illnesses. The mother and sister live together in the family home in a neighboring town about 45 minutes away. Mary's husband is deceased, and there are few other family members to assist in the care of her sister and mother.

Mary feels that it is her duty to care for both her sister and mother. The sister and mother want to remain in their home, even though neither is able to maintain the house, drive, or perform routine housekeeping and cooking chores. The mother suffers from dementia and the sister from a mental disability. Currently Mary's mother and sister seem unsafe living alone and lack good judgment to maintain safe living conditions.

As a coworker, you notice Mary is consumed with meeting the expectations for her frail, elderly family members. During the week she makes many trips to take care of their "emergencies." She also expresses that her phone rings "night and day" with requests for assistance, reassurance, and for visits or needed outings. You have also noticed that Mary has unplanned weight loss, and she does not have time for routine personal care such as hair appointments or grocery shopping. She frequently skips meals because she is either "too exhausted to cook or just too tired to eat."

Recently, Mary has adjusted her part-time work schedule at the church to meet the constant demands of her family members. This sometimes means she comes in late or leaves early before the work is completed. However, she always makes up her lost time by either working late on some days or working on her days off. You notice that Mary does not complain even though she occasionally comes in to work with little or no sleep. In spite of her personal problems, Mary continues to serve the members of the congregation as an FCN, teacher, and leader as well as ministering to her friends' needs.

Unfortunately, Mary has lost her radiant appearance, and the cadence of her step has slowed. She often appears worn, stooped and tired. Although she usually smiles and has a very positive attitude, it seems that she has lost her enjoyment of life.

Questions:
1. What kind of symptoms do you see in Mary?
2. How might you be helpful to Mary?
3. Is there anything you need to do for Mary, even though she is part of the ministry team and a peer?
4. How can you emphasize the importance of self-care to Mary?
5. Discuss any personal situations that are similar to Mary's.

Bath Teas or Salts Self-Care Exercise

Instructions:

1. This exercise can be done alone or with a partner. When done alone the focus is self-care. When done with a partner it is a simple, inexpensive ministry to relax, reflect, and show appreciation. Be sure to assess sensitivities and allergies before using scented salts or lotions; it may be best to use aroma-free materials.

2. Choose a packet of bath salts and soak the fingers of one hand in a bowl of warm water with bath salts for 5–10 minutes.

3. Dry the hand.

4. Rewarm the water and repeat the process with the other hand.

5. Dry the hand.

6. Apply herbal scented lotion to both hands.

7. Note: Be mindful of the difference in your skin, relaxation level, and mood. Think about when you might use this routine in daily life to create a mini-Sabbath.

Question:
What do you think might be the benefits of this kind of self-care?

Suggested answers:
- stimulates natural circulation for improved health
- relaxes tense, aching muscles and joints
- relieves tired, aching muscles
- eases body tension
- draws out impurities in skin
- soothes itching, burning and bites
- soothes skin irritations
- smoothes and softens skin
- encourages skin to renew itself
- provides deep relaxation
- restores moisture balance to skin
- promotes restfulness

Comfort Scriptures

Instructions:

1. In a retreat setting, create signs in various places (tree trunks, benches, rocks) with Comfort Scripture references (below) for healing and comfort. Place Scripture verses on small cards or pieces of paper, enough for each participant to have one each from each site, and place cards in a small container at each site. The number of sites will determine the time allotment for this activity.

2. Make sure participants have Bibles. Instruct the group to "wander" around the setting to discover the Scripture verses, look them up, and read them.

Question:

How could you use these Scripture passages for ongoing self-care or in your ministry?

Comfort Scriptures

Psalm 23:4	Comfort in need
Psalm 71:21	Comforted again
Psalm 119:50	Comfort in promises
Psalm 119:76	Comfort in love
Isaiah 40:1	A people comforted
Isaiah 51:3	Comfort and joy
Isaiah 61:2	Comfort all who mourn
Isaiah 66:13	A mother's comfort
Jeremiah 31:13	Joy and comfort
Matthew 2:13–18	Comfort refused
Matthew 5:4	Comfort in mourning
2 Corinthians 1:3–6	Comfort in trouble
2 Thessalonians 2:16	Eternal comfort

Meditation

Instructions:

1. Provide copies of "A Way to Sanctity and Happiness."

2. Allow time for individual meditation.

Question:

Depending on your group, you may ask for participants to share their personal reflections.

A Way to Sanctity and Happiness

If every day for five minutes you will keep your imagination quiet, shut your eyes to all things of sense and close your ears to all sounds of the earth, so as to withdraw into the sanctuary of your soul which is the temple of God and speak there to God saying:

"Oh God, Soul of my soul, I adore You. Enlighten, guide, strengthen and console me. Tell me what I ought to do and command me to do it. I promise to be submissive in everything that You permit to happen to me, only show me what is Your will."

If you do this, your life will pass happily and serenely. Consolation will abound even in the midst of troubles. Grace will be given in proportion to the trial as well as the strength to bear it, bringing you to the gates of paradise full of merit.

From *To Jesus Through Mary*, compiled by Christopher Cross
(http://www.catholicholyland.com/cms/prayer-book)

Spiritual Assessment

Instructions:
1. Allow time for participants to take the adult assessment below, pointing out that the adult assessment may also be used as a tool in their ministries.

2. Encourage participants to record reflective personal answers to these questions.

Question:
Do any of these questions cause you concern? Are there any negative or uncertain responses that may indicate that a conversation with a trusted colleague or spiritual leader could help you work through the issues of your life? A good listener can often help you find God's peace.

Spiritual Assessment—Adult

- What can you offer your family or your community that would benefit their lives?
- What gives your life meaning or purpose?
- Is God important to you?
- What does God do for you personally?
- Do you have particular beliefs or practices that are important to your sense of well-being?
- What is your source of strength and hope?
- What makes you happy?
- Do you experience any of the following: anger, confusion, denial, fear, anxiety, helplessness, or emotional flip-flops?
- Does anger or resentment block your peace of mind?
- Do you feel that God or life has treated you unfairly?
- Have your feelings toward God changed because of your present situation?
- What has given you the courage to cope with the trials in your life?
- Who do you turn to when you are afraid or in need?
- How do you feel about your relationship with your church?

Used with permission from Trinity Regional Health System.

Crossing the Line

Instructions:

1. Review boundary problems and have participants discuss the different patterns and identify the pattern of the person whose name is in bold on the boundary scenarios.

2. Ask participants to discuss in small groups the following boundary scenarios. Depending on your time, you may assign each group one or more scenarios.

Each of us needs to take responsibility for what is within our boundaries such as our feelings, attitudes, beliefs, behaviors, choices, thoughts, values, limits, talents, desires and love. Boundary problems come in different patterns that we can recognize. They are as follows:

- *Compliants* say yes to bad things because they haven't learned how to say no, or even that it's okay to say no to the bad.
- *Avoidants* say no to the good. They aren't able to ask for help; their boundaries keep people and even God out. Needs, problems, and legitimate wants seem bad and destructive.
- *Controllers* hear no as simply a challenge to change the other person's mind. Controllers can't respect other people's limits.
- *Nonresponsives* neglect the responsibilities of love by not responding to other people's needs.

Boundary problems also arise when an individual can't distinguish between *functional boundaries*, the ability to complete a task, project or job, and *relational boundaries*, the ability to speak truth to those with whom we are in relationship.

Very often it is easier to diagnose someone else instead of yourself. As you look at the following six scenarios, make your diagnosis of the person whose name appears in bold. Your choices are: *Compliant, avoidant, controller, nonresponsive,* or a combination of these categories. Then answer the questions that follow.

Summary of Boundary Problems (Cloud and Townsend, 2007)

The *compliant* feels guilty and/or controlled by others; can't set boundaries.
The *controller* aggressively or manipulatively violates boundaries of others.
The *nonresponsive* sets boundaries against responsibility to love.
The *avoidant* sets boundaries against receiving care from others.

BOUNDARIES SCENARIO 1

Cindi began to see a pattern in her life. If someone asked her to take on organizing a project in her spare time or to spend hours listening to someone's troubles, **Cindi** couldn't seem to say no. But if she needed just ten minutes of someone's attention, she felt like she couldn't ask for it.

Diagnosis: _____

Questions:
1. When is **Cindi** compliant? When is she avoidant?
2. Why would this cycle be draining?
3. What problems might being a compliant avoidant cause in relationships?

BOUNDARIES SCENARIO 2

Carol and **Sam** were relaxing at the end of a long day. Carol began to talk, admitting to feeling inadequate to lead a committee at their children's school. She feared making decisions that might disappoint other parents. Carol didn't like feeling inadequate and fearful. **Sam** looked up from the newspaper and said, "So don't feel that way. Just change your feelings. What's so hard about that?" He went back to reading the paper.

Diagnosis: _____

Questions:
1. What is the difference between being a good listener and trying to fix another person? Which is more supportive? Why?
2. What problems might **Sam's** non-responsiveness cause in his marriage?

BOUNDARIES SCENARIO 3

Jackson was the youngest of three children in his family. His sisters were three and five years older than he was. Until he was in the seventh grade, they had the habit of poking and pinching him until he bruised. Twice his sisters gave **Jackson** a black eye. But if **Jackson** defended himself and one of his sisters protested or got hurt, his parents punished him, saying, "Boys don't hit girls. It's bad manners." He grew up thinking that protecting himself was unacceptable.

Diagnosis: _____

Questions:
1. What were **Jackson's** parents teaching him about boundaries? (What did your parents teach you with their words and actions?)
2. Why do some people say yes to bad things?

BOUNDARIES SCENARIO 4

"Women's ministry will fall apart without you." **Donna**, a member of the staff of the faith community, looked at Belinda. "You can't quit." Belinda had been a star volunteer for almost six years, spending most Saturdays accomplishing a list of tasks **Donna** assigned to her. When she started using personal vacation days from her paid job to keep up with the goals **Donna** set, it was time for change. Several times Belinda tried to talk with **Donna** about the way **Donna** seemed to shift her staff responsibilities onto volunteers—mainly Belinda. When **Donna** responded by asking Belinda to do even more, that was the last straw.

Diagnosis: _____

Questions:
1. What responsibility is **Donna** avoiding?
2. In what ways is **Donna** being controlling through the use of manipulation?

BOUNDARIES SCENARIO 5

The women in the prayer group had been meeting together for six months. One night, one of them became more transparent, and others followed. The conversation deepened beyond the usual complaints about being too busy to genuine sharing about relationships, tearful parenting challenges, and difficult decisions. When people invited their hostess, **Mary**, to share, she cleared her throat. "God is calling me to support all of you in your struggles," she said. "Each of you will be on my prayer list. Why don't I pray for you now, and then we'll enjoy some dessert?"

Diagnosis: _____

Questions:
1. What has **Mary** learned about boundaries? What has she learned about her problems and probably about her God-given needs?
2. What problems might **Mary's** avoidance cause in her relationships?

BOUNDARIES SCENARIO 6

Brad and his wife, Allison, had made plans for a much-needed getaway as a couple, but the date happened to fall on Brad's mother's birthday. When **Andrea**, his mother, heard about the plans, she complained about how selfish Brad was being and how unappreciated he was making her feel. When he tried to explain that Allison was carrying a heavy load and really needed the break, **Andrea** refused to listen to Brad's concerns for his marriage. Reluctantly, the couple cancelled their plans and visited Brad's mom instead.

Diagnosis: _____

Questions:
1. How is **Andrea** both nonresponsive and controlling at the same time?

2. What problems might being a controlling nonresponsive—like **Andrea**—cause in relationships?

Boundary Building ... On Your Own

Instructions:
1. How would you describe your own struggles with boundary issues? How would you describe the boundary responses of one or two people with whom you are struggling most today?

2. Do you have good functional boundaries, but poor relational boundaries? Or do you have good relational boundaries, but poor functional boundaries? Why do you think your boundary strengths and weaknesses are what they are?

References

Required Textbook

American Nurses Association and Health Ministries Association. (2012). *Scope and standards of practice: Faith community nursing* (2nd ed.). Silver Spring, MD: Nursesbooks.org.

References

Ascension Health. (2007). Everyday discernment: A call to lead, inspired to serve.

Babbel, S. (2012). Compassion fatigue: Bodily symptoms of empathy. *Somatic Psychology.* http://www.psychologytoday.com/blog/somatic-psychology/201207/compassion-fatigue. Retrieved June 10, 2014.

Brown, A. & Roy, M. (2010). Does evidence exist to include dietary therapy in the treatment of Crohn's disease? Expert Reviews in *Gastroenterology & Hepatology, 4*(2), 191–215.

Church Health Reader Editors. (Spring 2013). *The model for healthy living.* Memphis, TN: Church Health Center.

Cloud, H. & Townsend, J. (2007). *Boundaries: When to say yes, how to say no, to take control of your life* (Participant guide). Grand Rapids, MI: Zondervan.

Davis, W. (2012). *Lose the wheat, lose the weight.* New York: Rodale.

Eswaran S., Goel, A., & Chey, W. (2013). What role does wheat play in the symptoms of irritable bowel syndrome? *Gastroenterology & Hepatology, 9*(2), 85–91.

Green. R. (Spring 2013). Application of the self-care deficit nursing theory: The community context. *Self-Care, Dependent-Care & Nursing 20*(1), 5–14.

Hyman, M. (2012). *The blood sugar solution.* New York, NY: Little Brown and Company.

Johnstone, B., Yoon, D.P., Cohen, D., Schopp, L. H., McCormack, G., Campbell, J., Smith, M. (2012). Relationships among spirituality, religious practices, personality factors, and health for five different faith traditions. *Journal of Religion and Health.* Dec; 51(4):1017–41. doi: 10.1007/s10943-012-9615-8 accessed April 21, 2014.

Laugsand, L. E., Strand, L. B., Platou, et al. (2013). Insufficient rest or sleep and its relation to cardiovascular disease, diabetes and obesity in a national, multiethnic sample. *European Heart Journal* doi: 10.1093/eurheartj/eht019. Available at: http://eurheartj.oxfordjournals.org.

Mearin, F. Pena, E., & Balboa, A. (2014). Importance of diet in irritable bowel syndrome. *Gastroenterologia & Hepatologia, 37*(5), 302–310.

O'Brien, M. E. (2014). *Spirituality in nursing.* Burlington, MA: Jones and Bartlett Learning.

Simmons, S. Striving for work-life-balance. *American Journal of Nursing, 112*(1), 25–26.

Additional References

Baab, L. M. (2005). *Sabbath keeping: Finding freedom in the rhythms of rest.* Downers Grove, IL: InterVarsity Press.

Blanchard, M.H., (2012). Work-life-balance? *Obstetrics and Gynecology, 119*(1), 177–179.

Boa, K. (2010). Discerning the will of God. Accessed April 22, 2014 at https://bible.org/article/discerning-will-god

Buchanan, M. (2006). *The rest of God: Restoring your soul by restoring sabbath.* Nashville, TN: W. Publishing Group.

Cross, C. *To Jesus through Mary.* Huntersville, NC: Published by the Author. http://www.catholicholyland.com/cms/prayer-book

Dawn, M. J. (1989). *Keeping the sabbath wholly: Ceasing, resting, embracing, feasting.* Grand Rapids, MI: Wm. B. Eerdmans Publishing.

Droege, T. A. (1996). *The healing presence: Spiritual exercises for healing, wellness, and recovery.* Bloomington, MN: The Youth & Family Institute.

Harper, B. (2012). *The skinny rules.* New York: Ballantine Books.

Holtz, K. and Matthews, M. (2012). *Dust & breath: Faith, health, and why the church should care about both.* Grand Rapids, MI: Wm. B. Eerdmans Publishing.

Jones, K. *Addicted to hurry: Spiritual strategies for slowing down.* Valley Forge: PA., Judson Press.

Jones, K. (2003). *Rest in the storm: Self-care strategies for clergy and other caregivers.* Valley Forge: Judson Press.

Melander, R. & Eppley, H. (2002). *The spiritual leader's guide to self-care.* Herndon, VA: Alban Institute.

Morris, S. (2011). *God, health, and happiness.* Uhrichsville, Ohio: Barbour.

Perlmutter, P. (2013). *Grain Brain.* New York, NY: Little, Brown and Company.

Remen, R. N. (1996). *Kitchen table wisdom: Stories that heal.* New York: Riverhead Books.

Remen, R. N. (2000). *My grandfather's blessings: Stories of strength, refuge, and belonging.* New York: Riverhead Books.

Rubietta, J. (1997). *Quiet places: A woman's guide to personal retreat.* Minneapolis, MN: Bethany House Publishers.

Rupp, J. (2005). *Walk in a relaxed manner: Life lessons from the Camino.* Maryknoll, NY: Orbis Books.

Soni, P. (2013). The struggle to juggle: Work-life balance at a private company in Durban, South Africa. *Journal of Management & Administration, (11)*1, 34–56.

Sulmasy, D. P. (1997). *The healer's calling: spirituality for physicians and other health care professionals.* Mahwah, NJ: Paulist Press.

Thomas, K. R. (2001). *New every morning: A daily touch of God's faithfulness.* Phoenix, AZ: ACW Press.

Warren, R. (2013). *The Daniel plan.* Grand Rapids, MI: Zondervan.

Weaver, J. A. (2000). *Having a Mary heart in a Martha world: Finding intimacy with God in the busyness of life.* Colorado Springs, CO: Waterbrook Press.

Online Resources

Musical Acupuncture, Musical Massage, Bathed in Baroque. http://www.rhythmicmedicine.com

National Center for Complementary and Alternative Medicine. http://nccam.nih.gov/health/whatiscam

Rhythmic Medicine, Therapeutic Music by Janalea Hoffman.

Songs for the Inner Child (CD, Shaina Noll) www.shainanoll.com/music/songs-for-the-inner-child/

Wrap-Up and Evaluation

Measuring Competency

This chart can be used to assess the individual outcomes in this module.
- A copy of this chart is attached to the Participant Module, so that each participant can complete this short evaluation.
- Have participants read each outcome and then place an X in the box that best matches their opinion about the objective being met.
- Encourage each participant to write a short reflection about this module in the space provided at the bottom of this chart.
- Use this data to make any necessary changes.

Outcome	Not Met	Somewhat Met	Met
1. Develop a deeper intimacy and personal connection with God through care of one's own body, mind and spirit.			
2. Discern the will of God.			
3. Engage in the practice of Sabbath, keeping it integral for care of mind, body, and spirit.			
Reflection: *In one paragraph, write a reflection on this module.*			

Appendix A

Model for Healthy Living
Assessment Wheel

Circle the number on the wheel that best describes your satisfaction in each of these areas in your life or the life of your church (1- unsatisfied, 10- completely satisfied). Connect the circles. What areas would you like to improve?

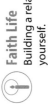 **Faith Life**
Building a relationship with God, your neighbors, and yourself.

1   2   3   4   5   6   7   8   9   10

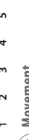 **Movement**
Discovering ways to enjoy physical activity.

1   2   3   4   5   6   7   8   9   10

 Medical
Partnering with your health care provider to manage your medical care.

1   2   3   4   5   6   7   8   9   10

 Work
Appreciating your skills, talents, and gifts.

1   2   3   4   5   6   7   8   9   10

 Emotional
Managing stress and understanding your feelings to better care for yourself.

1   2   3   4   5   6   7   8   9   10

 Nutrition
Making smart food choices and developing healthy eating habits.

1   2   3   4   5   6   7   8   9   10

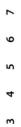 **Family & Friends**
Giving and receiving support through relationships.

1   2   3   4   5   6   7   8   9   10

Appendix B

Holmes and Rahe Stress Scale—Adults

According to the Holmes and Rahe Stress Scale, the number of "Life Change Units" that apply to events in the past year of an individual's life are added, and the final score will give a rough estimate of how stress affects health. Score of 300+: At risk of illness.

Life event	Life change units
Death of a spouse	100
Divorce	73
Marital separation	65
Imprisonment	63
Death of a close family member	63
Personal injury or illness	53
Marriage	50
Dismissal from work	47
Marital reconciliation	45
Retirement	45
Change in health of family member	44
Pregnancy	40
Sexual difficulties	39
Gain a new family member	39
Business readjustment	39
Change in financial state	38
Death of a close friend	37
Change to different line of work	36
Change in frequency of arguments	35
Major mortgage	32
Foreclosure of mortgage or loan	30
Change in responsibilities at work	29
Child leaving home	29
Trouble with in-laws	29
Outstanding personal achievement	28
Spouse starts or stops work	26
Beginning or ending school	26
Change in living conditions	25
Revision of personal habits	24

Trouble with boss	23
Change in working hours or conditions	20
Change in residence	20
Change in schools	20
Change in recreation	19
Change in church activities	19
Change in social activities	18
Minor mortgage or loan	17
Change in sleeping habits	16
Change in number of family reunions	15
Change in eating habits	15
Vacation	13
Christmas	12
Minor violation of law	11

Score of 300+: At risk of illness.

Score of 150-299: Risk of illness is moderate (reduced by 30% from the above risk).

Score <150: Only have a slight risk of illness.

Holmes and Rahe Stress Scale—Non-Adults

A modified scale has also been developed for non-adults. Similar to the adult scale, stress points for life events in the past year are added and compared to the rough estimate of how stress affects health.

Life event	Life change units
Death of parent	100
Unplanned pregnancy/abortion	100
Getting married	95
Divorce of parents	90
Acquiring a visible deformity	80
Fathering a child	70
Jail sentence of parent for over one year	70
Marital separation of parents	69
Death of a brother or sister	68
Change in acceptance by peers	67
Unplanned pregnancy of sister	64
Discovery of being an adopted child	63

Marriage of parent to stepparent	63
Death of a close friend	63
Having a visible congenital deformity	62
Serious illness requiring hospitalization	58
Failure of a grade in school	56
Not making an extracurricular activity	55
Hospitalization of a parent	55
Jail sentence of parent for over 30 days	53
Breaking up with boyfriend or girlfriend	53
Beginning to date	51
Suspension from school	50
Becoming involved with drugs or alcohol	50
Birth of a brother or sister	50
Increase in arguments between parents	47
Loss of job by parent	46
Outstanding personal achievement	46
Change in parent's financial status	45
Accepted at college of choice	43
Being a senior in high school	42
Hospitalization of a sibling	41
Increased absence of parent from home	38
Brother or sister leaving home	37
Addition of third adult to family	34
Becoming a full-fledged member of a church	31
Decrease in arguments between parents	27
Decrease in arguments with parents	26
Mother or father beginning work	26

Score of 300+: At risk of illness.

Score of 150-299: Risk of illness is moderate (reduced by 30% from the above risk).

Score <150: Only have a slight risk of illness.

Appendix C

Visualization

Many people find it helpful to use their imagination to create a mental "vacation" or a "private place" where they can go at any time to feel peaceful and relaxed.

1. Sit or lie down in a comfortable position. Try not to cross your legs. Leave your arms relaxed at your sides or in your lap.
2. Close your eyes.
3. Take a couple deep relaxation breaths.
4. Imagine yourself in a place that is comfortable, safe, relaxing, and beautiful for you. It can be a place you have been or an imaginary place.
    - an ocean beach
    - a forest
    - a garden
5. Now, fill in the details:
    - What do you *see* around you? In your mind look around you, create each detail—the colors of the leaves, the sun sparkling on the water, etc.
    - What *sounds* do you hear? Listen to the waves lapping against the shore, the birds chirping, and so on.
    - What do you *feel*? Feel the warmth of the sun on your skin and between your toes, etc.
    - What do you *smell*? Salt water? Flowers?
    - Is anyone with you? Are you alone?
    - Fill in any other details.
6. Build this image in your mind, and rest here. When you feel at peace and relaxed, slowly leave your special place and return your mind to the present.
7. Take a couple deep relaxation breaths.
8. Slowly open your eyes.

The place you create is yours alone, and you can return there whenever you need peace and relaxation.

Hint: Some find it helpful to create a transition to and from a relaxation place. For example, you could begin and end your visualization by walking down a hallway or a path to, then from, your place.

Quick Stress Reducer: You can also use visualization as a tool to help you prepare for a stressful situation. Preview the event in your mind. Imagine yourself doing the task perfectly. For example, if you are anxious about a speech, imagine yourself in front of the audience calm and confident. Hear yourself speaking with a strong and steady voice.

Used with permission from Trinity Unity Point Health and Trinity Parish Nurse Program.

Appendix D

Progressive Muscle Relaxation

Progressive Muscle Relaxation is a technique that trains your body to relax each muscle group, producing a feeling of deep relaxation. You will tense, and then relax the muscles of one area of your body at a time. It may feel awkward at first, but it gets easier and more effective with practice.

- Sit or lie down in a comfortable position.
- Take a few deep, quiet breaths.
- Use the list below as a guide. Tighten each muscle for a few seconds, then release. As you tense each muscle, notice how it feels. Feel the difference in the muscle as it relaxes.

Relaxation Sequence:
1. Pull toes up, hold, relax.
2. Turn ankles outward, hold, relax.
3. Stretch right leg, hold, relax.
4. Stretch left leg, hold, relax.
5. Squeeze thighs together, hold, relax.
6. Tighten buttocks, hold, relax.
7. Pull in abdomen, hold, relax.
8. Arch lower back, hold, relax.
9. Press lower back outward, hold, relax.
10. Breathe in deeply, hold, breath out.
11. Make a fist with your right hand, hold, relax.
12. Make a fist with your left hand, hold, relax.
13. Raise left shoulder toward ear, hold, relax.
14. Raise right shoulder toward ear, hold, relax.
15. Bend neck forward, hold, relax.
16. Purse lips, hold, relax.
17. Clench your teeth, hold, relax.
18. Open eyes wide, hold, relax.
19. Close eyes tightly, hold, relax.
20. Wrinkle your forehead and frown, hold, relax.
21. Lift eyebrows toward hairline, hold, relax.

After you finish, rest quietly. Take a couple deep breaths. Pay attention to how your body feels. When you are ready, open your eyes and get up slowly.

Progressive Muscle Relaxation Short Version

After you are comfortable with the process of Progressive Muscle Relaxation, you can try tensing larger groups of muscles in each step.

1. Relax your face muscles (lips, jaw, eyes).
2. Relax your neck muscles.
3. Relax your arm muscles (shoulder, arm, hand).
4. Relax your back muscles (upper, lower and buttocks).
5. Relax your tummy muscles.
6. Relax your leg muscles (thigh, calves, ankles).

Unit II
Professionalism

Unit II: Professionalism
Ethical Issues

Ethical Issues

Introduction

Learning Outcomes

Upon completion of this module, the participant will be able to:

1. Identify ethical issues in faith community nursing practice.
2. Apply the elements of ethical decision-making.
3. Examine ethical dilemmas using the Nursing Process Approach.
4. Incorporate ethical decision-making into faith community nursing practice.

Description

This module introduces ethical issues that occur in faith community nursing practice. The nature of ethical issues and the elements of ethical decision-making are discussed. A method of ethical decision-making that can be used in faith community nursing practice is introduced. The module provides the opportunity to apply ethical analysis and ethical decision-making to simulated faith community nursing practice situations.

Hours: 2

Research

Oh and Gastmans (2013) examined available quantitative evidence in the literature on moral distress experienced by hospital nurses. Upon review of 19 articles, the researchers noted that nurses experience a low *frequency* of moral distress but a moderately intense level of moral distress when it occurred. Nurses experienced moral distress more frequently when they perceived a more negative ethical climate, worked in a nursing shortage, in situations of futile care, and when a patient or family member directed inappropriate behaviors toward them. As a result, the nurses experienced higher levels of emotional exhaustion and depersonalization toward patients. The researchers reported that the negative coping strategies included leaving or considering leaving the workplace. Cumulative effects of unresolved moral distress may lead to "moral residue," which manifests as guilt, shame, and self-blame. These findings reflect the importance of recognizing signs of moral distress and residue, the significance of strong organizational leadership, and the need for positive ethical climates in nursing practice settings.

Faith Tradition

The Christian faith is concerned about (1) how we love and care for one another, as Jesus Christ loved and cared for us; (2) issues of social justice, such as access to health care, and distribution of scarce resources, such as nursing care; (3) advocacy on behalf of others to prevent harm and provide good to them; (4) suffering and healing; and (5) the morality expressed and lived out by Christians when addressing these concerns.

Key Terms

Code of ethics: a "conventionalized set of rules or expectations devised for a select purpose" (Johnstone, 2004, p. 19)

Ethical dilemma: a situation with at least two equally justifiable courses of action or judgments in which a person is uncertain which one to pursue or choose. Often it is not a "win-win" situation but one of "least loss"

Ethical issue: a matter in dispute between two or more parties because of a conflict of moral values

Ethical principles: guides for ethical decision-making and taking action

Ethical theories: systems of principles by which a person can determine what should or should not be done

Ethics: a branch of philosophy that involves clarification of the *shoulds* and *oughts* of individuals and society, or what is "right and wrong"

Values: worthwhile standards or qualities of a person or a social group

Reflection

"With what shall I come before the LORD, and bow myself before God on high?
Shall I come before him with burnt offerings, with calves a year old?
Will the LORD be pleased with thousands of rams, with ten thousands of rivers of oil?
Shall I give my firstborn for my transgression, the fruit of my body for the sin of my soul?"
He has told you, O mortal, what is good; and what does the LORD require of you but to do justice, and to love kindness, and to walk humbly with your God?
—Micah 6:6–8

The Beatitudes
"Blessed are the poor in spirit, for theirs is the kingdom of heaven.
Blessed are those who mourn, for they will be comforted.
Blessed are the meek, for they will inherit the earth.
Blessed are those who hunger and thirst for righteousness, for they will be filled.
Blessed are the merciful, for they will receive mercy.
Blessed are the pure in heart, for they will see God.
Blessed are the peacemakers, for they will be called children of God.
Blessed are those who are persecuted because of righteousness, for theirs is the kingdom of heaven."
—Matthew 5:3–10

Ethical Issues

Content Outline

OUTCOME 1

Identify ethical issues in faith community nursing practice.

Definitions to Understand Ethical Issues

Ethics is a branch of philosophy that involves clarification of the *shoulds* and *oughts* of individuals and society, or what is "right and wrong." It is the study of the choices by which we try to live a good life and how we understand the results of our choices.

Nursing Ethics is a system of principles concerning the actions of the nurse in his or her relationships with patients, family members, other health care providers, policymakers, and society as a whole.

Ethics is an integral part of the foundation of nursing (American Nurses Association, 2001, p. 5). In addition, ethics is an integral part of nursing's social contract with society.

Nursing ethics is a part of a broader system known as **biomedical ethics or bioethics**, the study of ethical problems in health care resulting from scientific advances.

An **ethical issue** is a matter in dispute between two or more parties because of a conflict of moral values.
- Resolving an ethical issue usually requires ethical deliberation or ethical decision-making.
- Ethical issues are often controversial topics that are value-laden, such as abortion, euthanasia, surrogate motherhood, or genetic engineering.
- An ethical issue is *not* the same as an ethical dilemma.

> **EXAMPLES**
>
> *It is not an ethical dilemma to save the life of a healthy individual who is experiencing ventricular fibrillation.*
>
> *It is an ethical dilemma to save the life of an individual with late stage Alzheimer's disease who is experiencing septic shock from aspiration pneumonia.*

An **ethical dilemma** is a situation where there are at least two equally justifiable courses of action or judgments but a person is uncertain which one to pursue or choose. Often it is not a "win-win" situation but one of "least loss."

The Role of Values in Ethical Issues

Understanding the role of values in ethical issues requires understanding where values come from, how values influence us, how values are classified, and what happens when values conflict.

What are values?
Values are worthwhile standards or qualities of a person or a social group. Values come from many sources.
- culture
- family
- peer group
- work group
- religious beliefs

Values are expressed in language or in standards of conduct that a person endorses.

How do our values influence us?
We organize our values into some system of prioritization of importance to us. Our value system changes as a result of life experiences and reassessment of one's values.

Values have motivational power to guide one's choices.
- Our choices, actions, and judgments often protect our values.
- The position we take on controversial issues is usually motivated by our values.
- In order to be a competent provider, the nurse must understand and seek a balance between science and technology and morality.

How are values classified?
Moral values relate to the moral interests that individuals have, such as being free from oppression, being self-determining, being free from pain or suffering, having a sense of well-being, being truthful, being honest, being kind, or compassionate. These impact choices about life with a view to do good for the sake of doing good.

Nonmoral values relate to personal preferences, beliefs, or matters of taste, such as cleanliness, being on time, choice of ice cream, or music genre.

Cultural values are the accepted and dominant standards of a particular cultural group. They function with belief systems and serve to give meaning and worth to the existence and experiences of the group. Cultural values often prescribe acceptable and unacceptable behaviors, social relationships, and rules of communication among group members; ethical values can be moral and nonmoral in nature.

Identifying values seemingly in conflict is the second step in preparing to make ethical decisions.

Religious values often are the product of the history and culture from which they have emerged and are learned from religious practices, often in childhood. They continue to influence a person even when one has abandoned the religious belief system.

These values can be acted out unconsciously because they are deeply embedded in the experience of the person; religious values can be moral and nonmoral in nature. These values impact choices about life with a view to please God, and command or teach beyond doing what is good for the sake of doing good.

Professional values are standards upheld by a particular professional group. Most codes of professional ethics list the basic values of the professional group and then the principles or guidelines that protect these values. The values can be moral and nonmoral in nature.

Personal values are values important to the individual. They usually are a combination of moral, nonmoral, cultural, religious, and professional values. Personal values often unconsciously influence our choices, judgments, and actions.

What happens when values conflict with one another?

All values can conflict with one another. Personal values conflict with professional values; religious values conflict with professional values; moral values conflict with nonmoral values.

It is especially difficult when personal, professional, cultural, or religious values conflict with moral values. When this happens, there is a need for ethical analysis and ethical decision-making.

There is no need for ethical decision-making if no moral values are in conflict with other values.

Ethical Issues in Faith Community Nursing Practice

There is an increasing complexity of ethical concerns as rapid changes in technology, economics, law, and secular influences interact in health care. Access to health care is becoming more difficult as the health care system takes on a business model. The growth of electronic records and social media has increased risks to patient privacy and confidentiality. Rapid technology changes challenge beliefs about the beginning and end of life, as well as quality and quantity of life.

Conflicts of values may surround …
- initiating, withholding or terminating life-sustaining treatments
- beginning-of-life decisions
- refusing treatment
- deciding who should be surrogate or proxy decision-makers

Protecting values may involve …
- deciding when it is no longer safe for elderly parishioners to live at home
- protecting parishioner confidentiality and privacy

Critical Thinking

How does the FCN use the knowledge about values in ministry?

- protecting parishioners from having their good will consumed by another parishioner
- understanding reproductive technologies

Justice and equality may affect ...
- access to treatment or the health care system
- developing outreach to homeless people in community
- treatment of gay and transgender congregational members
- treatment of persons with Human Immunodeficiency Virus (HIV) or Acquired Immunodeficiency Syndrome (AIDs)

OUTCOME 2
Apply the elements of ethical decision-making.

Ethical decision-making involves not only knowledge of personal values and beliefs but also knowledge of ethical theories and principles.

Ethical Theories

Ethical theories are systems of principles by which a person can determine what should or should not be done. The systems are categorized into various types (Hickman, 2006).

Utilitarianism makes decisions based on doing the greatest good (or allowing the least harm) to the greatest number of people. It is a Western world theory.
- Harm to the few is justified for the benefit of the majority.
- In US health care these decisions are made through a risk-benefit analysis. Are the benefits worth the risks?

Deontology emphasizes moral obligation in performing actions. This is a Western world theory.
- The focus is not necessarily on the outcome but on the ability to follow a rule.
- This becomes problematic when different systems of rules conflict.
- This includes Christian ethics that are *divine command* ethics—God's rules.

Virtue or Character Ethic has its roots in Aristotle (384–322 BC), the Greek philosopher who believed that everything we do aims at some good. It is not concerned with acts of goodness but in always *being good*.

Ethics of Caring involves relationship, connections, and mutuality.
- This is consistent with nursing practice and has strong links to faith community nursing practice.
- Early nursing theorists include Madeline Leininger, Jean Watson, and Patricia Benner.
    - Leininger wrote about caring as the essence of nursing.
    - Watson focused on caring as a moral imperative.
    - Benner addressed the primacy of caring in practice.

KEY TERM

Ethical theories *are systems of principles by which a person can determine what should or should not be done.*

Uustal (2003, pp. 14–17) described the ethics of caring from a Christian perspective. Christian nurses should:
- *Recognize that nursing is a calling from God.*
- *Believe that God has given them a special gift to serve others.*
- *View compassionate caring as an act of faith.*
- *Experience the ethic of care from God, who promises us, "Those who wait for the LORD shall renew their strength, they shall mount up with wings like eagles, they shall run and not be weary, they shall walk and not faint" (Isaiah 40:31).*

Ethical Principles

Ethical principles are guides to ethical decision-making and taking ethical action. They help to justify or provide sound moral reasons for a judgment or action. For example, the principle of autonomy guides one to respect individuals and their self-determined choices.

Beneficence is the obligation to do good or provide benefit for the patient, and to prevent or remove harm. *Good care* requires the provider to approach the parishioner in a wholistic manner (Aiken, 2004).

Scripture on **beneficence***:*

- ◆ *Isaiah 1:17*
- ◆ *Hebrews 13:16*

Nonmaleficence is the obligation to avoid harm or to protect one from harm. This is evident in laws to protect children, vulnerable adults, elderly, mentally incompetent, and those who lack capacity to make decisions.

Justice is the obligation to decide how benefits and burdens should be fairly distributed among patients.
- One way to do that is to treat equals equally and treat those who are unequal differently according to their needs.
- This means that those equal in health needs should receive the same amount of health care resources. It also means that when some people have greater health needs than others, they should receive a greater amount of health resources.
- This type of allocation is considered *just* because it distributes health resources according to need in a fair (or ethical) manner.

Scripture on **nonmaleficence***:*

- ◆ *Romans 13:10*
- ◆ *1 Corinthians 10:24*
- ◆ *Philippians 4:8–9*

Scripture on **justice***:*

- ◆ *Micah 6:6–8*
- ◆ *Proverbs 29:7*
- ◆ *Luke 18:6–8*

Autonomy is the obligation to respect individuals as self-determined choosers and to acknowledge their choices, which stem from personal values and beliefs of importance, unless those choices result in harm to others. It is based on human dignity and respect for the individual.
- Autonomy is not an absolute right, as limitations may be imposed if one's autonomy interferes with another's rights or well-being.
- This principle may be involved a conflict in matriarchal or patriarchal cultures or conservative religions.
- Western medicine and culture place a heavy emphasis on autonomy.
- Secular ethics places great emphasis on this principle.

Scripture on **autonomy***:*

- ◆ *1 Peter 2:18*

Veracity is the obligation to tell the truth and not lie or deceive others. Nurses are obliged to be truthful in culturally appropriate ways because not to do so may undermine the patient's or family's trust and the overall therapeutic effectiveness of the relationship.

Fidelity is the obligation to remain faithful to one's commitments. The commitments that usually fall within the scope of fidelity are obligations implicit in a trusting relationship between patient and nurse, such as keeping promises.

Scripture on **veracity***:*

- ◆ *Proverbs 12:19*
- ◆ *Zechariah 8:16*
- ◆ *Ephesians 4:15*

Confidentiality requires nondisclosure of private information shared within the trusting relationship between patient and nurse. An additional piece for the faith community is the *communal nature of a confessional community* (Solari-Twadell & McDermott, 1999). Nurses should be mindful of confidentiality in settings such as prayer chains and congregational prayer.

Sanctity of human life is the obligation to view human life as sacred and not to take human life even for noble reasons.

Scripture on **confidentiality**:
♦ *Proverbs 11:13*
♦ *Proverbs 17:9*
♦ *Proverbs 25:9*

Codes of Ethics in Health Care

Historically, a number of codes were adopted because of injustices against fellow humans.
- The **Nuremberg Code** of Ethics in Medical Research (1947) was developed after WWII because of the practices of Nazis in human experimentation.
- The **Declaration of Helsinki** (1964) further addressed informed consent for those who are legally incompetent.
- The American Hospital Association's **Patient's Bill of Rights** (1973) focused on the patient's role in choosing treatment options.
- **Institutional Review Boards** monitor biomedical research involving human subjects and assure that appropriate steps are taken to protect the rights and welfare of humans participating as subjects in research.
- **Codes** focus on respect for the autonomy of the individual, especially in secular bioethics. Christian bioethics add to one's obligation to a faith tradition's theology.

Scripture on **sanctity of human life**:
♦ *Genesis 1:27, 31*

KEY TERM
A **code of ethics** *is "a conventionalized set of rules or expectations devised for a select purpose."*

Ethical Standards for Nursing Practice and Faith Community Nursing Practice

A code of ethics is "a conventionalized set of rules or expectations devised for a select purpose" (Johnstone, 2004, p. 19).

The **first version of the code of ethics for nurses** in the United States was written in the late 1800s by Lystra Gretter, Farrand Training School for Nurses in Detroit, Michigan. Gretter felt that Florence Nightingale embodied the ideals of nursing so the first version of the code was named "The Nightingale Pledge."

THE NIGHTINGALE PLEDGE

In 1893, Mrs. Lystra Gretter and a Committee for the Ferrand Training School of Nurses in Detroit, Michigan, composed this modified Hippocratic Oath named for Florence Nightingale as a token of esteem for the founder of modern nursing.

"I solemnly pledge myself before God and in the presence of this assembly, to pass my life in purity and to practice my profession faithfully. I will abstain from whatever is deleterious and mischievous, and will not take or knowingly administer any harmful drug. I will do all in my power to maintain and elevate the standard of my profession, and will hold in confidence all personal matters committed to my keeping and all family affairs coming to my knowledge in the practice of my calling. With loyalty will I endeavor to aid the physician in his work, and devote myself to the welfare of those committed to my care."

American Nurses Association's *Code of Ethics for Nurses with Interpretive Statements* (2001) has three purposes (p. 5).
1. It is a succinct statement of the ethical obligations and duties of every individual who enters the nursing profession.
2. It is the profession's nonnegotiable ethical standard.
3. It is an expression of nursing's own understanding of its commitment to society.

This code provides guidelines for nursing practice, research, and education with nine provisions.
- The first three describe the most fundamental values.
- The second three address boundaries.
- The final three address aspects of duties beyond individual clients.

Canadian Nurses Association's Code of Ethics for Registered Nurses (2002) describes the ethical behavior expected of RNs in Canada.

International Council of Nurses (ICN) began working toward the development of a code of ethics for all nurses in the world at the 1923 ICN Congress held in Montreal, Canada. The fundamental responsibility of the nurse is to: promote health, prevent illness, restore health, and to alleviate suffering.

Most **codes of ethics for nurses** in the world agree on:
- practice competence
- protection of patient confidentiality
- nondiscrimination of patients
- ethical accountability of the nurse

Advocacy as a Central Nursing Ethic
Speaking on behalf of or helping the parishioner discuss needs, interests, and choices is an important part of every code of nursing ethics in the world. All professional organizations seem to give a special significance to the nurse's advocacy role.
- The concept of advocacy is consistent with the values expressed in the International Council of Nurses Code of Ethics for Nurses (2006). For example, the ICN Code states, the nurse "takes appropriate action to safeguard individuals when their care is endangered." The nurse is required to act to promote the wishes, welfare, and well-being of the patient.
- The nurse needs to avoid a paternalist approach (the father-knows-best way of thinking) when acting on behalf of a parishioner (Sanderson, 2013).
- In the setting of the faith community, advocating includes appropriate care for vulnerable populations, accessing adequate and appropriate health care resources, initiating referrals for care, and obtaining home care resources and equipment (ANA/HMA, 2012).

Additional Behaviors Needed by the Faith Community Nurse
- Know denomination teachings and faith beliefs. Read denomination documents, study the catechism or statements of denomination beliefs, or sit in on adult confirmation classes.
- Know the faith community's position on ethical issues, especially organ donations, issues of fertility, assisted reproduction, abortion, blood and withdrawal of life-sustaining treatments.
- Recognize that congregational members often face decisions that may conflict with their faith teachings.

Critical Thinking
Explain how the elements of ethical decision-making give you a framework that can be used with your faith community.

- Know what your role is as FCN to:
  - Support congregational members in their decisions.
  - Make sure congregational members are informed.
  - Provide the church's presence at a difficult time in the congregational member's or family member's life.
  - Offer spiritual support through readings, prayer.
- The FCN's role is helped when you (as the FCN):
  - Explore and identify your own faith beliefs.
  - Acknowledge where your own faith beliefs differ from the church in which you serve as faith community nurse.
  - Seek counsel and guidance from your pastor, priest, or faith community leader.
  - Know when to remove yourself from a situation because of a potential conflict of interest.

Integration of knowledge is necessary to begin ethical decision-making.

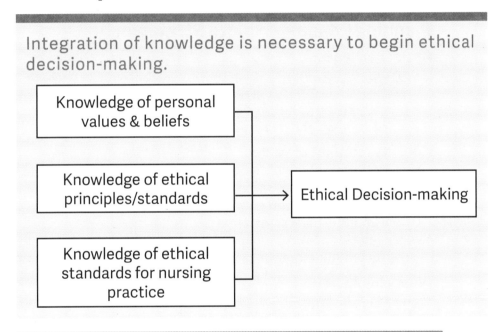

OUTCOME 3

Examine ethical dilemmas using the Nursing Process Approach.

The Nursing Process Approach is based on Burkhardt & Nathaniel (2008).

Assessment Phase—Gather Data

Uncover the **"story" behind the value conflicts.**

Gather
- the factual information from all parties. Identify who all the parties are. Who did what?
- scientific or technical facts.
- emotions, attitudes and opinions from all parties.
  - Why do the parties see the situation as an ethical problem?
  - Have each of the parties describe the conflicts of values they perceive.

- What are the parishioner's wishes?
- What are the family's wishes?
- intentional boundaries for self-care.

Clarify

- Have all parties clarify the conflicts and the values involved. The context within which the conflicts arose will be made explicit.
- What further information is necessary?

Diagnosis Phase—Articulate the Problem

Clearly **identify and describe** the ethical issue or dilemma. State it as succinctly as possible.

Identify the potential cultural, religious, personal, professional, and political origins of the values held by the parties involved.

Planning Phase—Explore Strategies

Assist parties to

- examine their values, and the values of others so that the parties can begin to negotiate.
- prioritize their values and preserve the most important ones in the process of decision-making.

Consider conflict of values.

This conflict might lead to a decision that affects several of the parties involved. For example:

- the quality of the person's life
- how long the person may live
- the emotional and psychological stress that parties to the conflict might experience

What should be done?

Explore all the ways in which the conflict of values might be resolved. Try to reach **consensus on "the right thing"** to do.

By their nature, ethical dilemmas produce differences of opinions and **not everyone will be pleased** with the decision. Be prepared for strong emotional responses.

The FCN should ask:

- What does it mean to care for this person?
- What are my faith community nursing responsibilities to this person?
- How do I, as a faith community nurse, maintain my ethical integrity in this situation?

Implementation Phase—Implement Strategy

Choose a course of action based on:

- the decision-maker's best judgment about what ought to be done
- consideration of the context of the value conflicts
- consideration of the values of the parties involved
- consideration of the ethical relevance of all values involved

Implement the decision or strategy. Be aware that in this phase emotions may be very strong.

Evaluation Phase—Evaluate Outcomes

Evaluate the outcome against the goal.
- Consider whether the process of ethical analysis could have been improved.
- Consider the implications of the ethical action implemented for future patient care situations.
- Assess the process that led to the decision.

Recognize that the **same or similar value conflicts may recur** time after time in a particular area of nursing practice:
- may be a result of the religious beliefs or cultural backgrounds of the parties involved
- may be a result of the personal or professional values of the nurse
- may require policy recommendations

OUTCOME 4

Apply ethical decision-making to faith community nursing practice.

Using the case studies in the Learning Activities, engage in small group discussions of **simulated situations** involving conflicts of value.

Use the **Nursing Process Approach** of ethical analysis to understand the values conflicts.

Propose **ethical actions** for the FCN using a knowledge of ethical theories, ethical principles, ethical concepts of nursing, and ethical standards for nursing practice.

Standards of Professional Performance for Faith Community Nursing

Standard 7. Ethics
The faith community nurse practices ethically.

COMPETENCIES

The faith community nurse:

- Uses *Code of Ethics for Nurses with Interpretive Statements* (ANA, 2001) to guide practice.
- Delivers care in a manner that preserves and protects the healthcare consumer's autonomy, dignity, rights, and spiritual beliefs and practices.
- Recognizes the centrality of the healthcare consumer and family as core members of any healthcare team.
- Upholds healthcare consumer confidentiality within religious, legal, and regulatory parameters.
- Assists healthcare consumers in self-determination and informed decision-making.
- Maintains a therapeutic and professional healthcare consumer–nurse relationship within appropriate professional role boundaries.
- Contributes to resolving ethical issues of healthcare consumers, colleagues, community groups, or systems, and other stakeholders.

- Takes appropriate action regarding instances of illegal, unethical or inappropriate behavior that can endanger or jeopardize the best interests of the healthcare consumer or situation.
- Speaks up as appropriate to question healthcare practice when necessary for safety and quality improvement.
- Advocates for equitable healthcare consumer care.
- Empowers healthcare consumers in developing skills for self-advocacy in support of their spiritual beliefs and practices.
- Incorporates ethical and moral theories, principles, and models in processes of care planning and delivery.
- Acknowledges and respects tenets of the faith and spiritual belief system of a healthcare consumer.

Learning Activities

Health and Healing Practices within Your Faith Tradition

Instructions:
The following questions are an opportunity to explore the health and healing practices of faith traditions. Use the question for a brief discussion as you introduce the module.

1. Is there a history of your faith community working in the health field or medical missions? Provide examples of your national denomination supporting health ministries.

2. What are your faith tradition's beliefs (social or policy statements) on health or health-related issues?

3. What are your faith tradition's views regarding the end of life? Euthanasia? Suicide? What are the implications for practice?
   - What are your faith tradition's views regarding conception and reproduction? What are the implications for practice?
   - Does your faith tradition have a statement on genetic research? What are the implications for practice?

Question:
What other statements or viewpoints might be distinct to your tradition? What are the implications for practice?

Values Identification Activity

Instructions:
1. Ask participants to pair up.

2. Ask participants to identify several values important to them.

3. Identify the types of values represented in this list.

Question:
Ask participants what they learned about the nature of values from this activity.

Case Discussion Activity

Instructions:
1. Break into groups of 3–4 people.

2. From the case situations, assign each group a different case to analyze.

3. Ask groups to use the steps of the Nursing Process Approach to ethical analysis to identify the values important to the case, the values conflicts, and the ethically important values.

4. Ask groups to recommend ethical action(s) for the faith community nurse.

5. Ask each group to select a "recorder" who will report on the discussion to the large group.

6. Allow 15 minutes for the group to discuss the case situation.

7. Allow 30 minutes for presentation of case studies to the large group.

Question:
Ask participants what they have learned about ethical analysis and ethical decision-making from this activity.

CASE 1
The Parishioner Who Is At Risk but Content with Her Circumstances

Sarah Smith, 80 years old, has been a member of her church for over 50 years. She provides care for her 60-year-old handicapped son in their three-room home. She has severe osteoporosis and uses a walker. She cannot attend church because she cannot leave her son alone. One of the members of her church visitation program has been seeing her once a week for a friendly chat and prayer.

The "visitor" has asked Marie Matthews, the FCN, to visit Mrs. Smith to determine whether her health and the health of her son are at risk in their present living environment. Mrs. Smith agrees to the FCN's visit. Marie knows that Mrs. Smith has a reputation for being extremely private and very independent.

On her first visit Marie notices that the home is very cluttered and has a strong odor from accumulation of dust, dirt, and mold. The home is heated with a space heater surrounded by stacks of old paperback books. There is little food in the pantry. After several visits Marie notices that Mrs. Smith has not changed her son's clothing or bathed him for a long time. However, Mrs. Smith seems to be comfortable with their lifestyle and does not see any reason to change their living arrangements. Her financial support comes from Social Security and a small pension. It is not clear when Mrs. Smith last saw her primary care provider, and she cannot recall when her son was last seen by his primary care provider.

The FCN, Marie, initially encourages Mrs. Smith to apply for services that could be available to her, such as homemaker services, a nutrition program, and financial management services. Marie also tells Mrs. Smith that more volunteers from the church would be willing to visit her and sit with her son while she attends church or sees her primary care provider. Mrs. Smith says that she does not want or need help from any more people and does not feel comfortable leaving her son with strangers.

Marie is concerned about the living arrangements of Mrs. Smith and her son. Marie is also wondering whether she should notify the Protective Services Unit of Elder Services that Mrs. Smith might be endangering not only herself but her son. However, this action could lead to Mrs. Smith losing her right to care for her son, or even to consideration of conservatorship and guardianship through the courts.

How far should Marie go in providing "good" for Mrs. Smith and her son, and who should decide what is "good" for them?

CASE 2
Protecting Parishioner Confidentiality

Mr. Dewey, 58 years old, is a respected leader in the church and serves on the governance and finance committees. Unfortunately, Mr. Dewey has a long history of alcoholism. This is known by other church members, but few talk about it because Mr. Dewey is considered an important community member. Last week he entered a local alcohol treatment program at his family's insistence and with help from the pastor and faith community nurse. He and his family were explicit in their discussions with the pastor and FCN that they did not want anyone to know that he is currently undergoing treatment for alcoholism.

Becky Smith, the 14-year-old daughter of another church member, is a teen volunteer at the local hospital. Several days ago, she delivered a flower arrangement to the substance abuse treatment floor, and she noticed Mr. Dewey's name on the card. She told her parents that Mr. Dewey was in the hospital. Her mother immediately called the church office and put his name and hospital room number on the prayer list, which is printed in the church bulletin.

Mr. Dewey's family is very angry with the pastor and the FCN. They say their privacy has not been protected and believe that the pastor and the FCN betrayed their confidence. The FCN soon finds out how the information was gained and transmitted. She asks the pastor to visit the Dewey home with her and explain how this mishap happened. She does not want anyone to think she or the pastor betrayed a confidence. The pastor, however, is not willing to do this. He advises her to "just let it blow over" and say nothing.

The FCN does not feel comfortable with this approach. What can she do?

CASE 3
Deciding What Is Fair and Just in Nursing Home Placement

Dana Green is the FCN at a faith congregation well known for its support of social justice issues and advocacy on behalf of the local community. In the past 15 years, this congregation has helped to build a state-of-the-art assisted living facility and a 60-bed nursing home for their members. Preference for placement in both facilities has always been given to members of the faith congregation. Members of the local community can apply for placement if there are available spaces and if they can pay for the services needed. The nursing home has beds for those who cannot pay, but they must be members of the faith congregation.

The FCN is on a local scholarship committee with Jane Albany, a family friend. Jane asks Dana for help in getting her elderly mother placed in the congregation's nursing home. Jane and her family are able to pay for all services needed by her mother, and they are sure that Dana can do something to support their cause. Dana, however, is aware that Fred Hobbit, a parishioner with few financial resources, is also applying for placement to the nursing home. Dana is torn between advocating for a family friend's mother or for the parishioner, Fred Hobbit, for placement in the one open bed at the nursing home.

What should the FCN do? What is the faith community nurse's obligation to both parties?

CASE 4
When a Pregnancy Reduction Is Recommended

A couple in the congregation, Jim and Alice Thomas, have been told that they are expecting four babies. The doctor is strongly recommending that the pregnancy be reduced to two babies. The joy of this long-awaited pregnancy is well known in this small, tightly knit congregation. However, no one except the couple, their parents, the faith community nurse, and the pastor knows about the recommendation.

The FCN does not personally oppose abortion but is well aware that the teachings of this faith community are against abortion. The pastor has met with the couple and their parents, who are long standing members of the congregation. He has reminded them of the church's teachings against abortion and is convinced that reducing the pregnancy amounts to abortion of otherwise viable fetuses.

The pastor asks the nurse to meet with all involved to help the couple to make the "correct" decision. He tells her that this is a very difficult ministry, but he knows the FCN will be helpful to the couple and their parents. Whatever is decided, he does not want to know. He will pray for the nurse and knows she will guide the couple to the morally right decision.

What is the role of the FCN in this situation, and what should be done?

CASE 5
Protecting a Parishioner from Another Parishioner

Gerry Post is the FCN at her church, a 300-member active faith community. In addition Gerry works as a nurse in a local health care agency. Dottie Small, a 68-year-old single woman, has been attending the church for about six months.

Over the next few months, Gerry learns that Dottie's partner died recently and that she does not have any family. She lives alone in a low-cost housing complex in the community and appears to be very lonely. Dottie soon begins to disclose that she has many diseases, including multiple sclerosis, cancer, ulcerative colitis, rheumatoid arthritis, a seizure disorder, and others. Because she works at the clinic where Dottie sees her primary care provider, Gerry knows that most of this information is not true as it is not in her medical history. It appears that Dottie claims being ill for attention and for the sympathy of others. Dottie calls 911 and goes to the hospital about once a month for various complaints, and no medical problems are ever found. Gerry suspects that Dottie might have a mental illness.

Dottie begins to ask Julie, another mid-60s single woman in the faith community, to lunch or dinner, and other social events at the church or in the community. She asks Julie to help her when she is ill or to drive her to doctor appointments and other activities. Gerry knows that Julie is also a very needy person who likes to be asked to do things. Julie begins to tell everyone that she and Dottie are friends and tells other parishioners that "poor Dottie" has a lot of illness and needs prayers and support.

Gerry begins to suspect that Dottie is grooming Julie to be her new caretaker and replacement for her lost partner. What should Gerry do to protect Julie and can she share any of the information she has about Dottie?

CASE 6
Homelessness—Responding to the Needs of Individuals Not a Part of a Faith Community

Cynthia Smith is a 23-year-old woman who was discharged from the hospital this morning. She delivered a three-pound five-ounce baby boy two days ago. He is premature and remains in the hospital due to medical issues. Cynthia arrives at the church with her husband seeking emergency shelter as it is mid-December, the local shelters are full, and it is 16 degrees below zero. Her husband, Michael, was a member of the local union employed at the sugar plant for almost eight years but has not been working for more than 16 months due to a lockout. As a result of complications due to her pregnancy, Cynthia also has not been able to work, so the couple lost their home. They slept in their car for several months and stayed with family or friends for as long as possible. Their home community is 45 miles from the metro area but they want to stay here at this time to be close to their son and because they do not have any money for gas to travel between the two communities.

Lynn Smith is the FCN who is working at the registration table at the church and signs in the couple. When Cynthia learns that the sheltering in the church site has separate sleeping spaces for men and women she begins to sob. Michael tries to console her and desperately voices how stressful it is not to be able to sleep near his wife to comfort her at this very difficult time. When Lynn hears their story and observes that they are clinging to an empty infant carrier and one shared suitcase, Lynn starts to cry as well.

What are the ethical issues present in this situation? How should Lynn respond to the couple? What specific things will she want to be aware of in her own behavior in working with this homeless couple? What interpersonal attributes will be important in this situation?

Recognizing that the FCN provides wholistic care, what other dimensions (beyond the spiritual dimension) need to be addressed? Identify specific issues within these dimensions that need to be assessed.

CASE 7
Advance Directives

Mr. Eng is a 93-year-old retired engineer who was in excellent health prior to suffering a stroke three days ago. His physician has one file in his medical record—a living will, which Mr. Eng wrote ten years before. At that time he indicated that, should he ever suffer a stroke of any sort, he would not want heroic measures to be taken. He had watched his wife live as an invalid for four years in a nursing home after experiencing a stroke. Mr. Eng wanted to be sure he would never be exposed to such an indignity nor continue such a burden on others. The physician is not aware whether this continued to be the wish of Mr. Eng since signing the document because he never had a conversation about the living will with Mr. Eng. The stroke is a massive one and likely to leave Mr. Eng unable to speak and paralyzed on the right side. The physician believes Mr. Eng probably can be helped with the use of aggressive medical care. Mr. Eng's daughter has asked the physician to do everything possible to save her father.

Does this situation constitute an ethical dilemma? If so, how can it be resolved?

What obligation does the physician have to respect the wishes of Mr. Eng?

What obligation does the physician have to respect the wishes of Mr. Eng's daughter?

References

Required Textbook

American Nurses Association and Health Ministries Association. (2012). *Scope and standards of practice: Faith community nursing* (2nd ed.). Silver Spring, MD: Nursesbooks.org.

References

Aiken, T. (2004). *Legal, ethical, and political issues in nursing* (2nd ed.). Philadelphia, PA: F.A. Davis.

American Nurses Association (2001). *Code of ethics for nurses with interpretive statements.* Washington, DC: American Nurses Publishing.

American Nurses Association and Health Ministries Association (2012). *Scope and standards of practice: Faith community nursing* (2nd ed.). Silver Spring, MD: Nursesbooks.org.

Burkhardt, M. & Nathaniel, A. (2008). *Ethics & issues in contemporary nursing* (3rd ed.). Clifton Park, NY: Delmar.

Fry, S.T. (2004). Nursing ethics. In S. G. Post (Ed.). *Encyclopedia of bioethics,* 3rd ed. (pp. 1898–1903). New York: Macmillan Reference USA.

Fry, S. T. & Johnstone, M. J. (2008). *Ethics in nursing practice: A guide to ethical decision making.* Oxford, United Kingdom: Blackwell Publishing.

Fry, S. T. & Veatch, R. M. (2006). *Case studies in nursing ethics,* 3rd Ed. Boston: Jones & Bartlett Publishers.

Hickman, J. S. (2006). *Faith community nursing.* Philadelphia: Lippincott, Williams & Wilkins

International Council of Nurses (2006). *Code of ethics for nurses.* Geneva, Switzerland: ICN.

Johnstone, M. J. (2004). *Bioethics: A nursing perspective, 4th Ed.* Sydney: Elsevier Australia.

Lovin, R. W. (2000). *Christian ethics: An essential guide.* Nashville: Abingdon Press.

Monsen, R. B. (Ed.) (2008). *Genetics and ethics in health care.* Silver Spring, MD: American Nurses Association.

Redman, B. K. & Fry, S. T. (2000). Nurses' ethical conflicts: What is really known about them? *Nursing Ethics, 7*(4), 360–366.

Sanderson, C. (2014). Ethical and bioethical issues in nursing and health care. In Cherry, B, and Jacob, S., Eds. *Contemporary Nursing: Issues, trends, and management* (6th ed,). St Louis, MO: Elsevier.

Shelly, J. (Ed.), (2003). Ethics at work. *Journal of Christian Nursing, 20*(4). (Classic reading: entire issue devoted to ethics in the workplace.)

Smucker, C., & Weinberg, L. (2009). *Faith community nursing: Developing a quality practice.* Silver Springs, MD: Nursesbooks.org

Storch, J. L., Rodney, P., & Starzomski, R. (Eds.) (2004). *Toward a moral horizon: Nursing ethics for leadership and practice.* Toronto: Pearson, Prentice-Hall.

Solari-Twadell, P., & McDermott, M.A. (1999). Parish nursing: *Promoting whole person health within faith communties.* Thousand Oaks, CA: Sage Publishing.

Uustal, D. (2003). The ethic of care: A Christian perspective. *Journal of Christian Nursing, 20*(4), 13–17.

Additional References

Batcheller, J., Davis, J., & Yoder-Wise, P. (2013). Hope for the future: Intensifying spirituality in the workplace. Nursing Administration Quarterly, *37*(4), 309-316.

Bentzen, G., Harsvik, A., & Brinchmann, B. S. (2013). "Values that vanish into thin air": Nurses' experience of ethical values in their daily work. *Nursing Research and Practice, 0,* 1–8. doi: 10.1155/2013/939153.

Doucette, J. (2013). Decision-making through the ethics lens. *Nursing Management, 44*(9), 46-50.

Evangelical Lutheran Church in America. (2003). A social statement on health, healing, and health care ... *Caring for health: Our shared endeavor.* Minneapolis: Augsburg Fortress.

Fadiman, A. (1997). *The spirit catches you and you fall down.* New York: Noonday Press.

Hoglund, B. (2013). Practicing the code of ethics, finding the image of God. *Journal of Christian Nursing, 30*(4), 228–233.

Hussain, A. (2006). Oil & water: *Two faiths—One God.* Kelowna, BC: CopperHouse.

Idliby, R., Oliver, S., & Warner, P. (2006). *The faith club: A Muslim, a Christian, a Jew—Three women search for understanding.* New York: Simon & Schuster, Inc.

Ivanov, L., & Oden, T. (2013). *Public health nursing,* ethics and human rights. Public Health Nursing, *30*(3), 231–238. doi: 10.111/ phn.12022.

Kangasniemi, M., Vaismoradi, M., Jasper, M., & Turunen, H. (2013). Ethical issues in patient safety: Implications for nursing management. *Nursing Ethics, 0,* 1–13. Advance online publication. doi: 10.1177/0969733013484488.

Oh Y., & Gastmans, C. (2013). Moral distress experienced by nurses: A quantitative literature review. Nursing Ethics, *0,* 1–17. Advance online publication. doi: 10.1177/0969733013502

O'Mathúna, D. (2011). The place of dignity in everyday ethics. *Journal of Christian Nursing, 28*(1), 12–20.

Picoult, J. (2004). *My sister's keeper.* New York: Washington Square Press.

Skloot, R. (2010). *The immortal life of Henrietta Lacks.* New York: Random House.

Online Resources

Five Wishes: *www.agingwithdignity.org*
Classic document on advance care planning.
Honoring Choices of Minnesota: *www.honoringchoices.org*
This is an excellent resource on faith, culture, and beliefs.
Muslim beliefs about illness and health practices: *www.islam-usa.com www.religionfacts.com/islam/beliefs/afterlife.htm*
Statement on Jewish Values and Health Care: *www.urj.org/life/community/health/bioethics*
Study guides on various bioethical issues can be ordered through this website.

Wrap-Up and Evaluation

Measuring Competency

This chart can be used to assess the individual outcomes in this module.
- A copy of this chart is attached to the Participant Module, so that each participant can complete this short evaluation.
- Have participants read each outcome and then place an X in the box that best matches their opinion about the objective being met.
- Encourage each participant to write a short reflection about this module in the space provided at the bottom of this chart.
- Use this data to make any necessary changes.

Outcome	Not Met	Somewhat Met	Met
1. Identify ethical issues in faith community nursing practice.			
2. Apply the elements of ethical decision-making.			
3. Examine ethical dilemmas using the Nursing Process Approach.			
4. Apply ethical decision-making to faith community nursing practice.			
Reflection: *In one paragraph, write a reflection on this module.*			

Unit II: Professionalism
Documenting Practice

Documenting Practice

Introduction

Description

Clear, accurate, and accessible documentation is an essential element of safe, quality, evidence-based faith community nursing practice. The faith community nurse (FCN) demonstrates quality by documenting the application of the nursing process in a responsible, accountable, and ethical manner. This module provides a comprehensive review of documentation within the context of faith community nursing practice. It emphasizes legal responsibilities and the importance of maintaining quality documentation and records to comply with practice standards. Faith community nursing is a relatively young nursing practice; thus, documentation is extremely important for the development and research of the practice. Nurses entering this specialty must be educated about the importance of documenting relevant data.

Hours: 2

Research

The level of expertise of the nurse is closely aligned with the quality of content contained in documentation. Thus, the ability of the FCN to document appropriately and comprehensively is an indicator of the quality of the content regarding the nursing process as well as demonstration of the practice (Wang & Hailey, 2011). The content of the documentation contains evidence of patient care and information critical for continuity and patient safety. The content also is critical for tracking patient outcomes. However, Dyess, Chase and Newlin's (2009) review of literature found a lack of outcomes captured in FCN documentation. Only 7 out of the 25 articles reviewed had content related to documentation and evaluation. The authors point to insufficiencies in documentation as barriers to demonstrating the legitimacy and effectiveness of the practice as a specialty. To improve the quality of documentation content, several research studies emphasize the use of standardized nursing language (Solari-

Learning Outcomes

1. Document in accordance with legal guidelines and practice standards.
2. Use accountable strategies to manage and maintain documentation records and client information.
3. Use the nursing process as the theoretical basis for documenting practice.
4. Use standardized nursing terminology in documentation.
5. Use systematic approaches to structure and format relevant data.
6. Communicate documented client information to other caregivers and the interprofessional team.

Twadell & Hackbarth, 2010; Wang & Hailey, 2011; Dyess, Chase & Newlin, 2009). Other recommendations for improving documentation include documentation education (Wang & Hailey, 2011), use of electronic documentation systems (Dyess, Chase & Newlin, 2009; Wang & Hailey, 2011), and application of nursing theory and emphasis on standards of practice or guidelines (Wang & Hailey, 2011).

Faith Tradition

In one faith community the FCN conducts a monthly blood pressure (BP) screening after each Mass with several levels of documentation. First, the nurse records the BP on the client's individual 4 x 6 card kept in a locked filing cabinet. Next, the FCN records the BP on the individual card the client keeps. This information is transferred to the monthly BP record, the quarterly report, and the annual report to the church council, as well as being forwarded to the hospital's FCN coordinator. As a result of this meticulous documentation, the FCN in this faith community has received an increase in her budget for the last three years.

Key Terms

Clinical Care Classification (CCC) System: a standardized, coded nursing terminology that identifies the discrete elements of nursing practice. CCC provides a unique framework and coding structure for capturing the essence of patient care in all health care settings.

North American Nursing Diagnosis Association (NANDA.org): developed a comprehensive list of nursing diagnoses that reflect client problems, concerns, or issues.

The Nursing Outcomes Classification (NOC): a comprehensive, standardized classification of patient or client outcomes developed to evaluate the effects of interventions provided by nurses or other health care professionals.

The Nursing Interventions Classification (NIC): a comprehensive, research-based, standardized classification of interventions that nurses perform. It is useful for clinical documentation, communication of care across settings, integration of data across systems and settings, effectiveness research, productivity measurement, competency evaluation, reimbursement, and curricular design.

The Omaha System: a problem-oriented, research-based, comprehensive practice and documentation standardized classification system designed to document client care.

SBAR Communication: a framework for guiding optimal communication of patient information between health care professionals. Components include: situation, background, assessment, and recommendation.

Reflection

"I too decided, after investigating everything carefully from the very first, to write an orderly account for you, most excellent Theophilus, so that you may know the truth concerning the things about which you have been instructed."
—Luke 1:3–4

Documenting Practice

Content Outline

Q. Why do we document?
A. Documenting demonstrates accountability to the ministry and the funding entities.

OUTCOME 1

Document in accordance with legal guidelines and practice standards.

Documentation is the written account of the care provided by the FCN, whether this care is to individuals, families, or groups. By documenting, the FCN demonstrates accountability to the ministry and the funding entities. For documentation purposes, the client can be an individual member of the faith community, a family, an organized group within the faith community, the faith community as a whole, or the community beyond the congregation.

- Documentation includes both qualitative and quantitative information.
- Documentation provides a framework for working with the client and guides the FCN's subsequent interactions with the client.

Legal compliance. Specific state and national laws impact documentation. The Health Insurance Portability and Accountability Act (HIPPA) exempts agencies that are not reimbursed for health care services, but the confidentiality of records may still be required. The FCN may also refer people to agencies that are covered by HIPPA; therefore, the FCN must be familiar with HIPPA regulations.

States have varying regulations on reporting child and elder abuse. The FCN must follow these laws. Accurate documentation is essential for reporting to outside agencies. See the module on Family Violence for specific observations that may indicate domestic violence and elder abuse.

Faith Community Nursing: Scope and Standards of Practice. Documentation is not only legally required by all state nursing practice acts, but it is also a professional responsibility outlined in *Faith Community Nursing: Scope and Standards of Practice* (2nd ed., 2012) for paid and unpaid FCNs.

Critical Thinking

How does Faith Community Nursing: Scope and Standards of Practice *(2nd ed., 2012) provide a framework for documentation?*

OUTCOME 2
Use accountable strategies to manage and maintain documentation records and client information.

Fundamentals of Documentation

Documentation is an integral part of the practice of faith community nursing and the quality of care provided by FCNs whether the FCN is in a paid or an unpaid position. Therefore, it is not optional and should not be neglected. Outcomes of nursing care and the processes that lead to those outcomes are evaluated based on documentation. Omissions, pointless duplications, and erroneous information lead to the following:

- The credibility of faith community nursing as a professional practice is undermined.
- How other health professionals regard the level of FCNs' contributions to health care is diminished.
- From a legal perspective, no FCN (paid or unpaid) can afford to be ignorant or careless with respect to the standards of practice for documentation (Taylor et al., 2011, p. 324).

The FCN is responsible for the documentation process. While the FCN may not do all the actual documentation, **the FCN is responsible for verifying that the information is recorded**. Volunteers also may be held responsible for documenting certain aspects of their services, such as blood pressure readings, information from home visits, or education programs. However, the FCN must check the information and make appropriate decisions concerning the information.

The documentation system should be developed when the FCN ministry begins. Policies and procedures should be in place from the start. The health ministry team (or overseeing committee), in conjunction with the FCN, is responsible to develop policies and procedures. The FCN provides the necessary information to the team for implementation of a complete documentation system.

Confidentiality. The records of the FCN are confidential. Use a **locked file cabinet** for individual records, which are stored in alphabetical order. An individual record may be for a person or family. The FCN has sole control of the key to the file cabinet.

If a computerized system is also implemented, this system must be **password-protected** and accessible only by the FCN. The computer files must be backed up on a regular basis, with the backup copy stored in a locked, fireproof cabinet.

Policies and procedures must address confidentiality of the records, storage of the records, backing up of computer records, and file transfer or release of records. Legal advice may assist with the policy and procedure development.

Ownership. Records are the property of the FCN and the client. **The client record should never belong to the faith community.**

Q. Who should document?
A. FCNs in both paid and unpaid positions should document care.

Critical Thinking
Florence Nightingale pointed out: "... despite the level of a nurse's devotion, it is useless if the observations are not noted." How is this statement applicable today?

HELPFUL RESOURCE
The ANA publishes a paper regarding the documentation aspect of the role of the nurse called, "ANA Principles of Documentation," which can be accessed at www.nursing world.org/principles.

Q. When should the FCN document?
A. While the FCN may not do all the documentation, the FCN is responsible for verifying that the information is recorded.

HELPFUL RESOURCE
See example of policies for the faith community nursing ministry in Durbin et al., 2013.

Q. Where are records maintained?
A. Protect confidentiality with a locked cabinet and password-protected systems.

HELPFUL RESOURCE

See Appendix for sample form: Authorization to Release Information from Faith Community Health Record to Third Party.

Critical Thinking

You hear an FCN say, "Caring for my client is more important than documenting, and besides I'm not paid, so it's not needed." How would you respond, and what is the rationale for your response?

Nurses are legally accountable for documenting their assessments and nursing responses" (Taylor et al., 2011, p. 291).

When the FCN leaves a specific faith community ministry, there are several possibilities for the individual records:

- The individual records are returned to the individual clients.
- The individual records are passed on to the next FCN.
- The FCN retains the individual records for the prescribed length of time, as indicated by state law (five years for adults; five years after the child has reached 18 years of age).
- If the FCN is paid or unpaid but working under the direction of an FCN coordinator, the records are retained by the health care agency, but not the church or sponsoring organization unless the agency is a health care service or hospital. A copy of the record is always available to the client.
- If the FCN leaves a position that is not part of a health care agency, the original record should remain with the nurse according to the statute of that state law, and a copy should be given to the client. If the client is deceased, the record remains with the nurse.

Disposition of group records, such as documentation of educational programs, should be addressed in the health ministry policy and procedures.

OUTCOME 3

Use the nursing process as the theoretical basis for documenting practice.

OUTCOME 4

Use standardized nursing terminology in documentation.

Client-Centered Care

Faith Community Nursing: Scope and Standards of Practice (2nd ed., 2012) specifies that each step of the nursing process must be documented. Documentation of the nursing process demonstrates that the FCN has clearly carried out his or her responsibility as a professional nurse. The client is at the center of care through the nursing process.

Assessment

This is the foundation of the nursing process; thus, it is critical that the FCN is skilled in performing comprehensive, systematic assessment based on a body systems framework (Taylor et al., 2011). Working in a non-clinical setting, the FCN needs to have expert skills in performing physical assessments, recognizing normal versus abnormal, and making judgments regarding findings.

Assessment data includes:

- physical, psychosocial, emotional, spiritual, environmental
- family support systems
- signs—objective information
- symptoms—subjective information

Diagnosis

The FCN formulates a nursing diagnosis based on the wholistic assessment data.

Nursing diagnoses should be prioritized according to the **level of threat to patient well-being.** *Maslow's Hierarchy of Human Needs* is a wholistic guide that can be used to prioritize patient needs before planning (Taylor et al., 2011). Also guiding prioritization are the patient's preferences and the nurse's knowledge of potential future patient problems. A nursing diagnosis:

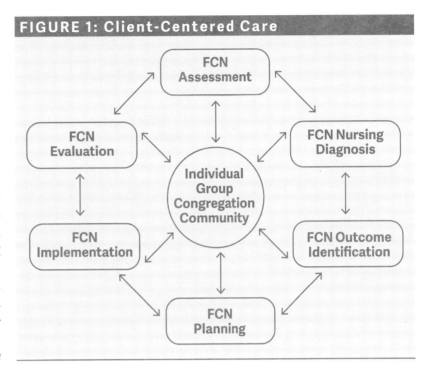

FIGURE 1: Client-Centered Care

- "Identifies actual, perceived or potential threats to health and spiritual well-being" (ANA-HMA, 2012, p.12).
- Must be validated with the client.
- Facilitates the determination of the expected outcomes and plan.
- For FCNs, recognizes spiritual care as central to the practice of faith community nursing. Examples of nursing diagnoses: Spiritual distress, risk for spiritual distress, and readiness for enhanced spiritual well-being.

The **North American Nursing Diagnosis Association** (NANDA. org) has developed a comprehensive list of nursing diagnoses that reflect client problems, concerns, or issues. Nursing diagnosis is a clinical judgment about actual or potential individual, family, or community responses to health problems or life processes. A nursing diagnosis provides the basis for selection of nursing interventions to achieve outcomes for which the nurse has accountability (http://www.nanda.org/nanda-international-glossary-of-terms.html).

"A nursing diagnosis provides the basis for selection of nursing interventions to achieve outcomes for which the nurse has accountability" (http://www.nanda.org/nanda-international-glossary-of-terms.html).

Outcome Identification

The FCN outlines specific outcomes for an individualized plan for the client. The client is involved in this process.

- The expected outcomes take into consideration the client's values, faith beliefs and practices, ethical considerations, and time estimates.
- The expected outcomes are documented as measurable goals—SMART goals.

KEY TERM

The **North American Nursing Diagnosis Association** *(NANDA.org) developed a comprehensive list of nursing diagnoses that reflect client problems, concerns, or issues.*

SMART GOALS	CHARACTERISTICS OF NURSING GOALS
Specific and individualized **M**easurable **A**ttainable **R**easonable **T**imed/dated	Patient-centered Address one response Observable and measurable Behavioral verb Target date or time
Example: The patient will make a visit to the primary care physician within 7 days after being discharged from hospital.	

"FCNs are often the only health care providers responsible for practice in a nontraditional setting" (ANA-HMA, 2012, p.14).

The **Nursing Outcomes Classification** (NOC) is a comprehensive, standardized classification of patient or client outcomes developed to evaluate the effects of interventions provided by nurses or other health care professionals. An outcome is a measurable individual, family, or community, state, behavior, or perception that is measured along a continuum and is responsive to nursing interventions (http://www.nursing.uiowa.edu/cncce/nursing-outcomes-classification-overview).

Take these precautions in developing outcome goals:
- Do not express outcome as a nursing intervention.
- Do not use verbs that are not clearly measurable, such as understand or learn.
- Do not have more than one patient behavior in short-term goals.
- Do not make vague outcome statements in which the goal of interventions is unclear.

These factors may affect patient outcome achievement:
- changes in patient's characteristics or situation
- changes in the FCN's knowledge of the situation
- resources (type, availability, access to, adequacy)
- standards of care, laws governing practice, ethical guidelines
- research findings or evidence-based factors

Planning

The plan of care, developed in conjunction with the client, is documented. Failure to include the client leads to inaccuracies and missing information in the assessment, nursing diagnosis, and outcomes identification.

It is imperative that FCNs use high-level **critical thinking skills** to plan effective health care. The FCN uses critical thinking for decision making in the following ways:
- prioritizing problems to address or delegate to others
- identifying the priority of problems to the client
- identifying the evidence of problem resolution from plan of care or interventions
- setting the time frame for resolution of problems
- identifying evidence that changes are needed in the plan of care, applying nursing science and evidence-based practice to the plan of care

- tailoring interventions to optimize the client's benefit (Taylor et al., 2011)

Nurses moving from the clinical setting into nontraditional faith community settings are required to shift their care planning focus from a medical model to whole-person health focus. Thus FCNs have issues unique to their practice:

- Clients' problems often go beyond the traditional medical focus.
- Work includes group activities.
- Work includes pastoral care and whole-person care.
- Faith communities normally do not have health records.
- Faith community nursing is both ministry and a specialty nursing practice.
- The spiritual dimension of care is not historically documented.
- At present, there has been no litigation against an FCN.
- At present, faith community nursing is not a reimbursable health care service.
- Documentation helps validate FCN boundaries.

Implementation

The FCN is responsible for implementing the plan of care and documenting the process, including any modification to the specified plan.

Implementing a plan includes documenting **Independent Nursing Actions**. Because FCNs work in nontraditional settings outside of health care agencies, almost all of their interventions are considered independent nursing actions.

Key to evidence-based practice are the theories that inform practice. Nursing uses theories from a variety of disciplines. Nursing theories provide a rationale for the practice that is validated through research (Hickman, 2006). FCNs' **documentation should demonstrate practice that is evidence-based.**

The **Nursing Interventions Classification** (NIC) provides specific interventions aligned with specific NOC and NANDA nursing diagnoses. NIC is a comprehensive, research-based, standardized classification of interventions that nurses perform. It is useful for clinical documentation, communication of care across settings, integration of data across systems and settings, effectiveness research, productivity measurement, competency evaluation, reimbursement, and curricular design (https://www.nursing.uiowa.edu/cncce/nursing-interventions-classification-overview).

NANDA, NOC, and NIC Alignment of Diagnoses

NANDA	At risk for infection related to inadequate primary defense: broken skin
NOC	Wound healing Knowledge: infection control
NIC	Infection protection Wound care

Critical Thinking
Are there other activities specific to faith community nursing specialty practice that may not be required in documentation in an acute care setting?

"Nurse-initiated interventions, or independent nursing actions, involve carrying out nurse-prescribed interventions resulting from their assessment of patient needs written on the nursing care plan or any other actions nurses initiate with the direction and supervision of another health care professional" (Taylor et al., 2011, p. 291).

"Evidence-based practice in nursing is a problem-solving approach to making clinical decisions, using the best evidence available—considered 'best' because it is collected from sources such as published research, national standards and guidelines, and reviews of targeted literature. It blends both science and art of nursing so the best possible patient outcomes are achieved" (Taylor et al., 2011, p. 80).

KEY TERM
*The **Nursing Interventions Classification** is a research-based classification of interventions that nurses perform.*

Critical Thinking

Describe the risks of incomplete documentation.

Consider the following table that demonstrates alignment of NANDA, NOC, and NIC classifications.

Evaluation

The FCN documents the results of the evaluation process. Determination of the client's response to care is key for evaluating the plan of care, goal achievement, and quality of care provided to the client.

Types of client data documented by the FCN to evaluate outcomes (Taylor et al., 2011) include:

- cognitive outcomes (client knowledge)
- psychomotor outcomes (client's new skill demonstrated)
- affective outcomes (changes in client's attitudes or beliefs)
- physiological outcomes (indicators from physical assessment)
- spiritual outcomes (indicators from spiritual assessment)

The evaluation centers on the **client's response** to the FCN's care plan for addressing problems or achieving goals:

- resolved, but other problems present
- prevented potential problems or risk factors
- remained ongoing or reduced
- ruled out (found not to be a problem)
- resolved, no new problems present
- goal met, unmet, or ongoing (more time required)

From the evaluation of the client's response, the following **actions** may result:

- continue same plan of care or client goals
- revise plan of care or client goals
- develop new plan of care or client goals
- no further care planning or goal setting needed

Other Documentation

Other types of documentation by the FCN may include:

- **Group-focused care**, such as educational programs, health fairs, support groups, and spiritual retreats. The policies and procedures should indicate what data is collected. Summary statistics should be aggregated related to each event.
- Results of **screening events**. While information about the entire event is collected, specific individual information must also be documented. Flow sheets may be helpful for this type of event.
- **Activities of the FCN**, such as office work, attending meetings or church functions, providing information to various community groups, and coordinating and supporting volunteer activities. Documentation as an activity report of the nurse is helpful in demonstrating to stakeholders (church leaders, funders, supervisors) the full activities and time investment of the FCN. Many hospital-supported faith community nursing programs use this type of report information to calculate community benefits based on the FCN's time.

Critical Thinking

How does the patient benefit when documentation is complete?

Patient Education

The FCN provides patient education throughout the continuum of care with patients. Many times patient education is fluid and gets overlooked in documentation; however, it is a critical element in quality patient care and promotes optimal patient outcomes. The FCN's documentation should include **planned and unplanned teaching**, any literature or materials used, method of teaching, other persons involved, and outcomes or follow-up of teaching (Taylor et al., 2011).

Informed choice guidelines, as set forth in the ANA Code of Ethics for RNs or FCN standards of practice, mean that FCNs must respect the patient's choices even if the patient chooses to participate in **risky behaviors.** Examples of risky behaviors include: acting contrary to medical advice, ignoring dietary restrictions, and refusing medications. FCNs should document objective and subjective descriptions of the patient's behaviors ("non-compliant" is an improper description) and the interventions performed by the FCN with the patient's response (Taylor et al., 2011). Extreme risky behaviors such as abuse, neglect, or threatening to harm oneself require the FCN to act in accordance with legal guidelines and to document.

OUTCOME 5

Use systematic approaches to structure and format relevant data.

When an FCN has an interaction with a new patient, a new **patient record** is opened for that individual.

- The FCN may collect background information for the record such as care provider, phone, e-mail, emergency contact, and address.
- The patient record includes the FCN's documentation of the details of initial and subsequent interactions with the patient.
- The contents of the record must demonstrate the plan of care, including patient problems, nursing diagnoses, goals or expected outcomes, interventions, and problem resolution or patient response to care (Taylor et al., 2011).

Oral or phone information exchanges (Taylor et al., 2011) generally should:

- be documented as verbal or phone information in the patient record by the FCN receiving the information
- note date and time of verbal or phone information
- note the name of person providing the information to the FCN
- verify accuracy of information with the person during the conversation

Q. How should data be documented?
A. A variety of systems and tools meet requirements for documentation as long as they include details of initial and subsequent interactions with the client.

HELPFUL RESOURCE
See Appendix for sample forms: Client Interaction, Brief Encounter, Demographic and Assessment, Physician Office Visit.

HELPFUL RESOURCE

See Appendix for sample forms: Blood Pressure Screening, Blood Pressure Monitoring, Generic Screening, Medication Sheet.

FCNs may use **flow sheets** when there is a series of encounters with patients either as part of an individual patient record or when the encounter is a part of a group screening, such as blood pressure screenings during a health fair. When using both flow sheet and narrative charting for an individual patient, FCNs must avoid double-documenting by placing information in the narrative that already has been documented on the flow sheet.

Methods of Documentation

The content of the patient record may take a variety of forms. Correct documentation will provide a record of the care, reflecting the ministry of the FCN to the faith community, the health care system, and potential or current funding agencies.

"Documentation should be consistent with professional and agency standards; complete, accurate, concise, factual, organized, and timely; legally prudent; and confidential" (Taylor et al., 2011, p.327). The Joint Commission's list of medical acronyms to avoid may be accessed at www.jointcommission.org/assets/1/18/Do_Not_Use_List.pdf.

Narrative Charting

Patient care is described over a chronological period of time. For FCNs this often entails a description of patient status, interventions, and patient responses during the time period that the FCN encounters a patient or patient's family member. FCNs using narrative notes need to be vigilant about including patient responses to their care. This is often an omission because, unlike other methods of charting, there is no cued reminder to follow up.

HELPFUL RESOURCE

See Appendix for sample form: Narrative Notes.

SOAP/IER Notes

This is a structured method of charting from a problem orientation using the following format:

S—Subjective. Information the patient or faith community tells the FCN.

O—Objective. Factual or observable information collected by the FCN during assessment of the patient or faith community.

A—Assessment. Conclusions of the FCN based on the collected subjective and objective data; formulated as patient problems or nursing diagnoses.

P—Plan. The FCN's strategy for relieving the patient's or faith community's problem, including immediate or short-term and long-term actions.

I—Intervention. Actions taken by the FCN to achieve an expected outcome.

E—Evaluation. Analysis of the effectiveness of interventions. If outcomes fall short of expectations, alternative interventions should be developed.

R—Revision. Any changes from the original plan of care.

Focus Charting

The FCN focuses on a concern of the patient or faith community that is identified during the assessment, utilizing the following organization:

- **Data**—subjective and objective information that supports the focus or concern of the patient or faith community
- **Action**—The FCN's interventions
- **Response**—The patient or faith community response to interventions

PIE Charting

The FCN's documentation focuses on evaluation of one or more problems identified during each encounter with the patient. "A" is often added to the acronym as "Assessment" before the problem is identified. This charting method streamlines documentation; however, FCNs should be aware that the planning step of the nursing process is omitted (Taylor et al., 2011).

- P—Problem
- I—Interventions
- E—Evaluation: response of patient

Classification Systems

While many FCNs may not be comfortable with **NANDA, NIC,** and **NOC**, these research-based, standardized nursing language systems allow this ministry to compare practices across the various models of faith community nursing in the multiplicity of locations.

Future research can validate the importance and contribution of faith community nursing practices if data are collected consistently using these standardized nursing languages. This will professionalize the documentation. NANDA diagnosis, NOC, and NIC serve as the foundation for nursing practice, education, and research wherever nurses practice. NIC and NOC provide terms for documenting nursing care and communicating nursing care across settings (https://www.nursing.uiowa.edu/cncce/facts).

The Omaha System is a problem-oriented system. The problem can move from general to specific. It is a research-based, comprehensive practice and documentation standardized classification designed to document client care from admission to discharge (http://www.omahasystem.org). There are three major sections:

- The **problem classification** includes the assessment data.
- The **intervention scheme** outlines the delivery system.
- The **problem rating scale** for outcomes encompasses the evaluation process and client changes.

The **Clinical Care Classification (CCC) System** is a standardized, coded nursing terminology that identifies the discrete elements of nursing practice. CCC provides a unique framework and coding structure for capturing the essence of patient care in all health care settings. Version 2.5 consists of two interrelated

HELPFUL RESOURCE

For a list of classification systems for nursing, see the "ANA Recognized Terminologies that Support Nursing Practice" available at http://nursingworld.org/npii/terminologies.htm.

"By using a common terminology that all people understand, this documentation system clearly communicates what parish nurses do" (Burkhart, 2002, p. 6).

KEY TERM

The **Omaha System** *is a research-based, problem-oriented classification system for documenting patient care.*

KEY TERM

The **Clinical Care Classification System** *uses coded nursing terminology to capture the essence of patient care.*

Critical Thinking

How can continuing education related to documentation for FCNs improve the quality of practice?

terminologies: the CCC of Nursing Diagnoses and Outcomes and the CCC of Nursing Interventions and Actions, classified by 21 Care Components to form a single system. The Care Components provide the standardized framework that links the CCC terminologies to each other and enables them to be mapped to other health-related classification systems (http://www.sabacare.com).

Computerized Documentation Systems

Advantages of computer-based documentation systems include:
- Documentation is quicker and more efficient.
- Data input on the various forms replaces handwritten entries.
- Evaluation of the data is enhanced as the system is able to aggregate data efficiently.
- Individual nursing diagnoses, outcomes, and interventions can be tracked as well as data from group activities.
- Quality of documentation is improved.

Perhaps the key advantage of computerized systems is that as more FCNs use electronic documentation systems, the practice will have increased opportunities in:
- research
- education
- quality improvement

HELPFUL RESOURCE

Lisa Burkhart (2002) has developed a complete non-electronic paper system, Integration—Parish Nurse Documentation System, which is free on her web page: http://www.luc.edu/nursing/about/faculty/name,34805,en.shtml.

Selecting a Documentation System

Questions to consider when selecting a system include:
1. Does it capture the spiritual dimension of care?
2. Does it meet legal requirements?
3. How easy is it to use?
4. Is it compatible with the practice of faith community nursing?
5. Does it capture useful summary data for the FCN and stakeholders?
6. Does the health care system already have a documentation system in place that will work for this ministry?
7. If the FCN is affiliated with a health care system, what are the obligations to the institution?

Critical Thinking

Select the most effective documentation formats for the FCN and give your rationale.

Can electronic documentation improve care or advance the overall practice of faith community nursing?

The FCN may wish to develop a documentation system unique to a faith community or practice. This should only be considered if none of the available systems meet the needs of the faith community. Questions to consider before starting are:
1. What data needs to be collected?
2. How much time will it take to put a new system in place?
3. Does the FCN have the expertise to develop such a system?
4. How will this system interface with other FCNs' practices?
5. What system will be used to aggregate the data?
6. Will this system be usable by other FCNs in this congregation?
7. Will a checklist work? What should be included?
8. How will the narrative be recorded?

Communicating Documentation Data

FCNs report two types of data: individual patient data and aggregate data.

Individual Patient Data

Individual patient data is communicated to persons other than the patient, such as family, primary caregiver, clergy, and other health professionals or agencies. Avenues FCNs may use to report patient data include:

- in person
- computer
- telephone
- shared patient records

ELECTRONIC SYSTEMS

Here are some examples of electronic systems designed specifically for faith community nursing documentation.

- *Henry Ford Macomb Hospital Faith Community Nurse Documentation System is an electronic, web-based documentation system for FCNs. This system uses NANDA, NOC and NIC classification. Find more information at www.fcndocumentation.com.*
- *Mercy Parish Nurse and Health Ministry Program Computerized Documentation System was developed by the Pittsburgh Mercy Health System. This system uses the CCC classification system. Find more information at www.pmhs.org.*

SBAR Communication is a framework for guiding optimal communication of patient information between health care professionals. Components include:

- situation
- background
- assessment
- recommendation

KEY TERM

SBAR Communication *is a framework for guiding optimal communication of patient information between health care professionals.*

Maintaining **appropriate and accurate documentation records provides a clear case history** of patient care. It also facilitates both continuity of care and communication between the FCN and other health care professionals. This is particularly important for the ongoing care of patients with chronic diseases.

Release of any patient information or records must be according to **legal and regulatory policies** that guide the release of patient information. FCNs should refer to the standards of practice and other state and federal practice guidelines.

When **reporting patient information to family**, friends, or others, keep in mind these guidelines.

HELPFUL RESOURCE

Description and guidelines for using SBAR can be found on the Institute for Health Care Improvement website: http://www.ihi.org/resources/Pages/Tools/SBARToolkit.aspx.

- Obtain patient approval of individuals or family members entitled to receive information.
- Obtain specifics of what information can or cannot be reported.
- Do not disclose any information without the patient's permission, preferably written consent.
- In case of an emergency situation where the patient is unable to speak or is unconscious, the FCN should use his or her best professional judgment.
- Always use honest, compassionate, and respectful communication.
- Document who, what, when, and how in regard to the report provided (Taylor et al., 2011, p. 350).

Aggregate Data

Aggregate data is communicated to stakeholders, including hospital leaders, faith community leaders, department reports, community benefit reports, grant or funding proposals, and oral or poster presentations. Receiving reports of care provided by the FCN assists stakeholders in understanding the practice of faith community nursing.

Aggregate data reports serve several valuable functions.

1. **Guide program development.** By providing aggregate data records of educational programs, the FCN can validate outcomes previously developed by the health ministries committee or congregation. These summary statistics guide program development and future decision-making. The faith community must also ensure that the work of the FCN is compatible with the mission of the church.

2. **Validate cost savings.** Resources are usually an important issue in faith community nursing practice. With proper documentation, the FCN can:
   - verify cost savings to the health care system.
   - show the integration of health and spirituality into the mission of the congregation, thus validating the cost.
   - demonstrate the time allocation of the work involved in the ministry.

3. **Gain future funding.** Statistical information is important for inclusion in funding requests; institutions that grant money are interested in the impact of the ministry.

4. **Evaluate quality of care.** Evaluation of quality in faith community nursing is based on documentation data.
   - Analyzing this data can help FCNs **improve the processes** of carrying out interventions, evaluating the plan of care, and determining the achievement of patient outcomes.
   - Evaluating **quality of care** is critical to the overall practice of faith community nursing because it **assures accountability** to the public, stakeholders, and clients.
   - In addition, it **ensures the ongoing existence** of faith community nursing practice, promotes adherence to moral ethical codes among FCNs, and helps FCNs uphold practice standards and regulation (Taylor et al., 2011).

Aggregated data reports can be disseminated in written, oral, video, electronic, and poster presentations, as well as brochures, articles, and other literature.

The goals of aggregate data reports may be to:
- Share best practices in faith community nursing.
- Demonstrate quality of care and outcomes of nursing care.
- Assess cost benefits and publicity or marketing impact.
- Identify individual or community or congregational needs.
- Advocate for a health issue or needed service.
- Demonstrate achievement of standards of practice.
- Evaluate ministry programs and facilitate planning.

OUTCOME 6
Communicate documented client information to other caregivers and the interprofessional team.

HELPFUL RESOURCE
See Appendix for sample form: Support Group Report form.

The FCN may not be able to address all the problems or concerns of the patient and therefore must confer with other health care professionals.
- Conferring entails seeking help by way of two avenues: consultation and referral (Taylor et al., 2011).
- Documentation supports conferring because it provides a complete picture to the interprofessional team and supports continuity of care.

Referral is the action of connecting the patient to another source of services or health professionals. Key to an effective referral is obtaining approval for the referral from the patient. The FCN must assure complete contact information and guidelines for the referral are provided to the patient or family (Taylor et al., 2011).

Individual consultation is the action of seeking advice or recommendations from another person or the patient. Thus, it is critical that the FCN first determine who has expertise or appropriate information for the situation or patient needs when consulting.

In a **team consultation**, the FCN works in alignment with a team-model ministry that supports social and spiritual needs of individuals and families.
- These ministries have several names (visitation ministry, care teams, congregational care, etc.).
- They tend to provide nonmedical support of individuals in the home setting, such as transportation, social contact, meals, and house repair.
- The FCN's role with these ministries can extend from being an integral member of the team to being a resource advisor for the team. The FCN often confers with the team regarding nonmedical needs of clients.

The combination of a team and FCN ministry can offer advantages for clients:
- It helps in aligning the ministries' resources and services with the nonmedical needs of the patient.
- It assures both medical and nonmedical needs are congruent.
- It supports coordinated, efficient care for the patient.

When working with team ministries, the FCN should consider these factors:
- The FCN is still accountable for maintaining the regulations of protected health information and confidentiality.
- Client consent should be obtained before the FCN shares documented information with the team or the team provides ministries.

Critical Thinking
What strategies can an FCN use when working with care ministry to uphold protected health information of the patient being served by the ministry?

- Documentation should include the FCN's contact or communication with the team in relation to addressing patient problems and concerns, as well as the patient's response to the team's care services.

Standards of Professional Performance for Faith Community Nursing

Standard 1. Assessment
The faith community nurse collects comprehensive data pertinent to the healthcare consumer's wholistic health or the situation.

DOCUMENTATION COMPETENCY
- Documents relevant data in a retrievable format that is both confidential and secure.

Standard 2. Diagnosis
The faith community nurse analyzes the assessment data to determine the diagnoses or issues.

DOCUMENTATION COMPETENCY
- Documents diagnoses in a manner that facilitates the determination of the expected outcomes and plan.

Standard 3. Outcomes Identification
The faith community nurse identifies expected outcomes for a plan individualized to the healthcare consumer or the situation.

DOCUMENTATION COMPETENCY
- Documents expected outcomes as measurable goals.

Standard 4. Planning
The faith community nurse develops a plan that prescribes strategies and alternatives to attain expected outcomes.

DOCUMENTATION COMPETENCY
- Documents the plan in a manner that uses standardized language or recognized terminology and is understood by all participants.

Standard 5. Implementation
The faith community nurse implements the identified plan.

DOCUMENTATION COMPETENCY
- Documents implementation and any modifications, including changes or omissions, of the specified plan.

Standard 5A. Coordination of Care
The faith community nurse coordinates care delivery.

DOCUMENTATION COMPETENCY
- Documents the coordination of care.

Standard 6. Evaluation
The faith community nurse evaluates progress toward attainment of outcomes.

DOCUMENTATION COMPETENCY
- Documents the results of the evaluation, including results from the faith or spiritual realm.

Standard 13. Collaboration
The faith community nurse collaborates with the healthcare consumer, family, and others in the conduct of nursing practice.

DOCUMENTATION COMPETENCY
- Documents referrals, including hospice and other provisions for continuity of care outside the faith community.

Learning Activities

Case Study: Absent Documentation

Instructions:
This case study focuses on the application of the legal and practice standards for documentation. After reading the case study, ask the participants to form small groups and discuss the provided critical thinking questions.

Case Study:
For five years an unpaid FCN worked about 10 hours per week in a 500-member faith community where about 40 percent of parishioners were over age 60. Most of her time was focused on hypertension control among parishioners. She provided BP screening and individual counseling sessions every Sunday evening. The FCN made home visits to follow up on parishioners with hypertension on weekdays. During that five-year period of time, none of the congregation members reported hospitalization for a stroke. However, the FCN did not document any other information related to her follow-up contact with parishioners except for the flow chart of blood pressures she maintained from her Sunday screening sessions.

Questions:
1. Although the FCN was in an unpaid position, was she required to document?
   - Yes: If so, what legal and practice standards were not met?
   - No: If not, why not? What legal or practice standards allow her not to document?

2. Can "no strokes" during the past five years be credited to the FCN's regular screening and focus on hypertension?
   - Yes: If so, explain rationale and evidence supporting it.
   - No: If not, why not?

3. What opportunities for evaluating the quality of care could have been performed if the FCN's documentation was complete?

Simulated Blood Pressure Records

Instructions:
This activity focuses on the application of documentation principles using group work.

Supplies:
10–15 4 x 6-inch index cards; monthly BP summary sheet, a quarterly report form for the local hospital (or other place where reports are sent), and a simulated annual BP report form for each participant or group.

Prepare the index cards by writing fictitious names and two recorded BPs with dates. On one or two of the cards write a short note, such as, "Client encouraged to have BP checked again the next day"; or "Client states Dr. changed BP meds but he can't afford them. Referred to City Free Clinic for free prescription filling."

Have each participant or group record the information from all the individual cards onto report forms. Bring the participants back together for a discussion about documenting BPs and any potential problems they envision in implementing this in their faith communities.

Question:
What would you recommend to improve this strategy for monitoring and documenting BPs?

Simulated Nursing Plans

Instructions:

Provide participants with NANDA, NOC, and NIC resources or lists of diagnoses. Ask participants to complete one or more of the nursing plans below in small groups. Bring groups back together to discuss their results.

Question:

For each case: What other NANDA, NOC and NIC diagnoses apply in the situation?

NURSING PLAN 1

The FCN visits a 19-year-old mom with a four-day-old baby. The mother says, "The baby isn't taking my breast. She's been fussy, and I feel like I haven't slept in days!"

NANDA_____

_____

NOC _____

_____

NIC_____

_____

Client Outcome Goal_____

_____

What other NANDA, NOC and NIC diagnoses apply in this situation?

NURSING PLAN 2

Mary, a 68-year-old client, lives alone and has a history of arthritis. She is on medication for high blood pressure. She states, "Caring for my garden is fine except on days when my arthritis flares up. So I saw a medication advertised on TV that I think will help control it on bad days. It sounds like just what I need."

NANDA_____

_____

NOC _____

_____

NIC_____

_____

Client Outcome Goal_____

_____

What other NANDA, NOC and NIC diagnoses apply in this situation?

NURSING PLAN 3

Mark is 65 years old and was recently told by his doctor that he has Type 2 diabetes. The doctor prescribed oral medication. Mark says to the FCN, "I have had other relatives with diabetes and they lost their eyesight and some are on dialysis. I've always been active. Now I can't do anything."

NANDA_____

_____

NOC _____

_____

NIC_____

_____

Client Outcome Goal_____

_____

What other NANDA, NOC and NIC diagnoses apply in this situation?

_____

Case Study: Unexpected Incident

Instructions:
This case study focuses on the application of quality and care improvements to documentation. After reading the case study, assign the participants to small groups. Encourage the participants to discuss the provided critical thinking questions.

The FCN was visiting an 800-member faith community. On this Sunday an elderly woman fell on the choir steps during service. Members rushed to her side and called upon the nurse to assist in the situation. The woman had injured her leg and had difficulty standing. After being seated in a chair she claimed to be fine: "I want to continue enjoying the service." After assessing the situation, the nurse advised calling an ambulance to transport her to the ER. However the woman refused. "I'm fine. I want to stay here for the service. I'm not going." After more cajoling and explaining the need for her to go to the ER by the FCN and other parishioners, the woman adamantly refused to go to the ER and continued participating in the service. Although the FCN was not a member of this congregation, she still fully documented the incident.

Weeks later, the church leaders were served with a notice of being sued for medical and hospital costs for the leg injury from the woman's fall. They were shocked and bewildered that a long-time member of the congregation was suing the church. The FCN's documentation was submitted as evidence in court and as a result the judge threw out the case.

Questions
1. The nurse was not working as an FCN for this faith community, so did legal and practice standards related to documentation apply in this situation?
    - Yes: If so, why?
    - No: If not, why not?

2. What data would have been critical for the FCN to document in this situation?

3. What method of documentation (SOAP/IER, narrative, etc.) would most likely provide the type of information that would help reconstruct the events surrounding the fall?

Expanded Activities Using Case Studies

Instructions:
This activity focuses on documentation principles, formats, and methods.

Gather case studies about FCNs providing care to clients, such as "Absent Documentation" or "Unexpected Incident" in this module or others. In small group, have participants practice documenting from the FCN's perspective. Have each group report back their documentation piece to the larger group.

Questions:
1. What documentation format worked best for each case study?

2. Does your group's documentation demonstrate the nursing process?
    - If yes, how?
    - If not, what information is needed?

References

Required Textbook

American Nurses Association and Health Ministries Association. (2012). *Scope and standards of practice: Faith community nursing* (2nd ed.). Silver Spring, MD: Nursesbooks.org.

References

American Nurses Association and Health Ministries Association (2012). *Faith community nursing: Scope and standards of practice.* Silver Spring, MD: NursesBooks.org

Dyess, S., Chase, S. K., & Newlin, K. (2010). State of research for faith community nursing 2009. *Journal of religion and health, 49*(2), 188–199.

Hickman, J. S. (2006). *Faith community nursing.* Philadelphia: Lippincott, Williams & Wilkins.

Solari-Twadell, P.A., & Hackbarth, D. P. (2010). Evidence for a new paradigm of the ministry of parish nursing practice using the nursing intervention classification system. *Nursing Outlook, 58*(2), 69–75.

Taylor, C.R., Lillis, C., LeMone, P., & Lynn, P. (2011) *Fundamentals of nursing: The art and science of nursing care.* Philadelphia: Lippincott, Williams & Wilkins. 7th Ed.

Wang, N., Hailey, D., & Yu, P. (2011). Quality of nursing documentation and approaches to its evaluation: a mixed method systematic review. *Journal of Advanced Nursing, 67*(9), 1858–1875.

Additional References

Burkhart, L. (2002). Integration: *A documentation system reporting whole person care.* Evanston, IL: Author.

Durbin, N. L., Cassimere, M., Howard, C., Lutz, M. & Wehling, B. (2013) *Faith community nurse coordinator manual: A guide to creating and developing your program.* Memphis, TN: Church Health Center.

Newcomb, P., Canclini, Cauble, D., Raudonis, B., & Golden, P. (2014). *Journal of Primary Care and Community Health* online first version of record accessed March 18, 2014. http://jpc.sagepub.com/content/early/2014/02/25/2150131914524441

Smucker, C. J., & Weinberg, L. J. (2009). *Faith community nursing: developing a quality practice.* American Nurses Association.

Online Resources

ANA Principles of Documentation. Accessed from www.nursingworld.org/principles

ANA Recognized Terminologies that Support Nursing Practice. Accessed from: http://nursingworld.org/npii/terminologies.html

Best Practices Modules: http://www.healthministries.info/modules/html

Clinical Care Classification (CCC) System: http://www.sabacare.com

Documentation systems:
- Henry Ford Macomb Hospital Faith Community Nurse Documentation System: www.fcndocumentation.com
- Integration—A Parish Nurse Documentation System: http://www.luc.edu/nursing/about/faculty/name,34805,en.shtml
- Mercy Parish Nurse and Health Ministry Program Computerized Documentation System: www.pmhs.org

Health Ministry Network of Minnesota

NANDA information:
- Website: www.nanda.org
- Glossary of terms: http://www.nanda.org/nanda-international-glossary-of-terms.html

National Clearinghouse on Abuse in Later Life. This website offers a PDF with the information on mandatory reporting of elder abuse: http://www.ncall.us.

National Outcomes Classification (NOC): http://www.nursing.uiowa.edu/cncce/nursing-outcomes-classification-overview

Nursing Interventions Classification (NIC): http://www.nursing.uiowa.edu/cncce/nursing-interventions-classification-overview

Omaha System: http://www.omahasystem.org/

SBAR Communication Technique: http://www.ihi.org/resources/Pages/Tools/SBARToolkit.aspx

The Joint Commission (TJC) Do Not Use Abbreviations List: www.jointcommission.org/assets/1/18/Do_Not_Use_List.pdf

Understanding Health Information Privacy: http://www.hhs.gov/ocr/privacy/hipaa/understanding

Wrap-Up and Evaluation

Measuring Competency

This chart can be used to assess the individual outcomes in this module.
- A copy of this chart is attached to the Participant Module, so that each participant can complete this short evaluation.
- Have participants read each outcome and then place an X in the box that best matches their opinion about the objective being met.
- Encourage each participant to write a short reflection about this module in the space provided at the bottom of this chart.
- Use this data to make any necessary changes.

Outcome	Not Met	Somewhat Met	Met
1. Document in accordance with legal guidelines and practice standards.			
2. Use accountable strategies to manage and maintain documentation records and client information.			
3. Use the nursing process as the theoretical basis for documenting practice.			
4. Use standardized nursing terminology in documentation.			
5. Use systematic approaches to structure and format relevant data.			
6. Communicate documented client information to other caregivers and the interprofessional team.			
Reflection: *In one paragraph, write a reflection on this module.*			

Appendix

Sample Forms

The following pages include these sample forms, which may be duplicated as needed:

- Authorization to Release Information from Faith Community Health Record to Third Party
- Client Interaction
- Brief Encounter
- Demographic and Assessment
- Physician Office Visit
- Generic Screening
- Blood Pressure Screening
- Blood Pressure Monitoring
- Medications Sheet
- Narrative Notes
- Faith Community Nurse Monthly Report
- Faith Community Nurse Education Program Documentation
- Faith Community Nurse Support Group Report

AUTHORIZATION TO RELEASE INFORMATION FROM
FAITH COMMUNITY HEALTH RECORD TO THIRD PARTY

Print Client's Name: _____

Daytime Phone Number: _____

I, _____ do hereby authorize

          Name of Client or Legal Guardian

_____ to release to _____

      Name of Faith Community Nurse   *Name of Third Party*

the following information:

concerning the care I received from the faith community nurse from
_____ **to** _____.

      beginning date   *ending date*

I understand that I may revoke this consent at any time in writing.

_____   _____
      Client Signature   *Date*

_____   _____
      Witness Signature   *Date*

CLIENT INTERACTION

Client Name: _____

Date of Interaction: _____ Time of Interaction: _____

Client Date of Birth: _____ Client Age or Age Range: _____

Client Gender: M F   Client Marital Status: _____

Client Address: _____

_____

Client Phone: _____

Emergency Contact

Name: _____ Phone: _____

Primary Care Physician: _____ Phone: _____

FCN Discharge Date: _____

Referred by: _____

Location of Contact (Circle):

Faith Community   Home Visit   Hospital
Office   Nursing Home Phone:

NURSING ASSESSMENT:

NURSING DIAGNOSIS (NANDA):

NURSING INTERVENTIONS (NIC):

NURSING OUTCOME (NOC, HOW INTERVENTIONS AFFECTED CLIENT):

NARRATIVE NOTES:

Faith Community: _____

Faith Community Nurse: _____

BRIEF ENCOUNTER

Client Name: _____ **Date of Encounter:** _____

Address: _____ **Phone:** _____

Age: __ 0–20 __ 21–59 __ 60–80 __ 80+   **Gender:**   M   F

Location of Contact (Circle):

Faith Community   Agency/Office   Phone

Hospital   Home   Nursing Home

Faith Community Status: **Name of Faith Community:**

__ Member __Other _____   _____

Referred by: _____

REASON/ACTION/OUTCOME: (NANDA, NIC, NOC)

_____

Faith Community Nurse Signature

DEMOGRAPHIC AND ASSESSMENT

Directions to home: _____ **Date:** _____

CLIENT INFORMATION

Client Name:
Last:_____First:_____Middle:_____Maiden:_____

Address: **Telephone:**
Street:_____ (H): _____

_____ (W): _____

City, State, Zip Code: _____ (Other): _____

_____

Birthdate: _____ **Race:** _____ **Gender:** _____

Language Spoken: _____

Highest level of education: _____ **Literacy:** _____

Marital Status: _____

Spouse/Significant Other Name: _____

Employment Status: _____ **Occupation:** _____

Income Source: _____

Special Job Skills: _____ **Veteran:** ____ Yes ____ No

_____

CONTACT(S) IN CASE OF EMERGENCY:

Name:_____ Phone: _____

Address:_____ Relationship: _____

Name:_____ Phone: _____

Address:_____ Relationship: _____

Living Arrangements: ☐ Home ☐ Apartment ☐ Facility ☐ Homeless

PHYSICIAN INFORMATION:

Physician Name:_____ Phone: _____

Address: _____

Physician Name:_____ Phone: _____

Address: _____

DURABLE POWER OF ATTORNEY:

Financial ☐ Yes ☐ No   Name: _____ Phone: _____

Health care ☐ Yes ☐ No   Name: _____ Phone: _____

INSURANCE:

Primary Insurance: _____ Group #: _____

Secondary Insurance: _____ Group #: _____

Household Member Name	Relationship	Age/ Date of Birth

_____   _____

Faith Community Nurse Signature   **Date**

MEDICAL HISTORY

Name: _____

Allergies:

Medications: _____

Foods: _____

Environment: _____

Alzheimer's Disease		**Nutrition:** Diet, Weight	
Arthritis		**Osteoporosis**	
Cancer		**Pain**	
Cardiovascular		**Renal Disease**	
Dementia/Confusion		**Respiratory**	
Depression		**Safety:** Home	
Diabetes		Relationships	
Eating Disorders		Other	
Epilepsy		**Skin**	
Gastrointestinal		**Sleep Difficulties**	
Hypertension		**Stroke/TIA**	
Mental Health		**Substance Abuse**	
Mobility Impaired		**Thyroid**	
Muscular: MS, MD		**Tobacco Use**	
Neurological		**Ulcers**	

Comments:

Surgery	Year

Hospitalizations / Reason	Date	Place

SPIRITUAL NEEDS

Name: _____

Parishioner: ☐ Yes ☐ No   Other Faith Community: _____

Faith Community activities (transportation, sacraments, other):

_____

_____

Bereavement Care: Spiritual Concerns:

_____   _____

_____   _____

Meaningful Religious Rituals: Spiritual Support:

_____   _____

_____   _____

PHYSICAL NEEDS

Blood Pressure: _____ Pulse: _____ Respiration:_____

Assistive Devices (prosthesis, disability equipment, magnifiers for participating at faith

community): _____

_____

_____

Transportation: ☐ Has own ☐ Family handles ☐ Needs coordination

Meals—needs assistance: ☐ Groceries ☐ Preparation ☐ Outside referral

Disabilities/problems:

_____

_____

Activities of Daily Living (ADL)—needs assistance with:

_____

_____

_____

_____

EMOTIONAL NEEDS

Fears/Concerns (safety, financial, health care):

_____

_____

_____

_____

Caregiver Relief/Support:

_____

_____

Support Group:_____ Phone Contact:_____

Emergency Plans:

_____

_____

SUMMARY OF ASSESSMENT

Physical:

Blood Pressure: _____ Pulse: _____ Respiration:_____

Environmental: _____

_____

Emotional: _____

_____

Spiritual: _____

_____

Nursing Diagnosis:

_____

_____

Nursing Interventions:

_____

_____

Nursing Outcome:

_____

_____

Nursing Diagnosis:

_____

_____

Nursing Interventions:

_____

_____

Nursing Outcome:

_____

_____

REFERRALS

Agencies Contacted:

Faith Community:_____ Date:_____

Comments: _____

_____

Community Agency:_____ Date:_____

Comments: _____

_____

Community Agency:_____ Date:_____

Comments: _____

_____

_____   _____

Faith Community Nurse Signature   **Date**

PHYSICIAN OFFICE VISIT

Faith Community Nurse Ministry at: _____

Physician Office Visit for: _____ Date: _____

My questions and concerns are:	1. 2. 3. 4. 5.

My current medications and their dosages are:	1. 2. 3. 4. 5.

Physician, your impressions are:	1. 2. 3. 4. 5.

Physician, your plan is:	1. 2. 3. 4. 5.

My Faith Community Nurse is: _____

He/She can be reached by phone at: _____

THANK YOU SO MUCH, DOCTOR, FOR BEING AN ACTIVE PARTNER IN MY HEALTH CARE.

GENERIC SCREENING FORM

Date: _____ Site: _____

Type of Screening: _____

I request participation in the _____ screening. I hereby release [insert name of organization] _____ from any liability which might arise as a result of this voluntary participation. I understand the data derived from this screening is preliminary, subject to error and is not conclusive. Some results may indicate a need for follow-up examination by a physician. I understand it is my responsibility to seek further medical care. Information acquired as a result of participation in this screening may be used by the organization for demographic and health-related purposes.

Name	Age	Results	Under MD Care?	Comment	FCN Initials
			Y N		
			Y N		
			Y N		
			Y N		
			Y N		
			Y N		
			Y N		
			Y N		
			Y N		
			Y N		

Participating Nurse Signature: _____ Initials: _____

Participating Nurse Signature: _____ Initials: _____

Faith Community: _____

Faith Community Nurse Signature: _____ Initials: _____

BLOOD PRESSURE SCREENING

Date of Screening: _____ Location: _____

Client Name: _____

Contact Information: _____

YOUR BLOOD PRESSURE TODAY IS _____/_____ .

BP type	Follow-Up Recommendations	Lifestyle Recommendations

☐ Normal
 	
☐ Pre-Hypertension
 	
☐ Stage 1 Hypertension
 	
☐ Stage 2 Hypertension
	☐ Recheck BP each year.
	☐ If on meds, recheck per medical professional or doctor directions.
	☐ If no meds, recheck BP in 1 month or earlier.
	☐ Recheck BP within one day.
	☐ See your medical professional or doctor within 1 week.
	☐ See your medical professional or doctor within _____ days.
	☐ Contact doctor or ER *without delay* for evaluation.
	☐ Other _____
		☐ **Regular exercise**
		  √ 3 times weekly for 30 minutes
		☐ **Well-balanced diet**
		  √ 5 servings of fruits and vegetables daily & low-fat dairy products
		☐ **Limit sodium**
		  √ About 2 grams salt per day *(1 teaspoon = 2.4 grams)*
		☐ **Healthy body weight**
		  √ Maintain Body Mass Index of 18.5 – 24.9 BMI = *(weight in lbs. x 703) ÷ (height in inches) ÷ (height in inches)*
		☐ **Limit alcohol**
		  √ 1 drink is one 12 oz. of beer or 4 oz. of wine
		☐ **Eliminate smoking**
		  √ Contact your medical professional or doctor for additional support
		☐ Other _____

Comments:		
FCN name:		

Participation in this screening is voluntary and may include a referral to physician and follow-up with nurse. All information obtained on this form will be kept confidential. Participation in this program cannot substitute for consultation with a physician or other medical professional for any medical or health-related condition.

BLOOD PRESSURE MONITORING

Name:		Standing		Sitting		Comments
Date:	Location:	Blood Pressure	Pulse	Blood Pressure	Pulse	
		/		/		
		/		/		
		/		/		
		/		/		
		/		/		

Name:		Standing		Sitting		Comments
Date:	Location:	Blood Pressure	Pulse	Blood Pressure	Pulse	
		/		/		
		/		/		
		/		/		
		/		/		
		/		/		

Name:		Standing		Sitting		Comments
Date:	Location:	Blood Pressure	Pulse	Blood Pressure	Pulse	
		/		/		
		/		/		
		/		/		
		/		/		
		/		/		

Name:		Standing		Sitting		Comments
Date:	Location	Blood Pressure	Pulse	Blood Pressure	Pulse	
		/		/		
		/		/		
		/		/		
		/		/		
		/		/		

MEDICATIONS SHEET

Client Name: _____

Pharmacy: _____ Phone: _____

Physician Name: _____ Physician Phone: _____

Known Allergies: _____

Name (Generic/Brand/OTC)	Dose	Frequency	Prescribed By	Purpose of Medication	Date and Initials

_____   _____   _____
Faith Community Nurse Signature   **FCN Initials**   **Date**

NARRATIVE NOTES

Client Name: _____   Date of Notes: _____

Faith Community Nurse: _____   Faith Community: _____

Location of Contact (Circle):   Faith Community   Agency/Office   Hospital
                                  Home   Nursing Home   Phone

Notes:

FAITH COMMUNITY NURSE MONTHLY REPORT

Faith Community or Agency: _____

Name of Faith Community Nurse: _____ **Month:** _____

INDIVIDUAL INTERACTIONS

Type of Content	Faith Community Nurse	Health Ministry Team Member
Telephone		
Faith Community		
Home		
Hospital		
Nursing Home		
Funeral/Wake		
Transportation		
Agency		
Physician's Office		
Other (specify)		

Age Groups			
0-20	21-59	60-80	80+

Type of Screening	Number Screened

PRESENTATIONS

Subject	Attendance	Support Groups	Monthly Attendance

REFERRALS TO:

Spiritual Leader: _____

Health Care Provider: _____

Community Agency (List agency and number of people referred):_____

_____

REFERRALS FROM:

Spiritual Leader: _____

Health Care Provider: _____

Faith Community Members: _____

Community Agency:_____

_____

MEETINGS (OPTIONAL):

List type and frequency of meetings: _____

_____

PERSONAL GROWTH (OPTIONAL):

Indicate subject, date, location, and value of your continuing education or personal growth attendance.

Spiritual Nourishment:_____

_____

Daily Practice of Reflection or Prayer: _____

_____

Mental Health Day: _____

_____

Retreat:_____

_____

Reading and Personal Study:_____

_____

Conference or Seminar:_____

_____

FAITH COMMUNITY NURSE EDUCATION PROGRAM
DOCUMENTATION

Title of Program: _____

Date: _____ Time: _____ Place: _____

Intended Audience: _____

_____

Number Attending: _____ Presenter(s): _____

Objectives: _____

_____

_____

_____

Content Outline (may be by attachment): _____

_____

_____

_____

_____

Evaluation (attach summary if written evaluation sheet used): _____

_____

_____

Attach following if used: attendance sheet, handouts, content outline, summary of evaluation, suggestions if program is repeating.

Faith Community Nurse: _____

Faith Community: _____

FAITH COMMUNITY NURSE SUPPORT GROUP REPORT

Name of Group: _____

Meeting Date: _____ Place: _____

Number in attendance: _____ Leader: _____

Comments: _____

_____

_____

_____

_____

Need for follow-up: _____

_____

_____

_____

_____

_____

_____

_____

_____

_____

_____

_____

_____

Faith Community Nurse: _____

Faith Community: _____

Unit II: Professionalism
Legal Aspects

Legal Aspects

Introduction

Learning Outcomes

Upon completion of this module, the participant will be able to:

1. Establish professional boundaries in faith community nursing practice.
2. Minimize exposure to liability in faith community nursing practice.
3. Analyze the major areas of accountability in faith community nursing practice using the ANA/HMA *Faith Community Nursing: Scope and Standards of Practice* (2nd ed., 2012) as a framework.
4. Practice faith community nursing according to guidelines in his or her specific state Nursing Practice Act.

Description

This module introduces the concept of professional accountability and responsibility of the registered nurse as outlined by the nurse's specific state Nursing Practice Act and its application to faith community nursing practice. Several specific denominations have strict beliefs about treatments offered in health care, many of which pose challenging issues within the health care setting. These range from refusal of blood transfusions, issues around testing and surgery, and issues specific to terminating pregnancies and end-of-life care. Accountability and responsibility are connected to stewardship and professionalism of the Faith Community Nurse Expectations for the faith community nurse (FCN) as described in ANA/HMA *Faith Community Nursing: Scope and Standards of Practice* (2nd ed., 2012), which provides the framework for issues of accountability.

Hours: 2

Research

As consumers have become more knowledgeable about health care, the number of legal cases naming nurses has increased. There have been no known cases involving faith community nurses (FCNs); however, since FCNs engage in an autonomous practice, they may be involved in a legal suit. Nursing journals have published a number of articles that either address the question of whether nurses should have malpractice insurance or describe the types of malpractice coverage the nurse should consider (Buppert, 2008); textbooks also discuss the issue of liability insurance (Mahlmeister, 2013). An increasing consensus appears to recommend that all nurses purchase malpractice insurance as a result of changes in the health care system, civil law, and insurance company policies.

Faith Tradition

The Christian faith is concerned about (1) how we love and care for one another, as Jesus Christ loved and cared for us; (2) issues of social justice, such as access to health care, and distribution of scarce resources, such as nursing care; (3) advocacy on behalf of others to prevent harm and provide good to them; (4) suffering and healing; and (5) the morality expressed and lived out by Christians when addressing these concerns.

Key Terms

Accountability: the acknowledgment and assumption of responsibility for actions

Malpractice: failure of a professional to meet the standard of conduct that a reasonable and prudent member of his or her profession would exercise in similar circumstances that results in harm. The professional's misconduct is unintentional.

Negligence: failure to act as an ordinarily prudent person would act under similar circumstances

Nursing Practice Act: statute in each state and territory that regulates the practice of nursing

Professional boundaries: the spaces between the nurse's power and the client's vulnerability

State board of nursing: appointed board within each state charged with responsibility to administer the Nursing Practice Act of that state

Reflection

"Now we know that whatever the law says, it speaks to those who are under the law, so that every mouth may be silenced, and the whole world may be held accountable to God."
—Romans 3:19

"True instruction was in his mouth, and no wrong was found on his lips. He walked with me in integrity and uprightness, and he turned many from iniquity."
—Malachi 2:6

Legal Aspects
Content Outline

KEY TERM

Professional boundaries *are the spaces between the nurse's power and the client's vulnerability.*

OUTCOME 1

Establish professional boundaries in faith community nursing practice.

Definition of Professional Boundaries

Professional boundaries are the spaces between the nurse's power and the client's vulnerability. The nurse's power comes from the professional position and the access to private knowledge about the client (National Council of State Boards of Nursing).

There is a need to establish professional **boundaries because these boundaries allow the nurse to control the power differential** between the nurse and the patient, which in turn assures a safe connection that allows the nurse to meet the patient's needs in the best way.

HELPFUL RESOURCE

A Nurse's Guide to Professional Boundaries from the National Council of State Boards of Nursing, https://www.ncsbn.org/ProfessionalBoundaries_Complete.pdf.

- While the nature of nursing work has a personal component, the relationship between the nurse and the client has as its foundation the purpose of preventing illness, reducing suffering, and protecting and promoting the health of the client.
- This foundation differentiates the relationship from relationships that are purely personal.

Guiding Principles for Maintaining Professional Behavior

1. The nurse's responsibility is to establish and maintain boundaries that support the professional relationship.
2. The nurse should work within the zone of helpfulness to the patient, not any personal benefit.
3. The nurse should avoid crossing the boundary between professional and personal interaction. Boundary violations can result when there is confusion between the needs of the nurse and those of the patient.
4. The nurse is mindful that the specific care setting, community influences, patient needs, and the nature of therapy affect the process of drawing boundaries.
5. The nurse should avoid excessive personal disclosure to the patient.

Critical Thinking

How does this information apply if the nurse is the FCN in a small faith community?

How can an FCN identify a potential boundary violation? Explain your answer.

6. The nurse needs to be cognizant of the potential boundary issues that exist in using social media to discuss patients, their families, or their treatment.
7. Professional sexual misconduct is an extreme form of boundary violation. This includes behavior or speech that a patient might reasonably interpret as being sexual in nature, seductive, sexually demeaning, or sexually harassing.

The nurse's challenges in avoiding boundary crossing are:
- Be aware.
- Be cognizant of feelings and behavior.
- Be observant of the behavior of other professionals.
- Always act in the best interest of the patient.

OUTCOME 2

Minimize exposure to liability in faith community nursing practice.

Tort Law

A **tort** is a **civil wrong** as opposed to a criminal wrong. It occurs between individuals and agencies. For instance, Mr. Smith is suing the nursing home for improper care of his wife resulting in her death.

There are two types of torts: an **unintentional tort** or wrong and an **intentional tort**. An unintentional tort is an unintended wrong against another person. The two most common unintentional torts are negligence and malpractice.

Negligence is defined as the failure to act in a reasonable and prudent manner. The claim of negligence is based on the accepted principle that everyone is expected to conduct themselves in a reasonable and prudent fashion. This is true of laypersons, student nurses, and licensed professionals. A more formal definition of negligence is the failure of a person to use the care that a reasonably prudent and careful person would use under similar circumstances (Griffith and Tengnah, 2008).

Malpractice, a special type of negligence, is the failure of a professional to meet the standard of conduct that a reasonable and prudent member of his or her profession would exercise in similar circumstances that results in harm (Iyer and Levin, 2007). The professional's misconduct is unintentional. As state Nursing Practice Acts have evolved to reflect the increasing professionalism of RNs, courts have begun to recognize the negligent acts of nurses as malpractice. Evidence of this change in perceptions is apparent in the increasing use of RNs as expert witnesses in malpractice cases.

Examples of Health Care Torts
- **Wrongful birth**—parents typically contend that they would have terminated the pregnancy had they known the child was going to be born with severe birth defects.

KEY TERM
Negligence *is failure to act as an ordinarily prudent person would act under similar circumstances.*

KEY TERM
Malpractice *is failure of a professional to meet the standards of a reasonable member of the profession in similar circumstances.*

The resolution of cases involving tort law are intended to:
- *preserve community peace*
- *establish culpability*
- *identify deterrence*
- *institute compensation or restitution*

- **Wrongful death**—filed by survivors of patients, alleging that the patient died because of the negligence of health care professionals or organization.
- **Assault**—any intentional act that creates reasonable apprehension of immediate harmful or offensive contact. No actual contact is needed.
- **Battery**—any intentional act that brings about actual harmful or offensive contact.
- **False imprisonment**—an intentional act or omission that confines or restrains another to a bounded area.
- **Loss of consortium**—alleged when relationships with spouses, children, or parents have suffered because of negligence.
- **Defamation of character**—saying or writing something that injures the reputation of another.
- **Emotional distress**—alleged when the wrongdoing, either intentional or negligent, of another causes emotional distress.
- **Intentional indifference**—failure to attempt to provide care that is consistent with the standard of care.
- **Breach of confidentiality**—sharing patient information with persons not authorized to have the information.
- **Invasion of privacy**—objectionable intrusion.

Four Elements of Negligence
For a legal finding of negligence, **all four** of the following elements must exist:
1. **Duty**—An obligation to conform to a recognized standard of care. Duty is usually established when a person accesses care given by a health care professional (for instance, the FCN).
2. **Injury**—The plaintiff must establish that actual damages have occurred.
3. **Breach of duty**—It must be shown that the health care professional deviated from the established standard of care, and that there was failure to adhere to an obligation.
4. **Causation**—An act that created a breach of duty must be the proximate cause of the injury. In other words, except for the breach of duty, the injury would not have happened. It must be shown that it was reasonably foreseeable that harm or injury would result from the act or omission. A **"Reasonably foreseeable" test** is whether a person of ordinary prudence and intelligence should have anticipated the danger to others caused by his or her negligent act.

Examples of Negligence Specific to FCNs Under the Concept of Duty to Care
Assessment failures include:
- failure to assess and analyze
- failure to document the assessment and analysis
- failure to act in accordance with patient's wishes for self-determination

Planning failure is the failure to appropriately use the patient's assessment for diagnosis and planning of care.

Implementation failures include:
- communication failures
- failure to take appropriate action
- failure to document findings and responses to interventions

Evaluation failure is the failure to act as a patient advocate.

Breach of duty is the failure to act consistently with:
1. Standards established by the Nursing Practice Act relating to the activities that are within the scope of practice for registered nurses.
2. ANA/HMA *Faith Community Nursing: Scope and Standards of Practice* (2nd ed., 2012) to show consistence between actions and standards.
3. Job description or contract detailing specific functions, policies, and procedures established by the organization.

Injury results when the person sustains actual damage resulting from negligence, such as developing a pressure sore.

To establish **causation**, it must be shown that the health care professional breached his or her duty to the patient, and this breach of duty was the proximate cause of the patient's injury.

Criminal Law

A crime is an offense against society, defined through written criminal statutes or codes. A criminal act is deemed to be conduct so offensive that the state is responsible for prosecuting the offending individual on behalf of society. Legal remedies for crimes include fines, imprisonment, and, in some states, execution (death penalty). Criminal acts are classified as either minor offenses (misdemeanors) or major offenses (felonies).

Misdemeanors that nurses are commonly charged with include the following:
- illegal practice of medicine
- failing to report child or elder abuse
- falsification of the patient's medical record
- assault and battery and physical abuse of patients

Felonies generally involve:
- drug trafficking
- fraud in billing for services of Medicare patients
- theft
- rape
- murder

A nurse found guilty of a felony generally serves time in prison and usually suffers the permanent revocation of his or her nursing license (Mahlmeister, 2013).

Critical Thinking

Should faith communities have malpractice insurance? Explain your answer.

What actions can the FCN take to protect himself or herself from malpractice liability?

Specific Legal Topics in Faith Community Nursing

FCNs need to understand professional boundaries in key circumstances that may expose them to legal action. These include:

- advance directives—living wills and durable power of attorney for health care
- health care agent or individuals holding medical power of attorney
- wills
- delegation of responsibilities to volunteer nurses
- volunteers
- Privacy/Health Insurance Portability and Accountability Act (HIPPA).

Legal Relationship between the FCN and the Employer

Legal relationships between an FCN and a faith community or agency may be characterized several ways:

- Employment by a health care system or institution.
- Independent contractor in an agreement with the faith community or health care institution.
- Unpaid position (no financial compensation other than expenses).

It is important to remember that no matter the nature of the relationship, the FCN faces potential exposure for legal liability. Adequate insurance coverage is essential.

Insurance for the FCN

Malpractice. With more states recognizing nursing malpractice as a legitimate claim in a civil suit, the question of whether nurses should carry **malpractice insurance** has become increasingly important.

- Nursing journals have published a number of articles that either address this question or describe the types of malpractice coverage the nurse should consider (Buppert, 2008); textbooks also discuss the issue of liability insurance (Mahmeister, 2013).
- An increasing consensus appears to recommend that all nurses purchase malpractice insurance as a result of changes in the health care system, civil law, and insurance company policies.
- Legal authors also are quick to note the fallacy of the assumption that having malpractice insurance increases the risk that the nurse will be targeted in a malpractice case. Lack of coverage will not discourage a lawsuit when there is a legitimate claim.

There are two basic types of malpractice insurance.

- *Occurrence-based polices* cover all incidents that arise during a policy year regardless of when they are reported to insurer.
- *Claims-made policies* cover only those claims made or reported during the policy year regardless of when they occurred.

Automobile. Since most FCNs use their personal vehicles in performing their responsibilities, **automobile insurance** is essential.
- The FCN's personal policy will be the primary automobile insurance.
- Policies vary by company, and the FCN may need to purchase a "rider" that provides coverage for an incident that occurs in connection to his or her position.
- Whether or not the FCN is paid, the faith community may or may not have a policy that covers liability in excess of the nurse's personal policy.

General Liability. Major insurance companies offer **general liability** or professional liability policies that offer protection in the event of a suit that claims the policyholder was negligent or made an error or omission while performing services.

Critical Thinking
How does the reality of risk affect the FCN's approach to providing care?

OUTCOME 3

Analyze the major areas of accountability in faith community nursing using the ANA/HMA Faith Community Nursing: Scope and Standards of Practice (2nd ed., 2012) as a framework.

What does it mean to be **accountable**? Accountability is the acknowledgment and assumption of responsibility for actions. Accountability is a belief and a value.

As an FCN, you are accountable to:
- **God**—accountability and responsibility are directly connected to stewardship
- **Recipients of the services** of the FCN
- **Faith community or health institution** where services are rendered (legal/contractual accountability)
- **Local and federal laws** concerning mandatory reporting and confidentiality, such as HIPAA
- **Professional authorities** such as:
  - Nursing Practice Act in your state
  - American Nurses Association's *Code of Ethics for Registered Nurses with Interpretive Statements* (2008)
  - American Nurses Association's Nursing: *Scope and Standards of Practice* (2010)
  - ANA/HMA *Faith Community Nursing: Scope and Standards of Practice* (2nd ed., 2012)

KEY TERM
Accountability *is the acknowledgement of responsibility for actions.*

Critical Thinking
How is accountability an expression of stewardship that honors God?

OUTCOME 4

Practice faith community nursing according to guidelines in his or her specific state's Nursing Practice Act.

Review and discuss the specific **Nursing Practice Act** for your state or the states represented by course participants. The Nursing Practice Act is a statute in each state and territory that

KEY TERM
The **Nursing Practice Act** *is a statute in each state and territory that regulates the practice of nursing.*

Critical Thinking

How is following established standards of nursing care a fulfillment of the FCN's responsibility to God? To others?

According to your state's Nursing Practice Act, what duties must the registered nurse (RN) not delegate?

regulates the practice of nursing. The **state board of nursing** is the appointed board within each state charged with responsibility to administer the Nursing Practice Act of that state.

Identify delegation of duties as outlined in the Nursing Practice Act of your state.
- The registered nurse is a professional who owes a minimum standard of care to all patients according to the state Nursing Practice Act.
- Criteria for lawful and safe delegation have been spelled out by state boards of nursing and professional organizations, such as the ANA and the NCSBN (ANA-NCSBN, 2005).
- These guidelines and a growing body of case law assist the nurse in making decisions about safe delegation of patient care (Mahlmeister, 2013).

Review the scope of practice as per the Nursing Practice Act of your state.
- FCNs always practice within the bounds of the ANA/HMA *Faith Community Nursing: Scope and Standards of Practice* (2nd ed., 2012).
- Review the Documentation Module for an overview of the FCN's responsibility regarding documentation.
- Discuss the scope of practice of the advanced practice nurse in a faith community setting.

Standards of Professional Performance for Faith Community Nursing

Standard 7. Ethics.
The faith community nurse practices ethically.

COMPETENCIES
- Upholds healthcare consumer confidentiality within religious, legal, and regulatory parameters.
- Maintains a therapeutic and professional healthcare consumer-nurse relationship within appropriate professional role boundaries.
- Takes appropriate action regarding instances of illegal, unethical, or inappropriate behavior that can endanger or jeopardize the best interests of the healthcare consumer or situation.

Standard 8. Education.
The faith community nurse attains knowledge and competence that reflect current nursing practice.

COMPETENCIES
- Participates in ongoing educational activities related to appropriate knowledge bases, professional issues, and spiritual care.
- Maintains professional records that provide evidence of competence and lifelong learning.

Learning Activities

Case Studies

Instructions:
1. These case studies are about professional boundaries, knowledge and understanding of the state Nursing Practice Act, and ANA/HMA *Faith Community Nursing: Scope and Standards of Practice* (2nd ed., 2012).

2. After reading or role playing the case studies, divide the participants into small groups. Encourage the participants to discuss the related questions provided.

Question:
After small group discussions, you may wish to have participants share insights with the larger group.

CASE 1
Mary Begins to Date

Mary is one of the FCNs at Our Lady of Hope United Methodist Church. Mary grew up in the town of 98,000 where she has attended the church since childhood. Mr. Larson and his wife, who recently died have attended the church for many years. Their two grown daughters and their families also attend the church. Mary visited the couple during Mrs. Larson's illness and provided support to the family after her death. In the past six months Mary, who has been divorced several years, and Mr. Larson have begun to date. One of his daughters resents their relationship and has severed all ties with the church and her father because of it.

1. Is this a boundary violation?

2. How would you respond to this situation?

CASE 2
Ellen Gets Personal

Ellen, an FCN, is having problems with her eldest daughter. She has begun to share her personal problems with one of the members who comes in for weekly blood pressure checks. The member likes her and is concerned about her situation. Ellen spends more and more time talking with this member. You are supervising Ellen and you are concerned about this situation.

1. What action should you take?

2. How can a situation like this be prevented from occurring in the future?

CASE 3
Tricia Starts Fresh

His Blessed Hope Church is a large faith community located in a large metropolitan city. The spiritual leaders have decided to begin an FCN ministry using an unpaid model. They know Tricia has attended a Foundations of Faith Community Nursing course and that she has a calling and a passion for the work. They have asked Tricia to be the FCN. She will be responsible for the development of the program.

1. How can Tricia use the *Scope and Standards of Faith Community Nursing* as the foundation for the program?

2. What processes should Tricia put in place to ensure that the program adheres to the state's Nursing Practice Act?

3. How should accountability be maintained?

4. What legal concerns should Tricia consider, and how will these be addressed?

CASE 4
Amber Faces the Law

A member of the Morning Glory faith community where Amber is the FCN has filed a lawsuit claiming he was not given appropriate care at the faith community when he came in to see Amber, and that he experienced complications because of it. Amber is unpaid. She and the chart have been subpoenaed.

1. How would you advise Amber to respond?

2. What concerns should she have?

3. Does the faith community have any liability in this case?

4. What is the faith community's responsibility for having a rider that adds a health care professional, paid or unpaid, to the faith community's staff?

Expanded Learning Activity

Invite a guest speaker who is an RN attorney to discuss the legal and professional responsibilities of the FCN.

Legal Issues Quiz

Instructions:
1. This quiz is an opportunity to process and integrate information from the module.
2. Administer the quiz individually or in small group discussions.
3. When everyone has completed their answers, lead the large group through discussing their responses.

Question:
Identify one or two legal issues in this module that shed new light on your ministry as an FCN.

Quiz
1. Give an example of ways the FCN might cross boundaries between professional and personal interaction.
2. Do FCNs need their own professional malpractice insurance policy? Why or why not?
3. In regard to legal liability, does it matter whether the FCN is paid or unpaid?
4. Give two examples of negligence under the concept of duty to care specific to FCNs.
5. How should the FCN respond to the spiritual leader who asks for information about the health status of individual members of the faith community?
6. Explain the relationship of documentation to legal liability of the FCN.
7. Where can the FCN find out to whom he or she can delegate?
8. Give an example of how the FCN could be accused of defamation of character.
9. How does the Health Insurance Portability and Accountability Act (HIPPA) impact faith community nursing practice?
10. What document should the FCN examine to determine rules and regulations and scope of practice for FCNs in his or her state of residence and practice?

References

Required Textbook

American Nurses Association and Health Ministries Association. (2012). *Scope and standards of practice: Faith community nursing* (2nd ed.). Silver Spring, MD: Nursesbooks.org.

References

American Nurses Association. (2010). *Nursing scope and standards of practice.* Washington, DC: American Nurses Association.

American Nurses Association. (2012). *Faith community nursing: Scope and standards of practice,* 2nd ed. Silver Spring, MD: American Nurses Association.

Buppert, C. (2008). Frequently asked questions and answers about medical malpractice, *Dermatol Nurs 20*(5) 405–406.

Fowler, M. (2008). *Guide to the code of ethics for nurses: Interpretation and application.* Washington, DC: American Nurses Publishing.

Griffith, R. & Tengnah, C. (2008). *Law and professional nursing.* Exeter, UK: Learning Matters.

Guido, G.W. (2005) *Legal and ethical issues in nursing.* (4th ed.). Upper Saddle River, NJ: Prentice Hall.

Iyer, P., Levin, B. (3rd ed. 2007). *Nursing malpractice.* Tucson, AZ: Lawyers & Judges Publishing.

Mahlmeister, L. (2014). Legal issues in nursing and health care. In Cherry, B. & Jacob, S. (Eds.). *Contemporary nursing: Issues, trends, and management* (6th ed.). St Louis, MO: Mosby.

Monarch, K. (2002). *Nursing and the law.* Washington, DC: American Nurses Publishing.

Additional References

Buppert, C. (2011). Three frequently asked questions about malpractice insurance, *J Nurse Pract 7*(1), 16–17.

Hanssen v. Genesis Health, WL 665318 (Iowa Appel. Ct., 2011)

Hickman, J. S., (2011) *Fast facts for the faith community nurse.* New York, PA: Springer Publishing Company.

National Council of State Boards of Nursing. A Nurse's guide to professional boundaries. Accessed April 21, 2014 at https://www.ncsbn.org/ProfessionalBoundaries_Complete.pdf.

Westrick, S. & Dempski, K. (2008). *Essentials of nursing law and ethics.* Sudbury, MA: Jones and Bartlett.

Nursing Practice Acts from various states

Online Resources

American Nurses Association: http://www.nursingworld.org

National Council of State Boards of Nursing: http://www.NCSBN.org

American Nurses Association and National Council of State Boards of Nursing joint statement on delegation: https://www.ncsbn.org/Delegation_joint_statement_NCSBN-ANA.pdf

Wrap-Up and Evaluation

Measuring Competency

This chart can be used to assess the individual outcomes in this module.

- A copy of this chart is attached to the Participant Module, so that each participant can complete this short evaluation.
- Have participants read each outcome and then place an X in the box that best matches their opinion about the objective being met.
- Encourage each participant to write a short reflection about this module in the space provided at the bottom of this chart.
- Use this data to make any necessary changes.

Outcome	Not Met	Somewhat Met	Met
1. Establish professional boundaries.			
2. Minimize exposure to liability in faith community nursing practice.			
3. Analyze the major areas of accountability in faith community nursing using the ANA/HMA *Faith Community Nursing: Scope and Standards of Practice* (2nd ed., 2012) as a framework.			
4. Practice faith community nursing according to guidelines in his or her specific state Nursing Practice Act.			
Reflection: *In one paragraph, write a reflection on this module.*			

Unit II: Professionalism
Beginning Your Ministry

Beginning Your Ministry

Introduction

Learning Outcomes

Upon completion of this module, the participant will be able to:

1. Evaluate the need for a faith community nurse ministry in the faith community.
2. Create an infrastructure for a beginning faith community nurse ministry.
3. Collaborate with spiritual leaders and members of the faith community to establish a health ministry.
4. Access resources within the faith community.

Description

This module addresses developing a health ministry in the faith community from early foundation work to the time of actually beginning the ministry. There are many considerations in this process, some related to faith community leadership, some to the health team, and some to the faith community nurse (FCN). The module also discusses realistic expectations and priorities of beginning a faith community nurse ministry.

This module is *not* all-inclusive for how to begin a ministry in the faith community. The entire Foundations of Faith Community Nursing curriculum is background information and part of the process. Without the foundational background of the curriculum, in its entirety, this module will only serve as procedure with no depth. Each of the standards in *Faith Community Nursing: Scope and Standards of Practice* (2nd ed., 2012) applies to faith community nursing and should be used to guide the FCN's practice as he or she develops ministry in the faith community.

The FCN should not be in the position of convincing the faith community that he or she is worthy to be there. Rather he or she should explain how an FCN ministry can help live out the mission of the faith community.

Hours: 2.5–4

Research

Dandridge (2014) conducted an integrative literature review of 22 articles published 2008–2013 to determine the value of the FCN in health promotion and disease prevention. This research revealed that FCNs are providing a wealth of interventions to diverse populations, but are not consistently evaluating outcomes. The concept of health ministry has existed for centuries. However, today, the increased costs, complexity and ongoing changes in health care have led to an increasing need for health ministries in faith communities. Faith community nurse programs are stepping up to help fill the gaps in health care, particularly with the vulnerable and underserved.

Faith Tradition

The beginning of faith community nursing traces back to Granger Westberg, a Lutheran minister, and his connections with Lutheran General Hospital in Park Ridge, Illinois. His original idea was to locate medical clinics in churches with physicians, nurses, and clergy working together to provide wholistic care to members of the faith community. This project evolved into placing nurses within a faith community, connecting the hospital with churches through faith community nursing. The beginning of this ministry has its roots in the Christian tradition; however, it can be adjusted to fit the needs of other faith traditions (Jewish, Buddhist, Muslim, etc.) if the nurse and faith community wish to use this as a model of wholistic health.

Key Terms

Faith community nurse (FCN): a registered professional nurse who is actively licensed in a given state and who serves as a member of the staff of a faith community. The FCN promotes health as wholeness of the faith community, its groups, families, and individual members through the practice of nursing as defined by that state's Nurse Practice Act in the jurisdiction in which the FCN practices and the standards of practice set forth in the ANA/HMA *Faith Community Nursing: Scope and Standards of Practice* (2nd ed., 2012).

Faith community nursing: the specialized practice of professional nursing that focuses on the intentional care of the spirit as well as the promotion of wholistic health and prevention or minimization of illness within the context of a faith community.

Health and wellness team: may also be called a health cabinet, a health and wellness committee or commission. The team should be made up of professionals as well as laypeople from the faith community who are committed to the concept of a ministry of health and wellness.

Politics: the practice and theory of influencing other people on a civic or individual level.

Reflection

"To start a ministry you begin. The compassion of Christ is the activating force."
—Carl Goere *(The Start of a Housing Ministry)*

See Scripture Reflections *in the Learning Activities for passages and discussion questions on health ministry themes.*

Review The Road of Life *(Appendix A).*

Beginning Your Ministry

Content Outline

OUTCOME 1

Evaluate the need for a faith community nursing ministry in the faith community.

Gather Leadership for Exploration

Begin by **identifying faith community leadership** who should be part of a discussion about an overview of a faith community nursing ministry.

- This will vary in each faith community. Begin by talking with someone from the ministerial staff.
- Prepare to explain **faith community nursing** and how this ministry could serve the faith community's needs. Review "Ministry Is…" in Appendix B. Review ANA/HMA *Faith Community Nursing: Scope and Standards of Practice* (2nd ed., 2012).
- **Faith community nursing** is the specialized practice of professional nursing that focuses on the intentional care of the spirit as well as the promotion of wholistic health and prevention or minimization of illness within the context of a faith community.
- **Faith community nurse (FCN)** is a registered professional nurse who is actively licensed in a given state and who serves as a member of the staff of a faith community. The FCN promotes health as wholeness of the faith community, its groups, families, and individual members through the practice of nursing as defined by that state's Nurse Practice Act in the jurisdiction in which the FCN practices and the standards of practice set forth in the ANA/HMA *Faith Community Nursing: Scope and Standards of Practice* (2nd ed., 2012).

The Relationship between the Community and the Nurse

The people who gather for an exploratory meeting will have a wide range of questions about faith community nursing, including these likely categories:

- The criteria or role of an FCN (see Position Requirements in Appendix D).
- Job description (see samples in Appendix E).
- Paid or unpaid models—advantages and disadvantages of each in regard to: empowerment issues, necessary time commitments, organizational structure, imminent educational needs of the FCN as well as ongoing educational needs.
- Which faith community leader will complete the FCN's annual evaluation?
- Resources available for programs—is this a line item in budget, or will it depend on fundraisers?
- Legal concerns—review church insurance policy to determine coverage of the FCN and volunteers.
- If the decision is made to have an FCN, then who will recruit the interested person, and what is the time frame for doing so?
- Investigate the possibility of having an FCN mentor (see Appendix G for sample mentor checklist). Health Ministries Association (HMA) also has a mentoring program available. Often, mentoring is provided by the educator or agency providing the Foundations of Faith Community Nursing course.
- Determine how the FCN will remain connected with colleagues. Will the faith community pay for travel expenses or conference registration?
- Malpractice insurance—availability of personal policies.

How this exploratory group proceeds will depend upon the structure in the faith community and whether local resources include a hospital system, a loose network of FCNs, the availability of a mentor, and other variables.

HELPFUL RESOURCE

The FCN will want to become part of the professional community of nurses by joining a professional organization such as the Health Ministries Association, Faith Community Nurses International, and local and state nurses associations, the American Nurses Association, or a specialty organization.

Critical Thinking

Discuss the importance of advance preparation as part of the process of beginning an FCN ministry in the faith community.

OUTCOME 2

Create an infrastructure for a beginning faith community nurse ministry.

What happens first? **Begin with prayer.**
- Ask for guidance and the key people who will be faithful and committed.
- Invite the spiritual leader, faith community, family and friends to also pray for you, the FCN, during the initial discernment period (30 days is recommended).
- Reflect on personal spiritual growth: define your reflective pattern and how you will begin or maintain your own prayer life (time alone, worship, Bible studies, prayer labyrinth).

Talk with your family and significant others about the FCN ministry expectations and possible changes in your life and theirs.

The C.U.R.E. model can serve as a guide for building a health ministry. (http://www.sih.net/about/community-benefits/health-ministry/health-cabinet/)

The role of the health and wellness team or health cabinet is to provide guidance and support to this important ministry.

*The **health and wellness team** is a group of professionals and laypeople who are committed to the concept of a ministry of health and wellness.*

Jill Westberg McNamara's Stronger Together: Starting a Health Team in Your Congregation *(2014) provides guidance for beginning a health ministry without getting overwhelmed.*

C—**Contact** the key people.
U—**Understand** the needs of the congregation.
R—Build **Relationships** and gather **Resources.**
E—**Evaluate** your ministry.

Step 1 of the C.U.R.E. Method: C—Contact Key People

If the faith community does not already have a **health and wellness team**, consider establishing one.

- This group may also be called a health cabinet, a committee, or a commission.
- This group will help you discover the individuals in the faith community who want to take an active role in improving health in the faith community.
- The people who agree to work with you—and each other—will be the health and wellness team.
- Be sure to include both people with professional experience in health-related fields, such as physicians, pharmacists, dietitians, as well as people with skills in other areas, such as a financial advisor, attorney, or project organizer.
- The role of the health and wellness team or health cabinet is to provide guidance and support to this important ministry. Their involvement, and the programs that result, will empower individuals in the faith community to move toward greater wholeness of body and spirit. Recruit people who are excited about making health changes, who want to know more about whole-life health, and who are willing to meet on a regular schedule to plan activities for the faith community.

How will you find these key people?

- Talk with your spiritual leader to discover whether he or she is aware of individuals with a special interest in health.
- Think back over your own conversations about health with people in the faith community.
- Invite people to come forward. Post a notice on the faith community bulletin board and in normal faith community communications, including the bulletin, newsletter, bulletin boards, presentations to committees, announcements during worship. Your notice might look like this:
  - Are you interested in improving your health?
  - Do you want to help others live the abundant life?
  - Do you have a heart for health?
  - Contact _____ to talk about being part of the health and wellness team.
- Provide basic education on the role of a health and wellness team, such as:
  - plan health programs for the faith community
  - place healthy messages in the bulletin
  - listen to the faith community's health concerns

  - report good news of improved health to the faith community
- Make personal contact with people you would particularly like to see contribute to the team.

Not everyone who initially expresses interest will join the team. Be flexible with your expectations while stirring up interest and awareness of health matters.

Once your key contacts form a team:
- Thank everyone for being willing to serve.
- Let the faith community know what the team will be called and that team members are available to hear their health concerns and suggestions for programs.
- Consider hosting an event, such as a fellowship time following worship, and ask team members to be present for conversation with members of the faith community.
- Offer healthy refreshments as a role model for healthy living.

The Health Team and the Faith Community
- The team represents various groups within the faith community, such as marrieds, singles, adults, youth, seniors, health care professionals, business people, and homemakers.
- The team is well-informed about health ministry on behalf of the congregation.
- The team envisions the potential of health ministry in the faith community.
- The team develops a mission statement and establishes short- and long-term goals to carry out within the faith community or larger community.
- The team communicates the concept of health and wellness ministry through the communication channels available within the faith community.
- The team assesses what is already being done related to health and wellness, what needs are not being met, and what resources are available within and outside the faith community.
- The team plans, implements and evaluates health ministry.
- The team organizes a commissioning service for health and wellness team members, validating the ministry and raising awareness within the faith community.
- The team asks for God's blessing and guidance.

The Organizational Structure of the Team
- Review the current ministerial staff structure in your faith community and in your denomination: Where does the FCN fit into the structure? Who does the FCN report to or who supervises the FCN?

Critical Thinking

Why is the FCN's relationship with the spiritual leader important to launching a ministry?

A key decision is whether the FCN will be a member of the health team or whether he or she will lead the team. Ensure that team members have a clear understanding of wholistic health and the role of the FCN in health promotion. Providing a copy of Stronger Together: Starting a Health Team in Your Congregation *by Jill Westberg McNamara (2014) is a good place to begin developing a common mindset within the team.*

Consider the characteristics of the faith community you serve and whether your team represents it well.
- *Do you have a youth representative on the team?*
- *Do you have a team member familiar with mental health issues or who is living with a mental illness or disability?*
- *Have you included members living with physical disability or chronic illness?*
- *Are there other lifestyle issues among members of your faith community that should be reflected in the team?*

Critical Thinking

Why is establishing a health and wellness team so important to the success of an FCN program?

KEY TERM

Politics *is the practice and theory of influencing other people on a civic or individual level.*

- What title will the FCN use? This may be faith community nurse, faith community minister, health minister, or other title given by your faith community or denomination. Determine what title is best and appropriate for both you and your faith community.
- If one is not already in place, create a position description: Use *Faith Community Nursing: Scope and Standards of Practice* (2nd ed., 2012) as a guideline and see Appendix E for sample job descriptions.
- Discuss and clarify relationships within the faith community. **Politics** is the practice and theory of influencing other people on a civic or individual level, and the dynamic happens in faith communities as well. Be realistic about the politics that exist in the faith community. Remember that all faith communities have politics.

Common Issues for Structure and Politics
- Are there clear expectations of spiritual leaders, the governing body, the faith community, and the broader community?
- Does the health team have access to secretarial or other staff support?
- Does the team have access to and collaboration with other groups within the faith community? Be sure to talk to each group about your FCN ministry.
- What is the level of support from leadership? Be sure to gain support early in the development process.
- Determine if the FCN position is paid or unpaid. As a matter of stewardship, sometimes the assumption is that the FCN will act as a volunteer if he or she is a member of the faith community.
- Ask whether professional development activities, such as continuing education conferences and the annual Westberg Symposium, will be covered and at what amount.
- Be aware that it is easy to get caught up in politics; remember that is not your focus.
- Build the ministry a little at a time and have ongoing assessment and evaluation. Don't let this become your ministry. It belongs to the faith community!
- Remember, "If you have affected only one person, then you have done your job, and done it well."

Practicing in a Faith Community Other than Your Own
- It may take longer to learn the culture of the faith community.
- Determine which individuals are the formal and informal leaders.
- Attend as many activities as possible in order to meet people in different situations.
- Don't participate in church gossip; it's always good to say, "I really don't know."
- Maintain confidentiality.

Critical Thinking

How does infrastructure support spiritual care?

OUTCOME 3

Collaborate with spiritual leaders and members of the faith community to establish a health ministry.

Establishing a Health Ministry Office

A key point in establishing a health ministry is establishing a **health ministry office.**

- Establish office hours and communicate your hours to the spiritual leader and the faith community.
- Determine and set up a documentation system. See the Documentation Module.
- Put necessary policies in place (blood pressure screenings and other screenings, documentation and records, volunteers).
- Set boundaries; be realistic about how many hours you will work and know the work hour expectations by the spiritual leader. Don't extend the number of hours you have negotiated. Review the Self-Care Module.

Step 2 of the C.U.R.E. Method: U— Understand the Needs of the Faith Community

Conduct a needs assessment for the faith community. Once you have gotten your health team together, you will want to know what activities, speakers, or programs are of interest to your congregation. In order to know what the faith community wants, you have to ask them. Pray for the health needs of your faith community.

Revise the Congregational Health Ministry Survey (Appendix I) for your congregation. Decide how long it should be. The length of the survey will determine when you ask the faith community to complete it (during worship, after worship, midweek Bible study, in small groups, online, and so on).

- Ask volunteers to review the survey and prepare a brief report for the health team and faith community about its appropriateness for your setting. Is it clear? Easy to complete?
- Use the most frequently requested health items as a guide for developing programs and activities for your health ministry calendar.
- Remember to make the assessment short and simple—as little as half a page. Have pencils available at the time you administer the survey. If the spiritual leader is present, ask him or her to talk about the importance of responding to the survey.
- Ask only what you need to know, such as:
  - Do you have a chronic illness (asthma, diabetes, etc.)?
  - Do you have someone in the home to help with your care?

SURVIVAL TIPS

Remember these important factors:
- *Connect, connect, connect!—with other FCNs, faith community leaders, community leaders.*
- *Communicate, communicate, communicate!*
- *Educate, educate, educate!*
- *Listen, listen, listen!*

HELPFUL RESOURCES

Sample surveys can be found in Appendix I and online at http://health.state.tn.us/ dmhde/pdf/ CongregationalSurvey.pdf. Resources for program implementation can be found in Exploration and Implementation Packet, *available through the Church Health Center Bookstore, http://www. churchhealthcenter.org*

- Do you have transportation to medical appointments and the faith community?
- Do you have special health questions?

Develop programs for the faith community. After you determine the needs and concerns of the faith community, the next step is creating the programs that will improve the health of all of your members while helping them develop health practices that will last a lifetime. Models of ministry that have been published in *Church Health Reader* include: Community Walking Group, Breast Cancer Support Group, Gardening and Mental Health, Supermarket-Style Food Pantry, Clergy Health Competition, and Congregationally-Based HIV/AIDS Advocacy (McNamara, 2014).

- Begin your ministry with familiar, nonthreatening, one-on-one activities.
- Blood pressure clinics often are a first choice because of the ease of organization and the positive results and referrals that can come from this simple activity.
- Write a wholistic health-related article for the church newsletter or bulletin on a regular basis.
- Display health literature on a bulletin board or other appropriate area.
- Implement an easy wholistic movement program, such as Sign Chi Do (www.signchido.com) or a chair exercise program,

Communicate with the faith community. Meet with church and community leaders, formally and informally. Remember *being* (presence) is more important than *doing*. Take it one step at a time.

Critical Thinking

How can collaboration with spiritual leaders affect a new ministry? Why do you think it is important to "start small and go slow"?

OUTCOME 4

Access resources within the faith community.

Step 3 of the C.U.R.E. Method: R—Build Relationships/Gather Resources

Consider the following categories of resources when beginning this ministry.

People

- Who sits in the pew next to you? A grant writer? Legal expert? Marketing manager? Cook and hospitality expert? Pharmacist? Facilitator? Academic dean?
- Who can help with blood pressure screenings? Health fairs? Fundraising?
- Is networking with other FCNs in the community a possibility? What about the ones in your Foundations class?
- How can the Faith Community Outreach office at the Church Health Center assist you in this new position?

- Explore with Church Health Center personnel how to become a *Friend of the Center* and receive information updates, such as the quarterly publication, *Perspectives*.

Finances

"Financial support is essential to establish and support the program. It is crucial to consider program structure, budget line items, financial responsibilities, funding sources, and budget maintenance. A faith community nurse program is a ministry, yet to ensure a solid foundation there must be a funding source and a clearly stated budget. The budget is a useful and necessary tool for every program on several points of practice: the most obvious being the structure and accountability for the finances of a program. It is the tracking system for the revenue and expenses of a department but also the snapshot for the institution's management that demonstrates a well-run program. Second, the line items or categories in a budget outline the activities that the program sees as essential to its operations. Last, it is a tool that fosters good stewardship through the monitoring of available resources for a program" (Durbin and Slutz, 2011).

- Will this be a paid or unpaid position?
- Who will the FCN be accountable to?
- Who is responsible for preparing the budget? What information is necessary to present to the finance committee? See Coordinator Manual or Smucker (2009, page 35) for typical budget expenses.
- Will your ministry be a line item in the budget?
- Are grants available from within or outside the faith community? What is the application process? (See Twadell & McDermott 2006, Chapter 25 for grant writing tips and Supplemental Module 6 *Sustaining and Nurturing the Parish Nurse Ministry*, 2005).
- Does the church allow you to ask for donations for specific causes?
- Place a donation box nearby when doing BPs, screenings, etc.
- Ask for gifts in honor or memory of faith community members to be given specifically to the FCN ministry.
- May endowment funds be used for continuing education?

Other Tangible Resources

- Who can donate items you might need, such as office equipment and supplies?
- Is there an Automated External Defibrillator (AED) on site or is there someone who might donate one?
- Plan ahead now for your continuing education—faith community nursing conferences, the annual Westberg Symposium, spiritual retreats or enrichment times. You must take care of and nurture yourself.

Critical Thinking
Why is it important for the FCN to build relationships?

Critical Thinking
What are the advantages or disadvantages for the faith community of the FCN being paid or unpaid?

<table><tr><td>

Critical Thinking

How does accessing resources apply to spiritual care?

</td><td>

Time
- God's time often is much different than ours; remember the importance of discernment, trust, patience and persistence. Ministry happens in God's time.
- Church time—often the work is very slow unless there is a champion, and even then there can be barriers.
- Business time puts a target on the calendar so the activity happens on a particular date.
- Your time must be carefully allocated. Don't overextend yourself. Self-care is really important! Your ministry will only be as wholistically healthy as you are.
- Don't forget to take time to celebrate milestones and accomplishments with special services or gatherings.

</td></tr></table>

Step 4 in the C.U.R.E. Process: E—Evaluate Your Ministry

"You have a successful health ministry. People have changed their lifestyles: improved their eating, exercise 3–4 times a week, stopped smoking, and are making important lifestyle changes that they can maintain for a lifetime. But how will you know what changes have been made if you don't keep records?
- Evaluate your programs so you will know what works and what programs were not helpful.
- Evaluate your programs so you will have results to inspire others to change their lifestyle."

(Tennessee Department of Health, Office of Faith-Based and Community Initiatives: http://health.state.tn.us/dmhde/growaministry.shtml)

Standards of Professional Performance for Faith Community Nursing

Each of the Standards is relevant for beginning a health ministry.

Learning Activities

Teaching Videos

Instructions:
Choose one of these two videos to view and discuss.
Option 1: *A Look at Parish Nursing* available through Church Health Center (www.churchhealthcenter.org)

Option 2: *The Spirit of Healing* available through Advocate Health Care (http://www.advocatehealth.com)

Question:
What main point did you take away from the video that will help your ministry?

Scripture Reflections

Instructions:
1. Distribute copies of the following Scripture passages or ask participants to read from the version of their choice.

2. In small groups, talk about the discussion questions.

3. Optional: Assign one passage to each small group and ask them to report to the larger group.

Question:
Engage the groups in a discussion about the points that struck them as most relevant to their own ministries.

Passage 1: Mark 2:1–12
When he returned to Capernaum after some days, it was reported that he was at home. So many gathered around that there was no longer room for them, not even in front of the door; and he was speaking the word to them. Then some people came, bringing to him a paralyzed man, carried by four of them. And when they could not bring him to Jesus because of the crowd, they removed the roof above him; and after having dug through it, they let down the mat on which the paralytic lay. When Jesus saw their faith, he said to the paralytic, "Son, your sins are forgiven." Now some of the scribes were sitting there, questioning in their hearts, "Why does this fellow speak in this way? It is blasphemy! Who can forgive sins but God alone?" At once Jesus perceived in his spirit that they were discussing these questions among themselves; and he said to them, "Why do you raise such questions in your hearts? Which is easier, to say to the paralytic, 'Your sins are forgiven,' or to say, 'Stand up and take your mat and walk'? But so that you may know that the Son of Man has authority on earth to forgive sins"—he said to the paralytic—"I say to you, stand up, take your mat and go to your home." And he stood up, and immediately took the mat and went out before all of them; so that they were all amazed and glorified God, saying, "We have never seen anything like this!"

- What does this passage say about the power of networking with others for health ministry?

- How does faith break down barriers to health?

- How can we help each other get past whatever paralyzes us (such as fear, lack of knowledge or experience)?

- How do you see yourself in this scenario?

Passage 2: Jeremiah 29:11–17

For surely I know the plans I have for you, says the LORD, plans for your welfare and not for harm, to give you a future with hope. Then when you call upon me and come and pray to me, I will hear you. When you search for me, you will find me; if you seek me with all your heart, I will let you find me, says the LORD, and I will restore your fortunes and gather you from all the nations and all the places where I have driven you, says the LORD, and I will bring you back to the place from which I sent you into exile. Because you have said, "The LORD has raised up prophets for us in Babylon,"—Thus says the LORD concerning the king who sits on the throne of David, and concerning all the people who live in this city, your kinsfolk who did not go out with you into exile: Thus says the LORD of hosts, I am going to let loose on them sword, famine, and pestilence, and I will make them like rotten figs that are so bad they cannot be eaten.

- What does this passage tell us about the context of health ministry?
- How do these verses help us understand the place of spirituality in wellness?

Passage 3: Proverbs 3:5–6

Trust in the LORD with all your heart,
*   and do not rely on your own insight.*
In all your ways acknowledge him,
*   and he will make straight your paths.*

- How do these verses apply to discerning God's call into health ministry?
- Consider the question: "Do I believe the Lord is guiding me in my decisions?"

Passage 4: Joshua 1:5–7, 9

No one shall be able to stand against you all the days of your life. As I was with Moses, so I will be with you; I will not fail you or forsake you. Be strong and courageous; for you shall put this people in possession of the land that I swore to their ancestors to give them. Only be strong and very courageous, being careful to act in accordance with all the law that my servant Moses commanded you; do not turn from it to the right hand or to the left, so that you may be successful wherever you go. ... I hereby command you: Be strong and courageous; do not be frightened or dismayed, for the LORD your God is with you wherever you go.

- How might God's instructions to Joshua relate to an FCN beginning a new ministry?
- What spiritual perspectives do you see in this passage that will encourage your work?

Elevator Speech

Instructions:

1. Prepare an "elevator speech"—a succinct statement that is descriptive and theoretical, but short enough to explain the work of faith community nursing in the time it takes to ride an elevator.

2. Brainstorm by listing the letters of **FAITH COMMUNITY NURSING** vertically on a page and finding appropriate words or sentences that describe you in relation to your FCN ministry.

3. Share your ideas with the entire class or with a smaller group of participants. Discuss how these words help us in talking to others about faith community nursing and establishing an FCN program in the faith community.

Expanded Learning Activities

Panel Discussion

Instructions:

1. Invite FCNs in your community to discuss their experiences in faith community nursing.

2. Make sure your instructions to the participating FCNs are clear in regard to what you want shared and time limit for each speaker. It is best to send written instructions and expectations to each panel speaker prior to the event.

3. Suggested questions to use for panelists: What have you most enjoyed about being an FCN? What has been your biggest struggle? How do you take care of yourself in the midst of caring for the entire faith community? Do you have a health team to support you?

Journaling

Instructions:
Provide a time for private journaling or reflection during the class. Have participants share their thoughts with the large group or a smaller group if they choose.

Small Group Discussions

Instructions:
Allow time for small group discussions about how to begin an FCN ministry. Then have participants share their thoughts with the large group.

Making a Poster

Instructions:
Have each participant make a tri-fold poster about important aspects of faith community nursing that can be displayed in their faith communities. Remember to have all of the necessary supplies on hand.

Applying the Information

Instructions:

1. First, divide the class into small groups to discuss what an FCN ministry means. Role-play can be used with observers offering insight.

2. In the discussion be sure to have the participants anticipate questions their pastor or faith community may ask when they return home.

3. Instruct each group to produce one short written document about the practice of faith community nursing. Be sure to have participants include plausible responses to the questions they may be asked.

4. Have participants share their thoughts with the large group.

5. Encourage participants to take notes as other groups present their ideas.

Guest Speakers

Instructions:
1. Invite guest speakers to the class, such as a human resources person to speak on the importance of job descriptions and how to write one; a team building speaker; clergy from other faith communities to understand their perspective of the FCN in their setting; a self-care expert.

2. Make sure your instructions to the guests are clear in regard to what you want shared and their time limit. It is best to send written instructions and expectations prior to the event.

Starter Plants

Instructions:
1. Purchase a packet of seeds, small pots, and potting soil. Be sure to have water on hand so the seeds can be watered after being planted.

2. In small groups, instruct the participants to plant their seeds. Encourage discussion during the planting using the analogy of the "growing seed" in relation to the analogy of "God's time." Remember to have the participants discuss the importance of trust, patience, and persistence in an FCN ministry.

3. Suggested questions: How important is God's timing to your ministry? How do the seasons of life relate to your ministry? What happens to the roots if you water too much or not enough?

Sample Job Description

Instructions:
Using the Components of a Job Description in Appendix C, work with a small group on writing a job description. Critique it with the larger group. Most faith communities will not have a job description for the FCN to follow. Many smaller faith communities may not have job descriptions for any staff member. The FCN can assist with this task. Even volunteers need job descriptions as a means of setting boundaries and having guidelines for practice. Share your work with the larger group.

Case Study

Instructions:

1. Read this story:

   Jane had a coworker tell her about faith community nursing. A Foundations Course for FCNs was scheduled for the next month. Her interest was sparked by all the potential ways she could get to know her faith community members better and care for them in a wholistic way. Jane attended the class with 12 other nurses. She was so excited, even though she felt overwhelmed and wasn't sure where to start and who to talk with first.

2. Outline a procedure for Jane's first steps. Who does she talk to in her faith community? Does she have or need a mentor?

3. What about taking 30 days to pray about the ministry? How important is this?

4. What will Jane need to do to take care of herself as she ministers to others?

5. What are some suggestions for beginning projects Jane can implement after she is established as the FCN?

6. Where can Jane find help as she continues this autonomous ministry?

Prayer in Motion

Instructions:

Prayer in Motion is one of the best wholistic methods for moving our bodies. The purpose of this program is to empower you with the tools that will help pave the way toward connecting mind, body and soul. All instructions are given on each DVD by Dr. Anne Borick, a physician in Arizona. This program has solid research and is particularly helpful for individuals who have had a stroke or Parkinson's disease. Purchase DVDs from *Sign Chi Do www.signchido.com*

References

Required Textbook

American Nurses Association and Health Ministries Association. (2012). *Scope and standards of practice: Faith community nursing* (2nd ed.). Silver Spring, MD: Nursesbooks. org.

References

American Nurses Association and Health Ministries Association, (2012). *Faith community nursing: Scope and standards of practice* (2nd ed.) Silver Spring, MD: Nursebooks. org

Bokinskie, J., & Kloster, P. (2008). Effective parish nursing: Building success and overcoming barriers. *Journal of Christian Nursing, 25*(1), 20–25.

Dandridge, R. (2014). Faith community/parish nurse literature: Exciting interventions. *Journal of Christian Nursing, 31*(2), 100–107.

Durbin, N. L., Cassimere, M., Howard, C., Lutz, M. & Wehling, B. (2013) *Faith community nurse coordinator manual: A guide to creating and developing your program*. Memphis, TN: Church Health Center.

Durbin, N. L. & Slutz, M. Budgets, funding, and grant writing. In *Faith community nurse coordinator manual: A guide to creating and developing your program* (2013). Church Health Center Inc., Memphis, TN.

Hickman, J. S. (2006). *Faith community nursing*. Philadelphia, PA: Lippincott, Williams & Wilkins.

McNamara, J. W. (2014). *Stronger together: Starting a health team in your congregation*. Memphis, TN: Church Health Center.

McNamara, J. W. (2002). *The health cabinet: How to start a wellness committee in your church*. St. Louis, MO: International Parish Nurse Resource Center.

O'Brien, M.E. (2003). *Parish nursing: Healthcare ministry within the church*. Sudbury, MA: Jones and Bartlett Publishers.

Patterson, D. L. (2003). *The essential parish nurse: ABCs for congregational health ministry*. Cleveland, OH: The Pilgrim Press.

Patterson, D. L. (2004). Parish nursing: A beneficial partnership for clergy. *The Clergy Journal*, ProQuest Religion, *80*(9), 32.

Smucker, C. J. (2009). *Faith community nursing: Developing a quality practice*. Silver Springs, MD: NurseBooks.org.

Solari-Twadell, P. A. & McDermott, M. A (2006). *Parish nursing: Development, education, and administration*. St. Louis, MO: Elsevier/Mosby.

Westberg, G. E. with Westberg, J. (1990). *The parish nurse*. Minneapolis, MN: Augsburg Publishing Company.

Additional References

Anderson, N., Daniels, M., Rastas, L. & Wescott, J. (2005). *Supplemental Module 6: Sustaining and Nurturing the Parish Nurse Ministry.*

Exploration and Implementation Packet, available through the Church Health Center Bookstore, http://www.churchhealthcenter.org

McNamara, J. W. (2014). *Stronger together: Starting a health team in your congregation*. Memphis, TN: Church Health Center.

Nouwen, H. J. *A spirituality of fundraising* (2010). Nashville, TN: The Upper Room.

O'Brien. M. E. (2014) *Spirituality in nursing: Standing on holy ground* (4th ed). Sudbury, MA: Jones and Bartlett Learning.

Steltenkamp, Mary Diane. (2013). *The blue book: A collection of stories about rituals*. Oklahoma City, OK: Catholic Charities: Archdiocese of Oklahoma City.

Wescott, JoVeta with Richard Johnson (2013). *Because I care: I am a parish nurse.*

Online Resources

Advocate Health Care: http://www.advocatehealth.com

Australian Parish Nurse Resource Center: http://www.apnrc.org

Canadian Association for Parish Nurse Ministry: http://www.capnm.ca

Carle Foundation Hospital: http://www.carle.org

Church Health Center: http://www.churchhealthcenter.org

Faith Community Nurses International: FCNInternational.org

Health Ministries Association: http://www.health ministriesassociation.org

Health Ministry Outreach Toolkit from National Health Network of Libraries of Medicine. Outreach tools to assist faith-based organizations in developing, implementing and assessing health outreach programs that meet the needs of their unique communities. http://guides.nnlm.gov/ministry

International Parish Nurse Resource Center: http://www.parishnurses.org

Kansas Parish Nurse Ministry, Inc.: http://www.Kansas ParishNurseMinistry.org

Ministries and Mission of the Presbyterian Church (U.S.A.): http://www.pcusa.org

National Episcopal Services: http://episcopalhealthministries.org

Northwest Parish Nurse Ministries: http://www.npnm.org/welcome_to_npnm0.aspx

Sign Chi Do: http://www.signchido.com

Tennessee Department of Health Office of Faith-Based and Community Initiatives: http://health.state.tn.us/dmhde/growaministry.shtml

National Network of Libraries of Medicine Health Ministry Outreach Toolkit: http://guides.nnlm.gov/ministry Outreach tools to assist faith-based organizations in developing, implementing and assessing health outreach programs that meet the needs of their unique communities.

Wrap-Up and Evaluation

Measuring Competency

This chart can be used to assess the individual outcomes in this module.
- A copy of this chart is attached to the Participant Module, so that each participant can complete this short evaluation.
- Have participants read each outcome and then place an X in the box that best matches their opinion about the objective being met.
- Encourage each participant to write a short reflection about this module in the space provided at the bottom of this chart.
- Use this data to make any necessary changes.

Outcome	Not Met	Somewhat Met	Met
1. Evaluate the need for an FCN ministry in the faith community.			
2. Create an infrastructure for a beginning FCN ministry.			
3. Collaborate with spiritual leaders and members of the faith community to establish a health ministry.			
4. Access resources within the faith community.			
Reflection: *In one paragraph, write a reflection on this module.*			

Appendix A

The Road to Life

At first I saw God as my observer, my judge keeping track of the things I did wrong, so as to know whether I merited heaven or hell when I die. He was out there, sort of like a president. I recognized his picture when I saw it, but I really didn't know him.

But later when I met Christ, it seemed as though life was rather like a bike ride, but it was a tandem bike, and I noticed that Christ was in the back helping me pedal.

I don't know just when it was that he suggested we change places, but life has not been the same since.

When I had control, I knew the way. It was rather boring, but predictable ... and it was the shortest distance between two points. But when he took the lead, he knew delightful long cuts, up mountains and through rocky places at breakneck speeds. It was all I could do to hang on! Even though it looked like madness, he said, "Pedal."

I worried and was anxious and asked, "Where are you taking me?" He laughed and didn't answer, and then I started to trust.

I forgot my boring life and entered into the adventure, and when I'd say, "I'm scared," he'd lean back and touch my hand.

He took me to people with gifts that I needed, gifts of healing, acceptance and joy. They gave me their gifts to take on my journey, my Lord's and mine.

And we were off again. He said, "Give the gifts away; they're extra baggage, too much weight." So I did, to the people we met, and I found that in giving I received, and still our burden was light.

I did not trust him, at first, in control of my life. I thought he'd wreck it; but he knows bike secrets, knows how to make it bend to take sharp corners, jump to clear high rocks, fly to shorten scary passages.

And I am learning to shut up and pedal in the strangest places, and I'm beginning to enjoy the view and the cool breeze on my face with my delightful, constant companion, Christ.

And when I'm sure I just can't do anymore, he just smiles and says, "Pedal."

—Author Unknown

Appendix B

Ministry Is ...

Listening, when you'd rather fix the problem.
Searching for the joy, when it's easier to say, "It's not fair."
Helping, when you feel like you're the one that needs the help.
Telling God, "Use me," when you'd rather ask to be rescued.
Encouraging, even when you don't understand God's reasoning.
Hugging when it feels awkward.
Saying, "Let's pray right now" instead of "I'll pray for you."
Serving when you doubt you have anything left to give.
Comforting, by being the flicker of light in others' dark caverns.

—Author Unknown

"Ministry happens when you participate in the mystery of being with.
You can't solve the world's problems, but you can be with people."

—Henri Nouwen

Job or Ministry?

A job is at your choice.
A ministry is at Christ's call.

In a job you expect to receive.
In a ministry you expect to give.

In a job you give something for a return.
In a ministry you return something that has already been received.

A job depends on your abilities.
A ministry depends on your availability to God.

A job done well brings you praise.
A ministry done well brings honor to Christ.

—James N. Spurgeon

Appendix C

Components in a Position Description for an FCN

Title: What is most appropriate or acceptable in your faith community to refer to this position? Faith community nurse? Health minister? Other?

Description of the Position: This is a brief statement of one or two sentences, not a list of duties. The description may include rationale for the position, such as Scripture, faith community's mission statement, and denominational recommendations. Position descriptions also do not contain qualifications. Qualifications may be listed separately. When writing qualifications, consider how they will be demonstrated. For example, how will you determine if the person has "good written communication skills"?

Position in the Faith Community: Who will the FCN report to or be supervised by? What is the relationship of the FCN with other staff, volunteers, or governing bodies? Who will evaluate the FCN? An organizational chart may be helpful.

Functions and Responsibilities: It is better to list general areas of responsibilities rather than specific tasks. You may wish to subdivide this section by the roles of the FCN: educator, counselor, advocate, and referral agent. Consider that this is a position description for future FCNs.

Time commitment: How many hours per week or month will the nurse work for the faith community? This may be a minimum amount rather than specific amount of time, especially if the position is volunteer, such as, "Will work a minimum of ten hours a week."

Benefits: Consider such things as: salary, professional insurance, mileage, and continuing education conferences. Will the position be paid? Will insurance be included? Does it include paid vacation?

Length of Service: This provides an opportunity to renegotiate the position and the terms at a later date. The position and the position description should be re-evaluated yearly. It is not advisable to evaluate the position before at least six months.

Number of Positions: Will there be more than one FCN? Will every nurse use the term faith community nurse? Consider the implications for potential areas of responsibilities and influence. Who will have the leadership role in a dyad or triad FCN ministry? Will spiritual leaders and members of the faith community understand the delineation of responsibility?

Appendix D

Faith Community Nurse Position Requirements Minimum to Competent

	Competent Level Qualifications	Minimum Level Qualifications
Skills	• Organization skills • Basic computer skills • Excellent communication skills • Report writing skills	• Organization skills • Basic computer skills • Excellent communication skills • Report writing skills
Education and Experience	• BSN required • 5+ years experience in med-surg • Community health nursing experience desirable • Ability to do community assessments • Ability to do health counseling	• BSN preferred • 3 years clinical nursing experience • Assessment skills
Professional Preparation	• Current license as a registered nurse in the state where the faith community is located • Completion of a basic preparation course in faith community nursing based on the standardized core curriculum endorsed through the Church Health Center/IPNRC • Completion of CPE or theological education helpful for spiritual assessment of clients	• Current license as a registered nurse in the state where the faith community is located • Completion of a basic preparation course in faith community nursing based on the standardized core curriculum endorsed through the Church Health Center/IPNRC
Special Job Characteristics	• Spiritual leadership as evidenced by experience in congregational ministries, lay leadership, theological education, and other related spiritual development • Substantial weekend and evening work; could be consulted in emergency situations involving a member(s) of the community or staff • Works well independently and as part of a team • Has a good understanding of spirituality and religiosity	

Appendix E

Sample Faith Community Nurse Job Descriptions

Sample 1

Job Description for the Ministry of Faith Community Nursing Practice

This position is designed to provide whole person, health promotion, disease prevention services with an emphasis on spiritual care. The major accountabilities and job activities of the faith community nurse role are integrator of faith and health, health educator, personal health counselor, referral agent, developer of support groups, trainer of volunteers, and health advocate.

I. Accountabilities

Integrator of faith and health

1. Assesses faith community's assets and needs incorporating an understanding of the relationship between faith and health.
2. Participates as a staff member of the faith community, attending all meetings of the staff of the faith community.
3. Identifies opportunities to enhance the understanding of the relationship of faith and health within the faith community.
4. Fosters, promotes, and provides opportunities for spiritual care to be discussed and integrated into the faith community, documenting spiritual care of groups and individuals.
5. Participates in the planning and providing of prayer and worship life of the faith community.
6. Teaches and models the integration of faith and health into daily life.

Health Educator

1. Utilizes information from asset and needs assessments of the faith community and surrounding community in planning for education programs.
2. Prepares, develops and/or coordinates educational programs based on identified needs for healthier lifestyles, early illness detection and health resources.
3. Maintains records of educational programs, including objectives, content, evaluation, attendance and budget.
4. Documents individual educational assessment, diagnosis, interventions and outcomes.
5. Provides the pastor, health committee of the faith community, and other designated parties

a summary evaluation of educational programs noting attendance and response of participants.
6. Networks with appropriate resources in the community to secure educational program resources.
7. Provides consultation and acts as a health resource to other staff of the faith community.

Personal Health Counselor

1. Provides individual health counseling related to health maintenance, disease prevention or illness patterns.
2. Encourages the client through presence and spiritual support to express their faith beliefs and utilize them regularly, especially in time of crisis and despair.
3. Documents client assessment, nursing diagnosis, interventions, and outcomes while maintaining confidential client records in accordance with the policy on documentation.
4. Makes visits to clients as needed providing health counseling, education, and spiritual presence and support.
5. Promotes stewardship of the body, emphasizing self care of the whole person.
6. Collaborates with pastoral staff to plan for health education programming.
7. Communicates with other health professionals as needed to meet the health needs of clients.

Trainer of Volunteers

1. Identifies and recruits professional and lay volunteers who can be available to respond to the health related needs of members of the faith community.

2. Facilitates and, when appropriate, trains individuals to assume volunteer responsibilities to meet identified needs of the faith community.
3. Works with staff, health committee, or others focusing on the integration of health into the life of the faith community.

Developer of Support Groups
1. Develops and/or facilitates support groups based on identified needs and resources.
2. Identifies available support groups in the community that could resource the faith community.
3. Refers and documents client participation in designated support groups.

Referral Agent
1. Provides and documents referrals to health care services and resources within the faith community and external community.
2. Collaborates with community leaders and agencies to facilitate effective working relationships while identifying new health resources.
3. Develops community contacts in order to secure resources and services to meet the needs of members of the faith community.
4. Networks with other faith community nurses and professionals.

Health Advocate
1. Encourages clients to avail themselves of services which will enhance their overall well-being, assisting the clients in identifying values and choices which encourage them to be more responsible for their health status.

2. Assists client and client families in making decisions regarding their health, medical services, treatments, and care facilities, as well as documenting assessments, diagnosis, interventions, and outcomes.
3. Identifies, communicates, and works cooperatively with community leaders, elected officials, and agencies to meet health needs of members of the faith community and surrounding community.

II. Job Activities
Management
1. Develops reports regarding faith community nurse activities as needed. Collaborates with others in developing and managing grant projects.
2. Coordinates all faith community nurse programming in the faith community.

Professional Development, Education and Research
1. Participates in continuing education programs to meet identified professional learning needs.
2. Participates in regular personal spiritual formation.
3. Acts as a preceptor to students from schools of nursing, seminaries and other disciplines as requested.
4. Develops and/or participates in research related to faith community nursing.
5. Develops and submits articles on experiences in faith community nursing for publication.

III. Job Requirements
(See chart on following page).

III. Job Requirements

	Competent Level Qualifications	Minimum Level Qualifications
Skills	1. Organizing skills 2. Basic computer skills 3. Excellent communication skills 4. Ability to develop reports	1. Excellent communication skills 2. Organizing skills
Education and Experience	1. BSN required 2. 5+ years experience in med-surg nursing 3. Community health nursing experience desirable 4. Ability to perform community assessments 5. Ability to provide health counseling	1. BSN preferred 2. 3 years clinical nursing experience 3. Assessment skills
Professional Preparation	1. Current license as a registered nurse in the state where the faith community is located	1. Current license as a registered nurse in the state where the faith community is located
Special Job Characteristics	1. Spiritual leadership as evidenced by experience in faith community ministries, lay leadership, theological education, and other related spiritual development 2. Substantial weekend and evening work	1. Works well independently and yet can function well as part of a work team 2. Has a good understanding of spirituality and religiosity

---

Sample 2

Faith Community Nurse (Paid)

Position Title: Faith Community Nurse (Paid)

Department: Faith Community Nurse Program

General Description
This position provides wholistic health services to the individuals affiliated with the assigned faith community. All services utilize spiritual care while identifying the health needs of the church; providing crisis intervention to parishioners; offering health education and promotional materials; supervising church volunteers in health-related activities; and providing patient advocacy through use of community agencies and patient empowerment.

Minimum Qualifications
Education, Training, and Experience: Must be a graduate of a state-approved School of Nursing, with a minimum of two years of experience in nursing. A Baccalaureate Degree with a major in nursing and community health experience are preferred. Completion of an approved faith community nurse educational program.

Knowledge, Abilities, and Skills: Has ability to assess health-related needs for each client. Demonstrates knowledge of teaching/learning principles. Possesses the ability to solve problems; to plan, organize, direct, and evaluate the health care of the client. Uses interpersonal and caring skills. Has the ability to understand and communicate the interrelatedness of body, mind, and spirit to health and wellness. Utilizes effective communication skills including oral and written skills. Has an understanding of and commitment to the church's vital mission in fostering wellness in today's society.

Licenses, Registrations, and Certifications: Current Registered Professional Nurse licensure in the state where the faith community or parish is located. Must maintain current CPR certification.

Job Relationships
Responsible to: Manager of Faith Community Nurse Department, church pastor

Workers supervised: Volunteers in the congregation

Inter relationships: Clients, physicians, hospital personnel, community agencies, church staff, and the general public

Working conditions: (list as institution requires)

Physical demands: (list as institution requires)

Patient Population Served
- Neonatal
- Pediatric
- Adolescent
- Adult
- Geriatric

Job Duties: Technical/Administrative/Clinical
Demonstrates competence in the skills (processes, procedures, and equipment) necessary to carry out assigned duties as identified below. Demonstrates competence in recognizing and responding to patients' physical, mental, emotional and developmental needs and is evaluated in relation to the patient populations served as appropriate for each responsibility.

A. Participates in the life and activities of the congregation as a member of the faith community staff. It is expected that the nurse's role will be determined by the unique needs of each participating organization; these may include, but are not limited to, the following:

1. Serves as a personal health counselor to members of the congregation
2. Serves as a resource to families in crisis
3. Serves as a liaison between clients and community/faith community resources and makes appropriate referrals
4. Implements classes on current health and wellness topics
5. Facilitates health screenings
6. Develops a Health and Wellness Committee or participates on a similar committee, which will serve as a resource in refining the nurse's role and function
7. Coordinates efforts with staff and groups within the church's organizational structure

8. Maintains statistical data to give evidence of functions and activities
9. Assigns appropriate activities to volunteers within the faith community
10. Notifies client's physician when appropriate

B. Demonstrates initiative in developing new concepts and maintaining the Faith Community Nurse Program

C. Implements the nursing process when applicable to the situation

D. Nursing Diagnosis: Identifies patient or family problems and needs, including potential problems

E. Planning
1. Identifies client's immediate needs
2. Collaborates with client, client's significant others, pastor, physician, other faith community nurses, and hospital or community agency personnel to assist with compliance of treatment and patient-centered goals
3. Collaborates with discharge planners when preparing client for a return to the home or living facility

F. Implementation
1. Demonstrates competence in the administration of faith community nurse interventions.
2. Implements health care in accordance with established faith community standards of care, policies, procedures, and state and federal laws.
3. Demonstrates teamwork in the implementation of client support and assistance.
4. Demonstrates leadership skills in the coordination and provision of client assistance.
5. Documents the client's compliance/response to recommended treatment.
6. Implements teaching guidelines in a timely manner and documents client/family understanding and effectiveness.

G. Evaluation
1. Incorporates information from client, family, health care and pastoral care staff to evaluate client's achievement of goals.
2. Consults with client, pastor, other faith community nurses, physicians, and other hospital and community agencies' staff to determine efficiency and effectiveness of support, health teaching, and assistance.
3. Initiates educational programs consistent with the needs of the faith community.
4. Develops minimum of one educational display, program, or newsletter article per quarter.
5. Identifies personal educational needs and takes responsibility for own professional development.
6. Participates in Quality Improvement Programs and Faith Community Nurse Program research studies.

H. Age-specific Criteria
Demonstrates the minimum knowledge, skills, and abilities necessary to provide care to clients across the lifespan, based on the physical, psychosocial, educational, safety, and related criteria identified below:
- knowledge of growth and development
- ability to assess age-specific data
- ability to interpret age-specific data
- ability to provide age-specific care
- possess communication skills necessary to interpret age-specific response to treatment
- ability to involve family or significant other in decision-making related to treatment

Personal and Professional Commitment
A. Attends all mandatory in-services
B. Assumes responsibility for personal growth and development and pursues opportunities for personal enrichment
C. Utilizes supplies and resources of the organization in a cost-effective manner
D. Maintains commitment to working scheduled hours

Used with permission from Trinity Medical Center, Rock Island, Illinois.

Sample 3

Faith Community Nurse (Unpaid)

Position Title: Faith Community Nurse (Unpaid)

Department: Faith Community Nurse Program

General Description

This position provides wholistic health services to the individuals affiliated with the assigned church. All services utilize spiritual care while identifying the health needs of the church; providing crisis intervention to parishioners; offering health education and promotional materials; supervising church volunteers in health-related activities; and providing patient advocacy through use of community agencies and patient empowerment.

Minimum Qualifications

Education, Training, and Experience: Must be a graduate of a state approved School of Nursing, with a minimum of two years of experience in nursing. A baccalaureate degree with a major in nursing and community health experience are preferred.

Knowledge, Abilities, and Skills: Has ability to assess health-related needs for each client. Demonstrates knowledge of teaching/learning principles. Possesses the ability to solve problems; to plan, organize, direct, and evaluate the health care of the client. Uses interpersonal and caring skills. Has the ability to understand and communicate the interrelatedness of body, mind, and spirit to health and wellness. Utilizes effective communication skills including oral and written skills. Has an understanding of and commitment to the church's vital mission in fostering wellness in today's society.

Licenses, Registration and Certifications: Current Registered Professional Nurse licensure in the state where congregation is located. Must maintain current CPR certification.

Job Relationships

Reports to: Director of Faith Community Nurse Program, congregation leader

Persons supervised: Volunteers in the congregation

Relates to: Faith Community Nurse Program Staff, other faith community nurses, Pastoral Care Department, hospital personnel, church staff, members of the congregation, and the general public

Principal Duties and Responsibilities

To the Church: The faith community nurse is expected to participate in the life and activities of the congregation as a member of the faith community staff. It is expected that the nurse's role will be determined by the unique needs of each participating congregation. These may include, but are not limited to, the following:

A. Serves as a personal health counselor to members of the congregation

B. Serves as a personal resource to families in crisis

C. Serves as a liaison to community/faith community resources and makes appropriate referrals

D. Teaches or coordinates classes on current health and wellness topics

E. Develops a Health and Wellness Committee or participates on a similar committee, which will serve as a resource in refining the nurse's role and function

F. Maintains client records and protects confidentiality of information

G. Maintains statistical data to give evidence of functions and activities

H. Gives and receives support from the faith community staff and committees

To the Hospital: The faith community nurse is expected to participate in the life and activity of the Faith Community Nurse Department and to be a living representative of the hospital's concept of wholistic health. Such activities may include, but are not limited to, the following:

A. Personal growth—to be involved in, and committed to the peer group and process designed to foster personal and spiritual development

B. Professional growth—to attend group sessions, which will be provided in response to the nurse's identified learning needs

C. Give and receive support from the peer group and hospital's multidisciplinary staff

D. Maintain client and statistical data and report monthly to the Project Faculty

E. Be available to the Project's Steering Committee and Faculty

F. Participate in an annual personal evaluation of faith community nurse activities, professional behavior, and spiritual support

Involvement of Unpaid Faith Community Nurse

A realistic approach must be made to developing a workload in keeping with the needs of the faith community and at the same time not over taxing the faith community nurse.

Used with permission from Trinity Medical Center, Rock Island, Illinois.

Sample 4

Faith Community Nurse

Job Title: Faith Community Nurse

Supervised by: (Title of faith community nurse program coordinator/manager/director)

Job Classification: Exempt

All duties and standards of this position will be performed according to established policies, procedures and guidelines for (name of sponsoring organization). These examples of work are not all-encompassing or restrictive and are expected to vary with changing needs and priorities. The duties for a specific position with this title will be defined and assigned by the site supervisor.

Statement of Purpose

The faith community nurse is responsible for working in consultation with the (title of faith community nurse program coordinator/manager/director), in accordance with a covenantal agreement between (sponsoring organization) and the church/agency. The faith community nurse plays a highly visible role in the life and activities of the congregation or community to which assigned, while actively participating in the mission, interpretation and promotion of faith community nursing.

Job Duties and Responsibilities

I. **Integrator of Faith and Health:** Seeks to promote an understanding of the relationship between faith and health by:
   A. Lifting up lifestyle practices as a matter of stewardship and faith.
   B. Participating in the worship life of the faith community.
   C. Providing spiritual care and guidance surrounding health issues.

II. **Health Educator:** Provides health education in the congregation and community by:
   A. Coordinating or presenting health-related classes or courses.
   B. Securing guest presenters for special courses.
   C. Providing articles for the church bulletin, newsletter or other publication as requested.
   D. Maintaining a health ministry bulletin board and/or literature rack at the church.
   E. Arranging for use of church facilities as appropriate for health education activities.

III. **Health Counselor:** Acts as a health consultant by:
   A. Wholistically assessing individuals in their homes and within the congregational setting.
   B. Assessing the health of the congregation and wider community and developing appropriate programming to address health-related needs.
   C. Accepting appropriate referrals.
   D. Providing health screenings.
   E. Assisting with visitation and follow-up in homes, hospitals and long-term care facilities.

IV. **Referral Advisor:** Acts as a referral source for members of the congregation and/or community served by:
   A. Referring individuals to pastor, physician, or community support services as needed.
   B. Acting as a liaison between congregation and community resources.
   C. Maintaining an awareness of the resources within the community.

V. **Health Advocate:** Acts as a health advocate by:
   A. Assisting people to understand and effectively use health care and social service systems.
   B. Serving as a resource person to other church committees and community organizations on health issues as requested.
   C. Making the church staff and congregation aware of social and legislative issues that affect health care.

VI. **Developer of Support Groups:** Acts as a developer of support groups by:

A. Assessing the need for support groups in various health-related areas.

B. Facilitating the development of support groups for the faith community and others served as needed.

C. Arranging for appropriate professional leadership for support groups as required.

D. Evaluating effectiveness of support groups in meeting health-related needs of participants.

VII. Health Ministry Volunteer Coordinator: Coordinates health ministry volunteer activity (may include student nurses or paid staff) by:

A. Recruiting volunteers for various health ministry activities.

B. Providing orientation and continuing education for volunteers.

C. Directing volunteer activities.

D. Evaluating volunteer performance and providing appropriate feedback and recognition.

VIII. Collegiality: Maintains a positive working relationship with others by:

A. Participating in regular meetings with the congregational pastor and staff.

B. Meeting with and providing staff support for the health cabinet or advisory board.

C. Actively participating in the meetings called by the (sponsoring organization).

D. Participating in the local faith community nurse network or other professional organization.

IX. Education: Acquires and maintains current knowledge in nursing practice, health promotion, and spiritual care by:

A. Participating in continuing education in-service programs and other educational activities authorized by the congregation and (sponsoring organization).

B. Attending any program deemed mandatory by the (sponsoring organization).

X. Quality Assurance: Systematically participates in evaluation of quality and effectiveness of practice by:

A. Evaluating the program on a continuing basis with appropriate parties.

B. Providing the congregation and (sponsoring organization) with appropriate statistical data in a timely fashion.

C. Documenting services provided according to congregation and/or (sponsoring organization) requirements.

D. Participating in quality assurance activities initiated by the congregation or (sponsoring organization).

XI. Job Requisites

A. Education and Training
1. Graduate from an accredited School of Nursing
2. BSN preferred
3. CPE or theological education helpful

B. Licensing/Registration/Certification
1. Currently licensed as a registered nurse in the state of (name of state in which congregation is located)
2. Minimum of three (3) years of experience preferably in one or more of the following areas: public health, health education, public school nursing, medical/surgical and/or emergency room outpatient nursing

C. Skills and Abilities
1. Excellent communication skills and teaching techniques
2. Knowledge of current nursing and health care issues in health promotion as related to lifestyle
3. Knowledge of health services and resources in community
4. Demonstrated knowledge of organizational dynamics of the denomination to be served
5. Excellent organizational skills
6. Participation in church and community activities that contribute to professional growth and to promotion of wholistic health philosophy

An individual without the requisites stated above may present a written justification explaining the relevance of his or her background for a specific vacant position. Depending on organizational needs and availability of more qualified applicants, an applicant may have some or all requisites revised or waived at the program's discretion.

Physical Requirements and Working Conditions
A. Manual dexterity, coordination, and skillful use of hands for working with required equipment
B. Ability to receive and express detailed information through oral communication, visual acuity and the ability to read and understand written direction
C. Ability to physically perform necessary documentation in writing or through use of tape recorder
D. Ability to occasionally lift and transport items weighing up to 10 pounds

Machines/Equipment/Tools
A. Primary: Telephone, Information system within the faith community
B. Secondary: Fax, Copy machine
C. Motor vehicle for travel within the community

Blood-Borne Pathogens Category:
Non-Exposure

Employee Acknowledgement:
I have reviewed and I understand the job duties and expectations outlined in this job description. I agree to perform the work in a manner acceptable to my immediate supervisor and within guidelines defined by the (sponsoring organization).

I also understand that continued employment will depend on my demonstrated ability to perform the work as expected.

Employee:_____ Date _____

Adapted from Patterson, D. (2003). The Essential Parish Nurse: ABCs for Congregational Health Ministry.

Appendix F

Faith Community Nurse Position Requirements Minimum to Competent

	Competent Level Qualifications	Minimum Level Qualifications
Skills	• Organization skills • Basic computer skills • Excellent communication skills • Report writing skills	• Organization skills • Excellent communication skills
Education and Experience	• BSN required • 5+ years experience in med-surg • Community health nursing experience desirable • Ability to do community assessments • Ability to do health counseling	• BSN preferred • 3 years clinical nursing experience • Assessment skills
Professional Preparation	• Current license as a registered nurse in the state where the faith community is located • Completion of a basic preparation course in faith community nursing based on the standardized core curriculum endorsed through the Church Health Center/IPNRC • Completion of CPE or theological education helpful for spiritual assessment of clients	• Current license as a registered nurse in the state where the faith community is located • Completion of a basic preparation course in faith community nursing based on the standardized core curriculum endorsed through the Church Health Center/IPNRC
Special Job Characteristics	• Spiritual leadership as evidenced by experience in congregational ministries, lay leadership, theological education, and other related spiritual development • Substantial weekend and evening work; could be consulted in emergency situations involving a member(s) of the community or staff • Works well independently and as part of a team • Has a good understanding of spirituality and religiosity	

Appendix G

Faith Community Nurse Mentor Program Checklist
(Informal Self-Evaluation)

Rating Scale: 1—Some understanding; 2—Understanding and experience; 3—Consciously incorporates into practice		1	2	3
Standard 1. Facilitation of Spiritual Care		**1**	**2**	**3**
1a.	Ability to draw from and reflect upon one's personal experience of faith, spirituality, theology and religion.			
1b.	Recognition of diversity within worship settings, and an ability to structure meaningful responses to diverse worship needs (e.g. children's time, use of silence, use of drama, etc.).			
1c.	Knowledge and skill in the areas of active listening, grief counseling, health counseling, and conflict resolution.			
1d.	Ability to engage others in conversation about their faith and faith development, including being able to share prayerfully together.			
1e.	Demonstrates valuing and respect for individuals in his or her care and colleagues with whom he or she works.			
Standard 2. Establishing a Faith Community Nurse Ministry				
2a.	Ability to conceptualize and articulate how to establish a faith community nursing ministry within a faith community.			
2b.	Understanding of the principles and procedures of church or temple polity and management within the uniqueness of a particular faith tradition.			
2c.	Knowledge of group processes and ability to work within group settings.			
2d.	Identifies the strengths and resources of the community of care to determine resources for health promotion.			
2e.	Knowledge of budget, financial accountability and grant writing.			
2f.	Ability to integrate theory with practice in a faith community nurse setting with the support of a faith community and an experienced faith community nurse mentor.			

	Standard 3. Health Promotion and Advocacy			
3a.	Ability to carry out nursing care in a holistic way with skills in assessment and intervention in physical, emotional, mental, social and spiritual dimensions of people's health.			
3b.	Ability to conceptualize and communicate the meanings of health, healing, and wholeness and health promotion as these relate to persons in a faith community setting.			
3c.	Invites individuals and groups to identify their own health issues and supports them in developing skills for self advocacy.			
3d.	Ability to refer to community health resources considering the readiness, values, and consent of the individual/community.			
3e.	Collaborates as a team member with health care providers, clergy, and volunteer support systems to meet the identified needs.			
3f.	Supports workplace wellness for the faith community nurse and the pastoral care team.			
	Standard 4. Professional Accountability			
4a.	Ability to reflect with peers and mentors on one's practice and vocational direction.			
4b.	Knowledge of appropriate and confidential documentation.			
4c.	Establishment of documentation system and reporting.			
4d.	Is accountable to maintain appropriate therapeutic boundaries.			
4e.	Maintains active registration with the state nursing regulatory body.			
4f.	Maintains Nursing Services Organization/Liability insurance.			
4g.	Actively identifies learning needs and seeks opportunities to enhance personal knowledge, growth and development.			

Faith Community Nurse sets goals (coordinating with the faith community pastor, leadership, or health cabinet):

- Establish Health Ministry: goals set within 60 days of completion of course.
- Health Outreach Plan: utilizing best practices within 90 days.
- Professional Accountability: documentation established within 6–12 months.

Used with permission from Interfaith Health & Wellness Association, a Program of Catholic Charities, Diocese of Palm Beach (2012).

Appendix H

Three Sample Services for Dedication or Commissioning of the Faith Community Nurse at a Faith Community or Health Care Institution

Litany of Dedication

This litany would be appropriate for use as part of a congregational worship service for the installation of a faith community nurse into the ministry of that congregation.

One: As people of healing and wholeness, we entrust our lives to the One who made us. We remind ourselves, each one of us, that we are not alone.

All: **As people of healing and wholeness, we entrust our lives to One who heals us. We remind ourselves, each one of us, that God's mercy is new each day.**

One: As people of healing and wholeness, we call forth one from among us to serve this congregation as a (parish nurse/faith community nurse).

(NAME), would you please come forward?

(NAME), you have been called to serve this congregation as a parish nurse/faith community nurse). Are you willing to accept this call?
If so, please say, "I am willing to serve."

(NAME), you have been called to care for the sick, comfort the afflicted, and encourage those who need support. Are you willing to care for those who are in pain?
If so, please say, "I am willing to serve."

You have also been called to be a leader in guiding the way to walk in paths that bring renewal and hope. Are you willing to serve in this manner, as well?
If so, please say, "I am willing to serve."

One: Sisters and Brothers, we are called together into ministries of care for the sick and encouragement for healthy living. Are you also willing to serve in this manner?
If so, please say, "We are willing to serve."

Unison Prayer

Loving God, we pray your blessing upon (NAME) this day as (she/he) begins (his/her) ministry as (parish nurse/faith community nurse) among us and with us on behalf of this congregation. Support, guide, and bless (NAME) as (he/she) seeks to answer the call to the ministry of faith community nursing, and grant (him/her) your strength, your wisdom, and your renewal. Help (NAME) to care for (his/her) own health and well-being, and help us all to work together to make ministries of caring central to our work, as we follow your call to preach, teach, and heal. Bless us as we minister together

to the hurting ones, the lonely ones, the wounded ones, and the weary ones, and help us take care of ourselves so that we may serve you all the days of our lives. It is in your precious Name we pray. Amen.

Suggested Hymn:

"Breathe on Me, Breath of God"
Words by Edwin Hatch 1886
Tune: TRENTHAM, S.M. by Robert Jackson 1894

Litany by Rev. Dr. Deborah L. Patterson.

Litany of Commissioning

This litany would be appropriate for use as part of a congregational worship service for the installation of a faith community nurse into the ministry of that congregation.

One: "There is an Indian proverb that says that everyone is a house with four rooms, a physical, a mental, an emotional, and a spiritual [room]. Most of us tend to live in one room most of the time but, unless we go into every room every day, even if only to keep it aired, we are not a complete person." (Rumer Godden)

All: **We dedicate the fruits of our labor to you, O God.**

One: "The lack of meaning in life is a soul-sickness whose full extent and full import our age has not as yet begun to comprehend." (Carl Jung)

All: **Bless our work that it may bring us purpose and satisfaction, and that it may bring our clients guidance and insight.**

One: "The great malady of our time, implicated in all our troubles and affecting us individually and socially, is 'loss of the soul.' When soul is neglected, it doesn't just go away; it appears symptomatically in obsessions, addictions, violence, and loss of meaning. Our temptation is to isolate these symptoms or to try to eradicate them one by one, but the root problem is that we have lost our wisdom about the soul, even our interest in it." (Thomas Moore)

All: **Bring healing to our world, O God. Bring peace in our time.**

One: "Healing is discovering how to live life in trust rather than in fear, how to relate to life as friend rather than enemy. It is about falling in love with life; learning to listen and respond to the longing impulses of the heart because these alone guide us to realize life's intention for us." (Anne Baring)

All: **Help us to teach trust, to teach courage, to teach love. Help us to listen, help us to respond, and help us to fulfill your plans for our lives.**

Prayer of Blessing (Unison)

Gentle and gracious God, bless each person gathered here today. Hear the groaning of our souls as we long for healing and wholeness in the world, in our communities, in every congregation and every home. Hear the tender entreaties of our spirits as we come to you with prayers for our families and for all the world. Hear us now as we lift up our silent joys and concerns to you. (A TIME OF SILENCE). **In your precious name we pray. Amen.**

One: (NAME OF FAITH COMMUNITY NURSE), would you please come forward? (NAME), you have been called as a (parish nurse/faith community nurse) to this congregation. This is a ministry of our entire congregation, but you have been entrusted with a special role in this work of healing and hope.

(NAME), do you promise to love God and serve God's people faithfully? If so, please respond, "I promise, with the help of God."

(TO THE CONGREGATION): Do you promise to love God and assist our faith community nurse in the ministries of healing to which we have all been called?

If so, please respond, "I promise, with the help of God."

Prayer of Commitment (Unison)

Loving One, bless us, whom you have called as disciples, that we may be a blessing to the frightened and the forgotten. Guiding One, help us to hear your voice and follow your paths in all that we do. Sheltering One, help us plant groves of knowledge that bear fruit in their season.

Help us teach wisdom and understanding. Help us preach justice and mercy. Help us bring the balm of love and compassion to a broken world.

Help us, our blessed Lord, always to feel your presence and strength, leading us through the trials and joys of life. Bless and sustain us all, and increase the ministries of healing that you are planting and tending. All this we pray in your precious and holy name. Amen.

Suggested Hymn:

There is a Balm in Gilead
For the Healing of the Nations
Lead Us from Death to Life
We Yearn, O Christ for Wholeness

Litany by Rev. Dr. Deborah L. Patterson.

Commissioning of New Faith Community Nurses

This commissioning service is suitable for use by a group of faith community nurses in a setting of a health system or faith community nurse program, or can be adapted to a congregational setting.

Gathering Music

Call to Worship

One:	Sisters (and brothers), entrust yourselves to the Rock of Ages, for you stand on Holy Ground.
All:	**Sisters, entrust yourselves to the Living Water, May it connect you, let you move, let your life flow.**
One:	Sisters, entrust yourselves to the warmth of the Spirit, May it bring you passion and love, let your inner fire glow.
All:	**Sisters, entrust yourselves to the breath of God's spirit, May it inspire you and refresh you and give you peace.**
Hymn:	"Breathe on Me, Breath of God"

Breathe on me, Breath of God, fill me with life anew
That I may love the way you love and do what you would do.

Breathe on me, Breath of God, until my heart is pure,
Until with you I will one will, to do and to endure.

Breathe on me, Breath of God, stir in me one desire:
That every earthly part of me may glow with holy fire.

Words by Edwin Hatch, 1886, alt.
Tune: TRENTHAM, S.M. by Robert Jackson, 1894

A Time of Silent Prayer

Scripture Romans 8:26b
"The Spirit intercedes for us with sighs too deep for words."

Meditation

Prayer of Blessing (Unison)

Gentle and generous God, bless each one gathered here this day, whom you have called as your disciples, that we may go forth to touch and bless all those among whom we minister. Guide us by your wisdom, so that we may be empowered to plant hope where it is most needed. Fill us with your courage, to speak the truth in love, and to act boldly on behalf of those who are in need of healing and understanding.

Touch each faith community nurse with tender comfort as they walk with those in pain and fear. When they are weary, hold each of them gently in your

loving arms, and plant within their spirits songs of hope and refreshment. Let each of them sing praises daily to you for your faithfulness and loving kindness to all Creation, we pray in your Holy name. Amen.

Hymn: "In Our Hearts and Neighborhoods"
Tune: Royal Oak ("All Things Bright and Beautiful")
Music by Cecil F. Alexander, 1848 (Public Domain)

Refrain: In our hearts and neighborhoods we sow the seeds of peace.
We would plant community, love's harvest to increase.

Verse 1: We work for hope and healing, we seek the lonely soul.
We stretch out hands in friendship, that God might make us whole.
Refrain

Verse 2: We pray for all the children, for youth who need our care,
For lonely homebound elders whose gifts they long to share.
Refrain

Verse 3: Oh, send us forth in courage, equipped with grace to know
Diversity's rich garden, God's love and care to grow.
Refrain

Words © 1996, Rev. Dr. Deborah L. Patterson

Benediction

Help us, loving Creator, always to feel your nourishing presence, calling us on. Bless and sustain the ministries of faith community nursing that you have called and are calling forth. We pray in your Holy name. Amen.

Dismissal to Serve

Litany by Rev. Dr. Deborah L. Patterson.

Preparing for Theological Reflection
Advocate Health Care Parish Nurse Ministry
Sample Process for
LECTIO DIVINA

God approaches us through Scripture.
- Select a Scripture text.
- Read Scripture aloud twice.
- Be silent for 3–5 minutes. Allow a word or phrase to choose you. Silently repeat the word or phrase on every breath as if each repetition is taking a step closer to God. The goal is not to think about God, but to draw near to God.
- Share your word or phrase without elaboration.

God speaks to us through our experience.
- Read Scripture aloud once.
- Be silent for 3–5 minutes. Allow the word or phrase to relate with your memories, hopes, dreams, feelings, and five senses. *Do not interpret.* If you find yourself analyzing, simply redirect the prayer with your repeated word.
- Share aloud your word or phrase, as well as your experiences associated with the word or phrase, as if you were merely describing something you observed. Use all of your feelings and all of your senses in your description. Invite others to relate to your story *without interpretation.*

God invites us into relationship.
- Read Scripture aloud once.
- Be silent for 3–5 minutes. Silently repeat the word or phrase on each breath. Allow your experience to relate to the group's experience.
- Offer interpretation for all that has been shared.

Some additional Lectio Divina resources:
- Casey, Michael. Sacred Reading: *The Ancient Art of Lectio Divina* (1966) is one of the best spiritual instruction books and the best on the topic of Lectio Divina.
- Websites: www.centeringprayer.com (Rev. Thomas Keating) and www.ocarm.org (Carmelite Sisters)
- Website for Scripture: www.biblegateway.com

Appendix I

Sample Faith Community Health Needs Survey

Thank you for taking the time to complete this survey. Please turn it in at the end of the service to a Wellness Committee member. By answering the following questions, a list of topics will be created for programming and education at (name of faith community) that you will find helpful.

Please indicate the number of family members living in your household:
___0–12 yrs___13–17 yrs___18–30 yrs___31–50 yrs___51–65 yrs___66–80 yrs___81 and older

1. Do you or any family members have any health problems? Please give a brief explanation.
   _____
   _____

2. Please list suggestions for health programs that you would like to have presented.
   _____
   _____

3. What time and day would you come to a health program?
   _____
   _____

4. What would you like to see the faith community nurse program do for the church community?
   _____
   _____

5. Do you have any experience in any health field that you would be willing to teach or share with the community of this church? (Explain.)
   _____
   _____

6. What do you do for your spiritual and emotional health?
   _____
   _____

7. Self-help groups may be developed to meet the interests and needs of the greatest number of people. Please indicate if you would participate in any of the following. You may mark as many as you would participate in.
   ____Multiple Sclerosis ____Living with Chronic Illness ____Loneliness ____Loss and Grief
   ____Caregiving to Chronically Ill   ____Arthritis   ____ Diabetes
   ____Cancer   ____Weight Control   ____Caregiving to Aged Relative
   ____Other _____

8. If a nurse were available in the congregation office on Sunday mornings, would you visit?
   ____Yes ____No

   Why or why not ? _____

9. If a library of self-help books were available, would you utilize it? ____Yes ____No
   If yes, what topics would be of interest?
   __Depression __Mental Illness __Stress __Grief __Healthy Lifestyle
   ___Other_____

Please remember this is a **CONFIDENTIAL SURVEY**. The information will be used only to set up programs to benefit the church. **No names will ever be used**.

You may drop this survey in any box at any church door or in the collection basket. Your prompt response will be greatly appreciated. Thank you for your help, and may God bless!

Name _____

Unit II: Professionalism
Communication and Collaboration

Communication and Collaboration

Introduction

Learning Outcomes

Upon completion of this module, the participant will be able to:

1. Incorporate active listening and presence in communication techniques.
2. Participate effectively in the ministerial team.
3. Participate in conflict resolution in the context of health care consumer care within faith community and/or health care settings.
4. Examine the impact of the faith community nurse's personality type and communication styles on functioning within the ministerial team.

Description

This module provides the fundamental principles of positive communication and an introduction to the role of collaboration with other members of the ministry group and the faith community. It will incorporate activities to assess communication styles; practice various methods of communication, including conflict resolution; and reflect on communication techniques of self and others.

Hours: 2

Research

An important role of the faith community nurse (FCN) is health risk assessment. Another role is to work in collaboration with other health care providers. Both of these nursing interventions are documented throughout Nursing Interventions Classifications (NIC) for nurses in various practice areas (Dandridge, 2014).

A literature review by Dandridge (2014) reveals that many interventions involved risk assessment and collaboration with other providers. To plan an osteoporosis prevention and management program in a faith community, a parish nurse, a family nurse practitioner, and a registered dietitian worked together (Foster-Burke, Ritter, & Zimmer, 2010). "Defy Diabetes!" partnered with a hospital system, certified diabetes educators, and parish nurses in multiple faith communities (Austin et al., 2013). Willis & Kricten (2012) reported on a collaboration between a community teaching hospital's trauma services and FCNs to increase awareness and provide resources for injury prevention in the faith community. Although not an intervention with individuals, a state university partnered with a large hospital-based parish nurse program to assess an underserved community for health risks and develop programming (Maitlen, Bockstahler, & Belcher, 2012).

Faith Tradition

Many denominations have a formal group in their faith communities, often called the health ministry team or care and concern team. This group is charged with the care of the people of the faith community. This can include, but is not limited to, visitation, transportation, meals, prayers, and cards. As the FCN will often be a member of this team, it is crucial for the FCN to have strong communication and collaboration skills, along with a fundamental knowledge of conflict management. This group also interfaces with individual members and other groups in the faith community, which requires skills in working with a variety of personalities and work styles.

Key Terms

Collaboration: the process whereby two or more individuals or organizations work together to achieve a task or common goal

Communication: interpersonal activity that involves the transmission of messages by a source to a receiver for the purpose of influencing the receiver's behavior

Conflict: strong disagreement between individuals or groups

Presence: the awakening that calls us into a conscious engagement with some aspect of the current moment

Therapeutic communication: interpersonal interaction between the nurse and the client during which the nurse focuses on the client's specific needs to promote an effective exchange of information (Videbeck, 2011)

Reflection

"Let the words of my mouth and the meditation of my heart be acceptable to you, O LORD, my rock and my redeemer."
—Psalm 19:14

"In one's family, respect and listening are the source of harmony."
—Buddha, Spiritual Leader 560–480 BC

Communication and Collaboration

Content Outline

KEY TERM

Communication *is an interpersonal activity that involves the transmission of messages.*

OUTCOME 1

Incorporate active listening and presence in communication techniques.

Definitions to Understand Communication

Appendices A, B, and C to this module offer further resources for effective communication.

Communication consists of interpersonal activity that involves the transmission of messages by a source to a receiver for the purpose of influencing the receiver's behavior.

The basic assumptions of communication include:
- It is impossible *not* to communicate.
- Faulty communication results in flawed feeling and actions.
- Feedback is the only way we know that our perceptions are valid.
- Linear communication involves a sender, a message, and a receiver.
- Communication is circular, transactional, and theoretical; it involves a linear context and includes feedback loops and opportunities for validation.
- Metacommunication involves nonverbal communication, such as body language, culture, facial expressions, gender, and appearance.

KEY TERM

Therapeutic communication *is interpersonal interaction between the nurse and the client focused on the client's needs.*

Therapeutic communication is interpersonal interaction between the nurse and the client during which the nurse focuses on the client's specific needs to promote an effective exchange of information (Videbeck, 2011). Therapeutic communication is not therapy, giving advice, or providing answers.

Characteristics of therapeutic communication include:
- goal-directed
- time limited
- focused

Considerations of therapeutic communication in the ministry of faith community nursing include:

- relationship between the FCN and the person ("being with" or presence)
- ethical considerations
- legal considerations and the Nursing Practice Act

Supportive Listening

Supportive listening is intentionally absorbing what the other person says. It takes practice, patience, and significant respect for the speaker.

- It is reflective and serves to hold up a mirror for the speaker to hear his or her words in a deeper, different way.
- The listener must relinquish control of the conversation; it is sometimes counterintuitive to give control to the speaker.

A member of the faith community who has just gone through a difficult experience may be overwhelmed and want to talk to someone. The person is not seeking advice, but connection, and a sense of relief from what he or she is going through.

- As a supportive listener, the FCN could invite this person to talk about the difficult experience and listen attentively, giving the person as much space as possible to talk.
- Occasionally the FCN would check in with the speaker, in a specific way, to reconfirm the connection and encourage the person to continue talking and thinking.

A supportive listener does not guess at feelings but rather works with what the speaker explicitly says. This may or may not include feelings. If it does not, be careful not to project feelings onto the speaker.

- In supportive listening, the common pattern is one of the speaker talking for a while, and then the listener quite briefly reflecting back in a specific way.
- Example: The FCN might say, "Tell me more about how it has been for you since your husband died." Then after listening to the individual describe the experience, the FCN might briefly say, "I can see this has been very difficult for you; please tell me more."

Active Listening

Active listening, a foundational communication technique, is a participatory conversation in which the FCN is listening with all of the senses, providing an active interpretation, giving feedback, and requesting validation from the person.

Nonverbal communication (both nurse and client) includes:
- physical: body movements, facial expressions, eye contact, gestures, posture, gait and clothing
- cultural setting
- gender differences
- generational differences

Methods of active listening include:
- repetition
- reflection

HELPFUL RESOURCE
See Appendix A, Characteristics of Therapeutic Communication, for more information on this topic.

Critical Thinking
In the context of the health care community and in the context of the faith community, how is language used?

How does an FCN learn the language of the community (vocabulary, grammar, syntax)?

Are we aware of the language that nurses speak, and the language that others speak to us?

KEY TERM

Presence *is the awakening that calls us into a conscious engagement.*

HELPFUL RESOURCE

See Appendix B, Communication Techniques, for more information on this topic.

HELPFUL RESOURCE

See Appendix C, Communication Blockers, for more information on this topic.

Critical Thinking

What stops someone from practicing Presence?

Where will the FCN use the skills of therapeutic communication?

How can the FCN teach others to use therapeutic communication?

- paraphrasing
- summarizing
- facilitating responses with open-ended questions
- buffering with "Tell me more."

Active listening is similar to supportive listening in that when the listener does speak, it is without advice, judgment or guidance.

- When using active listening, the FCN "listens for meaning" in the speaker's story, often in terms of a feeling to guess at the feeling and feed it back to the speaker.
- Example: "I heard you say that it has been a difficult and overwhelming time since your husband died. Is that correct?"

Presence

Presence is the awakening that calls us into a conscious engagement with some aspect of the current moment. It is being there or being with in a way that is meaningful to another person (Benner, 2014). It does not necessarily require long periods of time. Techniques include:

- clearing your own mind so that internal conversation ceases
- often just listening
- being invited by the person to share in the time of need
- using eye contact and touch as culturally appropriate
- maintaining boundaries

People with real presence are "comfortable in their own skin."

- Presence is a wholistic experience, where our entire being—mind, body and spirit—is engaged, not just our minds alone.
- Example: The FCN authentically engages the individual who is expressing feelings about an overwhelming, difficult situation by sitting close to the speaker, leaning in to hear, and maintaining eye contact with a soft, receptive gaze while listening.

Common **barriers to communication** include:
- preoccupation
- personal insecurity
- unusual speech patterns or behavioral mannerisms
- physical discomfort

OUTCOME 2

Participate effectively in the ministerial team.

Ministerial Team

Health ministry teams take many forms. However, the concept of a ministry team may be the most effective approach for health and wellness in faith communities (McNamara, 2014).

The strength of a team approach includes the following.
- A team assumes a group of people; you are much stronger working together!
- A team requires action and innovation. A team is not satisfied

with doing things "the way we've always done them."

- A team might assemble for a time limited project or it might live on for years to do many projects.
- A team's structure is flexible according to what works in your situation. It might be structured like a committee or it might be quite informal (McNamara, 2014, p. 21–22).

The **factors that form a cohesive working group** fall into several categories:

- Vocation: members of the group see work as a part of self and share deep roots in convictions of faith.
- Shared authority: decisions about goals of the group arise out of team deliberation.
- The work of ministry: the group has specific areas of focus but one common focus is service to the faith community.
- Characteristics that bind the group together:
  - shared vision
  - compatible energy level
  - complementary personalities
  - experience of trust and respect
  - sense of humor
  - sensitivity to other team members' life challenges
  - freely shared praise, thanks, and celebration

Types of Staff Structures

A **hierarchical structure** depends on the head of the ministerial staff of the faith community. In some cases, the denomination may drive the structure.

- *Advantages*: efficiency and sense of purpose
- *Disadvantage*: lack of investment in goals

In a **collaborative structure**, decisions are made by a staff team.

- *Advantages*: high level of ownership, enhanced creativity, healthy independence, sharing of responsibility
- *Disadvantages*: great deal of time, can inhibit individual initiative

In an **independent structure**, staff members function independently of each other.

- *Advantages*: creativity, freedom to work alone
- *Disadvantages*: conflict from individuals having competitive followings within the faith community, little expression of caring among the staff, lack of awareness of overlap with the work of other staff, lack of common goals

Practical Issues on the Ministerial Staff

The **spiritual leader's comfort, experience and skill** in personnel administration and supervision may vary.

A **job description** for each person is necessary to decrease ambiguity. It should include:

BUILDING THE MINISTRY TEAM WITH INDIVIDUALS IN THE FAITH COMMUNITY

BUILDING THE MINISTRY TEAM WITH INDIVIDUALS IN THE FAITH COMMUNITY

In addition to interacting with ministerial staff, the FCN often will interact with a ministry team focused on health ministry. The ministry team should consist not only of staff, but of individuals in the faith community who are interested in promoting the health of the faith community. A balance of health professionals and non-health professionals is ideal. An assessment of their skills and talents will ensure that they are working within their gifting, which will ultimately contribute to the success of the ministry team (McNamara, 2014).

KEY TERM

Collaboration *is the process whereby two or more individuals or organizations work together.*

Critical Thinking

Describe a plan for leading group meetings in your faith community, including ground rules.

Describe a plan for participating in a group meeting being led by the spiritual leader or senior staff.

How can the FCN engage in team building as part of the ministerial staff?

- major position objectives
- the scope of the position
- specific responsibilities
- lines of communication and supervision
- the evaluation process

There are **unspoken rules or unstated authority** in every faith community:
- "We have always done it this way."
- Examination of the history of the faith community and past leaders, both elected and non-elected, give insight into the "rules."

Coordination and Collaboration

It is important to have face-to-face contact with clergy and significant team members at a set time apart from the weekly worship time.
- Discuss "ground rules" for how you will use your time together.
- Establish clear start and ending times.
- If necessary, talk about what topics are off-limits, such as individuals or issues outside the scope of your group.
- Ask people to silence phones, pagers, and mobile devices and refrain from using them during the meeting.
- The health ministry's activities must fit with other priorities and programs of the faith community.

Collaboration is the process whereby two or more individuals or organizations work together to achieve a task or common goal.
- Mutual goal setting is important for success.
- Establish frequency and means of feedback, both from other staff and from the faith community in general.

Smucker (2009) suggests these steps for collaboration.
1. Review roles.
2. Examine work and see what tasks can be done independently and which should be in tandem with others.
3. Describe how the FCN can be integrated into present work being done by ministerial team members.
4. Consider having team members complete a personality inventory to learn more about each other's gifts and challenges.

Wei-Skillem & Silver (2013) suggest these principles for effective collaboration.
- Focus on mission rather than growth.
- Focus on trust rather than control.
- Focus on others rather than yourself.
- Focus on sharing resources rather than garnering resources.
- Focus on the whole rather than the particular.

OUTCOME 3
Participate in conflict resolution in the context of healthcare consumer care within the faith community and/or healthcare settings.

Conflict is strong disagreement between individuals or groups. Conflict occurs when individuals or group members feel obstructed or irritated by one or more other group members.

Understanding Conflict

We **learn about conflict** because:
- Conflict is essential to growth, learning, awareness, intimacy, effectiveness, positive relationships, and to having a true dialogue.
- There will always be conflict; the Old and New Testaments are filled with examples of conflict.
- Conflict is not inherently negative.
- The goal is to get people to embrace conflict as a natural occurrence that supports growth and change.
- Conflict is an inevitable by-product of intense human interaction.
- Successfully managing conflict is less dangerous than the repression of conflict.

Types of conflict may be internal or external.
- **Internal conflict** exists within and may be easier to resolve with self-control, self-awareness, maturity, and employing the strategy of "choosing your battles." Controlling internal conflict prevents escalation.
- **External conflict** may be either situational or interpersonal.
  - Situational conflict is temporary and exists in the moment; limited resources and incompatible priorities are examples of situations that can cause conflict. The sooner it is resolved, the less chance of escalation.
  - Interpersonal conflict is the most difficult to resolve. It often involves an ongoing struggle for power or control, differing goals, ideas, or interpretation.

KEY TERM
Conflict *is strong disagreement between individuals or groups.*

Responding to Conflict

If the FCN also happens to be a spouse of the clergy or member of the group having conflict, he or she may have to step back and let others step in to resolve the conflict.

The key concept is to recognize conflict quickly and remain objective.

Conflict Responses
- avoidance*
- forcing with power
- capitulation
- excluding a member
- assertiveness

- accommodation*
- compromise*
*Often the preferred responses of females or nurses.

Principles for Resolving Conflict

Use these principles and processes to work through conflict.

- awareness
- honesty
- listening
- open communication
- intention to resolve the disagreement in as peaceful and mutually beneficial way as possible
- willingness to divest oneself of "being right"

Causes of Conflict

Determine what is causing the conflict. Is it:

- failed communication?
- personality conflict at a power level?
- values or goals differences?
- differences over methods?
- lack of cooperation, responsibility issues, noncompliance with rules?
- authority issues?
- competition for limited resources?
- use of fair procedures?

Finding the Path to Take

Understand the culture and context of the conflict.

- self awareness
- awareness of others

Listen with your heart.

- be open
- be empathetic

Embrace and acknowledge **emotions**.

Search beneath the conflict **for hidden meaning**.

Separate what matters from what's in the way.

- not who is right
- engage in dialogue

Learn from difficult behaviors.

- empathy
- patience
- perseverance

Problem-solve creatively and negotiate collaboratively.

Explore resistance and mediate.

OUTCOME 4

Examine the impact of the faith community nurse's personality type and communication styles on functioning within a ministerial team.

Personality and Its Impact on Working within a Ministerial Group

Understanding Individual Preferences

Each individual has **preferences**, whether or not they can articulate them. Some people have a healthier sense of "differentiated self" than others—they can have different opinions or values, but remain connected emotionally.

Key members of the faith community will have different **personality types**. It may be useful for a group to use a tool to understand the personalities on the team.

The **DISC** behavioral instrument identifies different personality types as:

   D—dominant: direct, outspoken, results-oriented, problem-solver

   I—influencer: friendly, outgoing, talkative, optimistic, people-oriented

   S—steady: team player, stable, consistent, peacemaker

   C—conscientious: logical, organized, methodical, detail-oriented

Identify gifts of each personality type or communication style, and discuss the impact of personality type on leadership style.

Ideally, ministry groups will have a blend of personalities. Diversity creates beauty. The group may wish to consider all of the members taking one of the personality inventory tools and discussing the results during a routine meeting or retreat building experience. Knowing how group members process information will result in a stronger, more effective group.

HELPFUL RESOURCE
See Personality Inventories in the Learning Activities for links to tools a group might use to better understand each other.

Critical Thinking

What is my communication style while working in a group? What steps can I take to identify the styles of others in my team ministry?

Standards of Professional Performance for Faith Community Nursing

Standard 11. Communication
The faith community nurse communicates effectively in a variety of formats in all areas of practice.

COMPETENCIES

The faith community nurse:
- Assesses communication format preferences of healthcare consumers, families, and colleagues.
- Assesses his or her own communication skills in encounters with healthcare consumers, families, and colleagues.
- Seeks continuous improvement of his or her own communication and conflict-resolution skills.
- Conveys information to healthcare consumers, families, the interprofessional team, and others in communication formats that promote accuracy.
- Questions the rationale supporting routine approaches to care processes and decisions when they do not appear to be in the best interest of the healthcare consumer.
- Discloses observations or concerns related to hazards and errors in care or the practice environment to the appropriate level.
- Maintains communication with other providers to minimize risks associated with transfers and transition in care delivery.
- Contributes his or her own professional perspective in discussions with the interprofessional team.

Standard 13. Collaboration
The faith community nurse collaborates with the healthcare consumer, family, and others in the conduct of nursing practice.

COMPETENCIES

The faith community nurse:
- Partners with others to effect change and produce positive outcomes through the sharing of knowledge about the healthcare consumer and the situation.
- Communicates with the healthcare consumer, family, groups, spiritual leaders, hospital and hospice chaplains, and other healthcare providers regarding healthcare consumer care and the faith community nurse's role in the provision of that care.
- Promotes conflict management and engagement.
- Participates in consensus building or conflict resolution in the context of healthcare consumer care within faith community and healthcare settings.
- Applies group process and negotiation techniques with healthcare consumers and colleagues.
- Adheres to standards and applicable codes of conduct that govern behavior among peers and colleagues to create a work environment that promotes cooperation, respect, and trust.
- Cooperates in creating a documented plan focused on outcomes and decisions related to care and delivery of services that indicates communication with healthcare consumers, families, and others.
- Engages in teamwork and team-building processes.
- Documents referrals, including hospice and other provisions for continuity of care outside the faith community.

Learning Activities

Personality Inventory

Instructions:
Preview the personality inventories below and select one to ask participants to take. Because the process can take 15–45 minutes, you may prefer to ask each participant to take the test prior to this module. If you order the inventories prior to class and administer them to participants during the class, plan your time accordingly.

Concise Personality *Online Profile* **Summarized (Standard)** is available at uniquelyyou.com. Similar to DISC, this tool details human behavior and personality temperaments. It's as easy as taking a survey that asks a series of quick questions. Users receive reports immediately online after completing the questionnaires. (Price: $10.00)

https://www.uniquelyyou.com/results.php?pageNum_rsCWResults=2

The DISC personality test is available on a variety of sites, including **Personality Profile Solutions** (https://www.discprofile.com/products/?c=7) and Corexcel (www.corexcel.com/html/disc-profile.htm). Also, DISC Personality Testing (http://discpersonalitytesting.com/) offers a free abbreviated online test with immediate results.

www.yourpersonality.net. This site provides a number of online personality and close relationships tests, experiments, and demonstrations that help users learn more about themselves and how they relate to others.

http://personality-testing.info offers a range of tests, among them, the Open Extended Jung Scales. The result users receive will be similar to Myers-Briggs Type Indicator.

Each test is designed to provide customized feedback based on responses. Have each participant take a personality inventory to identify his or her personality type prior to teaching the module. Have all participants use their personality type to divide into groups from one end of the spectrum to the other for each area. A discussion can then take place regarding the particular area and how the group might process a particular ministry issue or the person's issue. Consider inviting a spiritual leader who will work closest with the FCN to join participants in this session and also take the inventory.

Question:
After small group discussions, you may wish to have participants share insights with the larger group.

Compare and Contrast

Instructions:
Provide Bibles in three different versions or copies of the following passages. Ask participants to work in groups to compare and contrast each passage from three different versions of the Bible.

James 1:19–20
Revised Standard Version: Let every man be quick to hear, slow to speak, slow to anger, for the anger of man does not work the righteousness of God.

The Message: Post this at all the intersections, dear friends: Lead with your ears, follow up with your tongue, and let anger straggle along in the rear. God's righteousness doesn't grow from human anger.

New International Version: My dear brothers and sisters, take note of this: Everyone should be quick to listen, slow to speak and slow to become angry, because human anger does not produce the righteousness that God desires.

Psalm 19:14
Revised Standard Version: Let the words of my mouth and the meditation of my heart be acceptable in thy sight, O Lord, my rock and my redeemer.

The Message: These are the words in my mouth; these are what I chew on and pray. Accept them when I place them on the morning altar, O God, my Altar-Rock, God, Priest-of-My-Altar.

New International Version: May these words of my mouth and this meditation of my heart be pleasing in your sight, Lord, my Rock and my Redeemer.

Matthew 7:12
Revised Standard Version: So whatever you wish that men would do to you, do so to them; for this is the law and the prophets.

The Message: Here is a simple, rule-of-thumb guide for behavior: Ask yourself what you want people to do for you, then grab the initiative and do it for *them*. Add up God's Law and Prophets and this is what you get.

New International Version: So in everything, do to others what you would have them do to you, for this sums up the Law and the Prophets.

1 Corinthians 13:4–6
Revised Standard Version: Love is patient and kind; love is not jealous or boastful; it is not arrogant or rude. Love does not insist on its own way; it is not irritable or resentful; it does not rejoice at wrong, but rejoices in the right.

The Message: Love never gives up.
Love cares more for others than for self.
Love doesn't want what it doesn't have.
Love doesn't strut,
Doesn't have a swelled head,
Doesn't force itself on others,
Isn't always "me first,"
Doesn't fly off the handle,
Doesn't keep score of the sins of others,
Doesn't revel when others grovel,
Takes pleasure in the flowering of truth,
Puts up with anything,
Trusts God always,
Always looks for the best,
Never looks back,
But keeps going to the end.

New International Version: Love is patient, love is kind. It does not envy, it does not boast, it is not proud. It does not dishonor others, it is not self-seeking, it is not easily angered, it keeps no record of wrongs. Love does not delight in evil but rejoices with the truth.

Question:
1. How do the words resonate with you?

2. Which version seems to go with your way of speaking and hearing?

3. In your ministry, how will you put this charge to good use?

4. What does this verse say to you about communication?

My Father and the Lima Beans

Instructions:
Have the class read aloud *My Father and the Lima Beans* (Underwood, 1995). Each participant (including faculty) should read one paragraph until the story ends.

Question:
Why is diversity in faith community groups necessary, and how does this story capture what diversity means to a community?

Diagram the Ministerial Staff Structure

Instructions:
Ask the participants to diagram the structure of their ministerial staff, showing relationships and indicating whether it is hierarchical, independent, or collaborative, or a combination.

Question:
Encourage reflection on how the structures that emerge fit with the participants' preferred ways of interacting.

It's Not About the Nail

Instructions:
Watch the video "It's Not About the Nail" on YouTube: https://www.youtube.com/watch?v=-4EDhdAHrOg

Question:
Identify different communication styles and barriers to communication presented in this video.

Case Study: Medical Emergencies

Instructions:
In the large group, review the following case study and discuss ways in which coordination and collaboration might happen: staff meeting, pastoral staff meeting, prayer chains, pastoral care book, minutes from committee meetings, e-mail, and so on. Reflect on the pros and cons of each scenario.

Case Study:
A faith community experienced several medical emergencies during their weekly services over a four-month period. The spiritual leader asked the FCN to develop a Medical Response Team (MRT) that would be on call during scheduled weekly services to respond to the emergencies. The FCN called a meeting of individuals with a health care background to discuss the vision and mission and potential policies and procedures for the MRT. Some of the individuals thought that each incident should be documented and the situation should be reported to the faith community staff in charge of ministry to the sick. Other individuals were adamant that there should be no record of the medical incidents. The FCN suggested that legal counsel should be obtained and agreed to follow up with spiritual leaders to obtain legal counsel. The group agreed to have a second planning meeting in two weeks to discuss next steps in developing the MRT team.

In the meantime, the group of individuals who did not believe that record keeping was needed approached other members of the planning team to insist that they agree with them at the next meeting, threatening to withdraw from the MRT if others did not agree with their position. Disagreement over the vision and mission of the MRT, and the potential policies and procedures to accomplish the vision, resulted in team members competing with one another rather than collaborating, questioning each other's motives, and failing to trust the FCN who was leading the effort to develop a MRT. As these differences became more apparent, gossip within the faith community and complaining to others created increased offense and separation between individuals who needed to work together to accomplish the task.

Questions:
1. What strategies should the FCN implement to resolve this conflict?

2. What positive outcomes might be gained if this conflict is resolved?

References

Required Textbook

American Nurses Association and Health Ministries Association. (2012). *Scope and standards of practice: Faith community nursing* (2nd ed.). Silver Spring, MD: Nursesbooks. org.

References

Austin, S., Brennan-Jordan, N., Frenn, D., Kelman, G., Sheehan, A., Scotti, D. (2013). Defy Diabetes! A unique partnership with faith community/parish nurses to impact diabetes. *Journal of Christian Nursing, 30*(4), 238–243. doi:10.1097/ CNJ.0b013e3182a35fcb

Benner, D. (2014). *Presence and encounter*. Ada, Michigan: Brazos Press.

Dandridge, R. (2014). Faith Community/Parish Nurse Literature: Exciting Interventions, Unclear Outcomes. *Journal of Christian Nursing 31*(2), 100–107. doi: 10.1097/CNJ.0000 000000000063

Foster-Burke, D., Ritter, L., Zimmer, S. (2010). Collaboration of a model osteoporosis prevention and management program in a faith community. *Journal of Obstetric, Gynecologic, & Neonatal Nursing, 39*(2), 212–219. doi:10.1111/j.1552-6909.2010.01111.x

Maitlen L. A., Bockstahler A. M., Belcher A. E. (2012). Using community-based participatory research in parish nursing: A win-win situation! *Journal of Christian Nursing, 29*(4), 222–227.

McNamara, J. W. (2014). *Stronger together: Starting a health team in your congregation*. Memphis, TN: Church Health Center.

Smucker, C. (2009). *Faith Community Nursing: Developing a Quality Practice*. Silver Spring, MD: American Nurses Association.

Underwood, P. (1995). *My father and the lima beans*. Bayfield, CO: A Tribe of Two Press.

Videbeck, S. (2011). *Psychiatric Mental Health Nursing* (5th ed). Philadelphia: Wolters Kluwer/Lippincott Williams & Wilkins.

Wei-Skillem, J, and Silver, N. (2013). Four network principles for collaboration success *The Foundation Review, 5*(1), 121-129.

Willis R. E., Krichten, A. E. (2012). Stopping the ouch of injury: Injury prevention for faith community nurses. *Journal of Trauma Nursing, 19*(1), 17–22. doi:10.1097/JTN.0b013 e318249fb55

Additional References

Cohen, M. H. (2008). Professional communication and teamwork. *Creative Nursing, 14*(1), 17–23.

Epner, D. E., & Baile, W. F. (2011). Wooden's pyramid: Building a hierarchy of skills for successful communication. *Medical Teacher, 33*, 39–43.

Judd, M. (2013). Broken communication in nursing can kill: Teaching communication is vital. *Creative Nursing, 19*(2), 101–104.

Lackey, S. A. (2009, April). Opening the door to spiritually sensitive nursing care. *Nursing 2009, (39)*4, 46–48.

Lenciono, P. (2011) *The five dysfunctions of a team*. San Francisco: Jossey-Bass.

Morris, G. S., Miller, S. M. A new day for faith community nursing. *Journal of Christian Nursing, 31*(2), 112–116. doi:10.1097/ CNJ.0000000000000064

Mueller, C. D. (2010, November-December). Create sacred space with stories: Storytelling as a formation tool and spiritual practice. *Health Progress*, 17–21.

Roberts, S. B. (2012). *Professional spiritual & pastoral care: A practical clergy and chaplain's handbook*. Woodstock, VT: SkyLight Paths Publishing.

Sroczynski, M. (2003). The art of managing difficult conversations. *Proceedings from the Eighth Annual Conference for Nurse Leaders and Managers*. Saint Anselm College, Manchester, NH.

Wagner, J., Liston, B., & Miller, J. (2011). Developing interprofessional communication skills. *Teaching and Learning in Nursing, (6)*97–101.

Weeks, H. (2010). *Failure to Communicate: How conversations go wrong and what you can do to right them*. Boston: Harvard Business Review Press.

Wright, S., & Neuberger, J. (2013). Spiritual expression: A manifesto for spirituality in health care, issued last year by Stephen Wright and Julia Neuberger, prompted passionate responses. *Nursing Standard, 27*(41), 16–18.

Online Resources

Boother, D. (2012). Gender benders: gender negotiation communication style differences.

http://www.negotiations.com/articles/gender-bender/.

Corexcel. www.corexcel.com/html/disc-profile.htm

DISC Personality Testing. http://discpersonalitytesting.com/

Harvard Law School. Free reports on team building strategies. Program on Negotiation at Harvard Law School. Retrieved June 3, 2014 from http://www.pon.harvard.edu/free-reports/

Personality Profile Solutions (https://www.discprofile.com/ products/?c=7)

Presbyterian Church USA. (1992). *Seeking to be faithful together: Guidelines during time of disagreement*. Retrieved June 3, 2014 from http://www.pcusa.org/resource/seeking-be-faithful-together/

Process of Communication videos: http://youtu.be/ uDwhQpSirOY or http://youtu.be/64MvcVq3

Wrap-Up and Evaluation

Measuring Competency

This chart can be used to assess the individual outcomes in this module.
- A copy of this chart is attached to the Participant Module, so that each participant can complete this short evaluation.
- Have participants read each outcome and then place an X in the box that best matches their opinion about the objective being met.
- Encourage each participant to write a short reflection about this module in the space provided at the bottom of this chart.
- Use this data to make any necessary changes.

Outcome	Not Met	Somewhat Met	Met
1. Incorporate active listening and presence in communication techniques.			
2. Participate effectively in the ministerial team.			
3. Participate in conflict resolution in the context of healthcare consumer care within faith community and/or healthcare settings.			
4. Examine the impact of the faith community nurse's personality type and communication styles on functioning within a ministerial team.			
Reflection: *In one paragraph, write a reflection on this module.*			

Appendix A

Characteristics of Therapeutic Communication

1. **Self-awareness.** Work at becoming aware of your personal communication style and how it affects other people. Keep focus on the individual or family, not on the FCN.

2. **Awareness of the needs of others.** Be sensitive to the needs of others. Send clear messages, affirming the individual or family and respecting their values.

3. **Use simple, clear messages.** Verbal and nonverbal messages must support one another; avoid words with complex or multiple meanings; exclude tangential and irrelevant details.

4. **Use a flexible communication style.** Continuously assess and adjust your style to meet the individual needs of the individual or family.

5. **Appropriate timing.** The same message delivered when the listener is tired or preoccupied with other matters will be received differently than in times of relative tranquility.

6. **Ask for feedback.** Use feedback to determine if the message received is the same as the message sent. This allows the speaker to correct misperceptions and distortions, or give more information to enhance understanding.

7. **Environment and physical factors.**
   - Quiet, calm setting that allows little chance for interruptions or distractions.
   - Awareness of personal space. Must be aware of nonverbal behaviors (shifting position, rapid eye movements, moving away) on the part of the individual that indicate a need for more personal space.
   - Use culturally appropriate eye contact.

8. **Active listening** is a "dynamic process whereby a person hears a message, decodes its meaning, and conveys an understanding about the meaning to the sender" (Arnold and Boggs, 2003). In the communication process, active listening is as important as talking.
   - It is possible to hear what someone is saying without really listening. Listening involves taking words and sounds that are sent and constructing meaning.
   - Through active listening, meaning derived from the listening process may be different from what the sender intended. This can be attributed to the values, expectations, and experiences that the listener assigns to the message.
   - Active listening involves listening for themes. What are the important thoughts and feelings underlying the other's words and nonverbal behaviors? What is explicitly stated as well as what is implicit in the message?

Appendix B

Communication Techniques

1. **Use of encouragers.** Simple leads integrated into a conversation such as "go on" or "tell me more," along with leaning forward, nodding, and smiling indicate interest.

2. **Use of questions** to elicit more information.
   - Open-ended questions are inquiries that allow the person to respond in a variety of ways. They begin with: what, how, when, can you tell me, or can you give me an example?
   - Closed-ended questions are those that can be answered "yes," "no," or with a one-word answer. These questions are restrictive but are very useful to obtain information quickly, such as, "Have you had these feelings before?"

3. **Restating** is repeating or rephrasing all or part of the other person's message. This is used for emphasis or clarity and should be used sparingly.

4. **Clarifying** is seeking to understand the message by asking for more information when the message is vague and difficult to follow. Example: "I'm sorry. I'm confused. Can you give me an example of what you mean?"

5. **Reflecting** is stating what was said in the same or different words. Example: "You've really had a tough time recently."

6. **Silence** allows the other person time to think about what has been said and is very helpful when powerful emotions are being shared; for instance, when the other is crying. A short silence can be followed by an empathetic statement such as, "This subject seems very painful to you." Silence is also useful following a point that needs to be emphasized.

7. **Summarizing** is similar to paraphrasing in that it makes a statement about the content of the communication. Summarizing synthesizes several messages and links themes and feelings. Example: "It sounds as if you would find it difficult to apply for that job because you don't have a resume, you lack confidence about the interview, and you are afraid you will not be able to explain your recent hospitalization."

8. **Appropriate verbal interventions include:**
   - *Identifying the strengths* of the other person, including personal characteristics, social support, and situational opportunities.
   - *Confronting.* The nurse must gently, but honestly, confront the individual with the reality of the behavior.
   - *Setting limits.* Sometimes the other person engages in "scapegoating," excessive self-blame or blaming others, emotional withdrawal, and aggressiveness to self or others. Such behavior needs to be addressed directly.
   - *Giving constructive feedback.* Feedback helps others change distorted patterns of thinking, feeling, and behaving. Reality-based communication allows the other person to clarify, expand, and reframe his or her experiences.
   - *Redirecting.* Redirection is used to refocus the person from a tangential train of thought to a more direct discussion of the topic.
   - *Modeling.* Modeling is a strategy that puts into words or actions behaviors to help the other see what the behavior looks like to others. Role-playing is an active, conscious form of modeling in which the person acts out desired patterns of behavior before using them in real-life situations.
   - *Reframing.* Reframing offers a different interpretation of a situation. When the nurse modifies the meaning of a situation through reframing, the individual is able to select from a broader field of options for changing behavior.
   - *Using humor.* Humor can be used to ease an overly intense moment and help to put things in perspective.

9. **Confirming responses** are designed to validate the individual. It is a way to acknowledge the person's feelings.

10. **Feedback** gives information to the person about their behaviors, ideas, and actions.

Appendix C

Communication Blockers

1. **Giving advice.** This prevents the person from expressing feelings about a situation.

2. **Blaming the client.** This forces the person to defend actions or non-actions and prevents the person from sharing weaknesses.

3. **Changing the topic inappropriately.** This communicates a lack of interest in what the person is trying to say.

4. **Defensiveness.** This places a barrier between you and the person and states that you are more interested in protecting your own position than in hearing their situation.

5. **False reassurance.** This devalues the fears and concern that the person is experiencing and says that you are not willing to hear their pain.

6. **Judging the client.** This places you in a position of authority over the person and prevents him or her from sharing weaknesses.

7. **Leading statements.** This limits what the person feels is of interest to you and does not create a space for them to truly express themselves.

8. **Moralizing.** This points out error or holds out a standard of conduct that is not person centered.

9. **Multiple questions.** This prevents clients from responding to your first question and increases pressure on them.

10. **Overuse of closed-ended questions.** This puts up an interrogation mode that limits responses to yes and no answers.

11. **Parroting.** This mindlessly repeats what they have just said and makes the person question your attention to them.

12. **Patronizing the client.** This is a "put-down" to people and indicates that you don't see them as fully equal humans.

13. **Placating the client.** This gives the impression that you want to say an easy answer and move on. It does not communicate real concern.

14. **Rationalizing feelings.** This means finding an easy excuse for the feelings the person is having. It devalues their experience.

15. **Stumped silence.** This is not the easy silence of presence but conveys that you do not know how to respond or direct the conversation.

16. *Why* **questions.** These questions are the basis for peoples' feelings and may make them feel invalid.

Unit III
Wholistic Health

Unit III: Wholistic Health

Health Promotion

Health Promotion

Introduction

Learning Outcomes

Upon completion of this module, the participant will be able to:

1. Use knowledge of various definitions of health to compose a personal definition of health.
2. Compare and contrast health promotion and disease prevention.
3. Provide health teaching for individuals or groups that addresses such topics as healthy lifestyles, risk-reducing behaviors, developmental needs, activities of daily living, preventive self-care, and spiritual practices for health and healing.
4. Use selected professional standards as a guide for developing health promotion programs.
5. Use health promotion and health teaching methods appropriate to the situation and the health care consumer's values, beliefs, health practices, developmental level, learning needs, readiness and ability to learn, language preference, spirituality, culture, and socioeconomic status.

Description

This module discusses the concept of health promotion as it relates to the practice of faith community nursing. "Health Promotion is the process of enabling people to increase control over their health and its determinants and, thereby, improve their health" (WHO, 2005).

This definition is based on the positive and inclusive concept of health (physical, mental, social and spiritual) as a critical human right and determinant of the quality of life everyone should have.

Hours: 2.5–3

Research

Odulana et al. (2014) conducted a survey of adult congregants (n = 1,204) of 11 predominantly African-American churches in North Carolina to determine willingness to attend health promotion activities. Congregants' belief in the church's role in health promotion and their desire to learn about healthy behaviors highlights the role of the African-American church as a partner in addressing health disparities and the need to capitalize on this expectation through stronger partnerships between medical and faith communities. The White House Office of Faith-Based and Neighborhood Partnerships offers the highest-profile markers of federal efforts. Formal partnerships between the faith-based and public health sectors are instrumental for achieving both domestic and global health promotion priorities (Levin, 2014).

Faith Tradition

The following excerpts from a statement of the Catholic Church prior to the passage of the Affordable Care Act indicate the church's support of health promotion.

"As Catholics, we are proud of the Church's health care contribution to the world. Indeed, the hospital was originally an innovation of the Catholic faithful responding to our Lord's call to care for the sick, 'I was sick and you took care of me, I was in prison and you visited me' (Matthew 25, v. 35–36). All individuals, including those who receive assistance for health care, must be given incentives for good preventative practices: proper diet, moderate exercise, and cessation or moderation of tobacco and alcohol use. The gift of life comes only from God, and to spurn that gift by seriously mistreating our own health is morally wrong.

"Following ... the sense of the life and dignity of every human person, it is vital to preserve, on the part of individuals and their families, the right to make well-informed decisions concerning their care. The needed change in health care must therefore flow from certain principles that protect the fundamental life and dignity of the human person and the societal principles of justice" (Naumann & Finn 2010).

Key Terms

Active learning: a planned series of actions or events to invite the participant to process, apply, interact and share experiences as part of the educational process

Disease prevention: measures not only to prevent the occurrence of disease, such as risk factor reduction, but also to arrest progress of disease and reduce its consequences once it is established

Health: a state of complete physical, mental and social well-being and not merely the absence of disease or infirmity (WHO, 1948)

Health promotion: the process of enabling people to increase control over their health and its determinants and thereby improve their health (WHO, 2005)

Reflection

"Are any among you sick? They should call for the elders of the church and have them pray over them, anointing them with oil in the name of the Lord. The prayer of faith will save the sick, and the Lord will raise them up; and anyone who has committed sins will be forgiven. Therefore confess your sins to one another, and pray for one another, so that you may be healed. The prayer of the righteous is powerful and effective."
—James 5:14–16

Health Promotion

Content Outline

KEY TERM

Health *is a state of complete physical, mental and social well-being.*

OUTCOME 1

Use knowledge of various definitions of health to compose a personal definition of health.

In the **medical model**, health has been defined primarily as an absence of physical and mental disease. The illness paradigm typically emphasizes disease rather than health and well-being.

In contrast, the most often cited definition from the **World Health Organization** (WHO) is: "Health is a state of complete physical, mental and social well-being and not merely the absence of disease or infirmity."

While this definition, first published in 1948, has remained unchanged, during the **Ottawa Charter for Health Promotion** in 1986, the WHO expanded the understanding of health to be "… a resource for everyday life, not the objective of living. Health is a positive concept emphasizing social and personal resources, as well as physical capacities."

- The Ottawa Charter further stressed that peace, shelter, education, food, income, a stable ecosystem, sustainable resources, social justice, and equity are necessary for health.
- This definition of health called for attention to socio-environmental conditions where war rather than peace is a certainty, areas ravaged by natural disasters such as earthquakes and floods, countries where infectious disease abounds, situations of widespread pollution, and locales where education is not available to everyone.
- Since few of us are in a complete state of physical, mental, social, and emotional well-being at all times, the WHO definition motivates us to grow in multiple ways.

The WHO definition of health is the most accepted definition, but numerous other definitions of health have been proposed. Some of these definitions **focus on individuals**.

- Health is a capacity for living (Carlson, 2003).
- Health is an optimal individualized fitness so that one lives a full, creative life (Goldsmith, 1972).
- Health is having a good quality of life (Brown et al., 1984).

Critical Thinking

What physical challenges, mental constructs, social obligations, or emotional feelings keep you from a wholistic sense of well-being as you live, love and learn?

- Health is an actualization of inherent and acquired human potential through goal-directed behavior, competent self-care and stratifying relationships with others ... while maintaining harmony with relevant environments (Pender, Murdaugh and Parsons, 2002).

Yet other definitions of health point to social and environmental contexts.

- Health is the state of optimum capacity to perform roles and tasks one has been socialized into (Parson, 1958).
- Health is the totality of life processes, which is evolving toward expanded consciousness (Newman, 1986).
- Health is an open process of becoming, a rhythmic coconstituting process of the individual—environment relationship, the individual's pattern of relating value priorities, an inter-subjective process of transcending with the possible and the individual's negentropic unfolding (Parse, 1981). http://currentnursing.com/nursing_theory/Rosemary_Pars_Human_Becoming_Theory.html
- Health is a dynamic state in the life cycle that implies adjustment to environmental stressors through optimum use of resources to achieve maximum potential for daily living (King, 1983, Raingruber, 2014).

Every individual's definition of health is unique, based on **cultural norms, faith beliefs, and values**. First, it is important for the faith community nurse (FCN) to consider a personal definition of health and then to determine how individual clients define their own health.

Every individual's definition of health is unique, based on cultural norms, faith beliefs, and values.

Critical Thinking

What are the basic components of health?

What is your personal definition of health?

OUTCOME 2

Compare and contrast health promotion and disease prevention.

This module will use the WHO definition from the Bangkok Charter for Health Promotion in a Globalized World (2005) which says: "Health promotion is the process of enabling people to increase control over their health and its determinants and thereby improve their health." This definition is based on the positive and inclusive concept of health (physical, mental, social and spiritual) as a critical human right and determinant of the quality of life everyone should have.

To facilitate that process, we must provide people with appropriate information. FCNs have a key role in providing that information to their congregations in the form of health teaching and education, advocacy, personal counseling, and utilizing community resources. This module focuses on the FCN's role of providing information in the form of health teaching and education.

FCNs are highly educated, experienced health professionals who bring accessibility and expertise to their faith communities.

KEY TERM

Health promotion *is the process of enabling people to increase control over their health and its determinants.*

Many insurance companies and some hospitals provide great examples of the value of access to the expertise of a nurse. Their clients can call in with a question, concern, or health issue and gain information while being advised of a plan of action right over the phone. FCNs can direct people to local resources and give out health and wellness information as well as be useful when parents seek well baby or well child information, information on vaccines, smoking cessation, addiction counseling, adolescent mental health resources, nutrition information, and so on. In these situations, access to accurate health information may enable people to increase control over their health.

The Meaning and Origin of Health Promotion

The concept of health promotion is generally believed to have developed in the last three decades. However, it has roots in ancient civilizations and in particular in **Greek antiquity**.

- As evident from medical and philosophical documents from as far back as the sixth to fourth centuries BC, "the ancient Greeks were the first to break with the metaphysical/ supernatural conceptions of health and disease that had so far dominated human societies" (Tountas, 2009).
- A physio-socratic school of thought, developed by the ancient Greeks, realized that maintaining good health and fighting illness were not metaphysical or supernatural, but depended on natural causes and that health and disease cannot be dissociated from particular physical and social environments, or from human behavior.

The concept experienced a **resurgence in popularity in the late 1940s** and has steadily gained attention in medical and political arenas.

- Through a series of international conferences, which began in Alma Ata, Russia in 1978 and continuing to the Helsinki, Finland 2013 Global Conference on Health, WHO has been the stimulus for globalized health promotion.
- As part of the global community, what affects one country affects other countries as well. Accepting this concept and the idea that the health of the population is a national asset, many governments acquiesced to actively support health policy initiatives that specifically address health promotion.

Healthy People 2020, the US's 10-year goals and objectives for health promotion and disease prevention, and "myHealthyPeople," a new challenge for technology application developers are examples of such initiatives.

- This plan was unveiled in December 2010 by the US Department of Health and Human Services.
- Healthy People has been committed to improving the quality of US health by producing a framework for public health prevention priorities and actions for the past 30 years.

Health Promotion and Disease Prevention Compared

Health promotion is sometimes used as a complementary term alongside disease prevention. Their definitions, while similar, are different.

Defining *Health Promotion*

The WHO statement from the Bangkok Charter for Health Promotion in a Globalized World (2005) is based on the positive and inclusive concept of health (physical, mental, social and spiritual) as a critical human right and determinant of the quality of life everyone should have.

Previous definitions of health promotion have focused on one or more of these elements.

1. **Health promotion as a goal or objective.** "Enhancement of health" includes positive health and enhancement of well-being; achieving health for all; and wholistic health (i.e., the inter-related domains of physical, mental, social and spiritual health).
2. **Health promotion as a process.** Health promotion empowers individuals and communities, which increases their control over decisions that affect their health.
3. **Health promotion as a perspective.** This relates to identifying and responding to health-related issues.
   - Health promotion takes a **sociocultural perspective**.
     - **understanding** the nature and origins of health-related issues or problems
     - **responding** to health-related issues/problems

     Health promotion focuses on the broader **socioeconomic environmental factors** that contribute to creating and enhancing inequities in health status. Strategies that are important in reducing the existence or impact of these social determinants of health include:
     - creating supportive environments
     - strengthening community actions
     - building healthy public policy
     - reorienting health services towards shifting balance of resources towards prevention, rather than clinical interventions
   - Health promotion focuses on **individual-level factors**.
     - developing/enhancing personal skills
     - influencing individual determinants of health-related behavior
     - behavior change (Bartholomew et. al 2011).
   - Health promotion interventions are also focused on the **population at large** and occasionally on high-risk environments. Unlike disease prevention, there is seldom a linear or direct relationship between cause and effect. Health problems have multiple interconnected causes and consequences.

HELPFUL RESOURCE
Theoretical models for explaining and directing health promotion have been used since the 1960s. See Appendix A, Health Belief Models.

The essence of health promotion is **empowerment**. Therefore, health professionals work in partnership with community members to empower people to take charge of their health by the following strategies.

- coalition development
- providing appropriate referrals
- advocacy
- teaching healthy lifestyles
- supporting lifestyle choices
- acting as a resource

As reflected in the strategies, community involvement is key when the socioenvironmental approach is used.

- An important aspect of the socioenvironmental approach is identification and support of cultural influences of the participants.
- Faith traditions or religious beliefs are also critical factors in changing behaviors. During assessment, the FCN should explore faith-based beliefs about health.

Defining *Disease Prevention*

Although there is frequent overlap between the content and strategies of health promotion and disease prevention, disease prevention is defined separately. Disease prevention is rooted in the medical model of health promotion, specifically the pioneering work of Leavell and Clark's model (1958) from their book *Natural History of Disease and the Application of Appropriate Preventive Measures*.

Disease prevention includes measures not only to **prevent the occurrence of disease**, such as risk factor reduction, but also to **arrest the progress of disease** and reduce its consequences once it is established.

Disease prevention in this context is considered action, which usually emanates from the health sector, dealing with individuals and populations identified as exhibiting identifiable risk factors, often associated with different risk behaviors.

The model has three levels of disease prevention.

1. **Primary prevention** is preventing a disease from occurring. It involves a plethora of interventions including teaching people about healthy behaviors.
2. **Secondary prevention** is the early detection and prompt treatment of disease and helping people change risky or unhealthy behaviors.
3. **Tertiary prevention** employs interventions to help the individual restore health, limit disability, and receive rehabilitation for disease sequelae.

Models explaining behavioral health and change may also be used.

- High-risk groups or people with unhealthy behaviors are the target group for interventions and strategies such as pharmaceuticals, screening for risk conditions, various

KEY TERM

Disease prevention *includes measures to prevent the occurrence of disease and to arrest the progress of disease.*

Critical Thinking

How can the FCN encourage individuals to take responsibility for their own health?

What health promotion strategies could you, as the FCN, implement to address a common health risk in your faith community?

therapies, surgery, and medical care for illnesses. Medical and allied health professionals manage care.

- The direct relationship between cause and effect often produce immediate dramatic, observable, measurable results. For instance, immunizing against the current strain of flu may result in fewer people infected each year.
- Cost benefit ratios for disease prevention interventions are easy to calculate compared to cost benefit ratios for health promotion measures.

The following table provides a comparison of key factors in disease prevention and health promotion.

Comparison of Disease Prevention and Health Promotion

Factor	Disease Prevention	Health Promotion
Target group of interventions	High-risk groups, which are defined as those with unhealthy lifestyles.	The population at large is the focus of interventions. Interventions also target high-risk environments.
Causes and effects	There is a direct relationship between cause and effect. For example, by immunizing against polio, the disease of polio is prevented.	There is no direct relationship. Each health problem has multiple causes that include a "web" of causes and a "web" of consequences.
Provider of care	Care is managed by the interprofessional team (physicians, nurses, physical therapists, social workers, and so on).	Professionals work in partnership with community residents to develop health initiatives.
Strategies used	Traditional medical interventions such as surgery, pharmaceuticals, screening for risk conditions, medical management, illness care, and therapies are used.	Interventions include establishing partnerships with community members, empowering citizens, advocacy, supporting lifestyle choices, developing coalitions, and acting as a resource.
Models employed	Included are specific approaches such as: (a) the medical approach including Leavell and Clark's disease prevention model (1958); and (b) the behavioral approach including the Health Belief Model, Pender's Health Promotion model (1982, 1986), or the Transtheoretical Model (1977).	In health promotion, the socioenvironmental approach is used. Community collaboration is key to implementing health strategies.
Types of data collected	Hard data such as drug use, incidence, and prevalence are gathered.	Soft data such as attitudes, behaviors, and awareness are collected.
When results are observable	Immediately measurable.	It may be a long time before the results of health promotion initiatives can be observed. It is often more than 10 years before one can measure the changes.
Cost-benefit ratio	Easier to measure than health promotion strategies. For example for every $1.00 spent on polio immunization, $6.00 is saved.	Hard to measure the cost benefit because of the long-term commitment.

OUTCOME 3

Provide health teaching for individuals or groups that addresses such topics as healthy lifestyles, risk-reducing behaviors, developmental needs, activities of daily living, preventive self-care, and spiritual practices for health and healing.

As an accepted and respected member of a congregation, the FCN embodies the integration of health promotion and wholistic care. The **functional roles of FCN ministry** promote faith and health through active involvement and visibility within the faith community.

- Presence, a substantial portion of the ministry, serves to deepen and strengthen relationships within the congregation over time. These relationships provide entry for the counseling role that includes listening and providing spiritual guidance from a wholistic perspective. With this perspective, the FCN can convey to others that a sense of well-being can be encouraged, even when medical healing cannot be achieved.
- The FCN is uniquely qualified to promote health not simply as the absence of disease but as spiritual, physical, social, and psychological well-being, and as a sense of harmony with self, others, the environment, and God.
- Health promotion-focused roles are central to faith community nursing practice. In the role of educator, the FCN disseminates information that supports optimal health and decreases health risks.
- The caring environment of the faith community is ideal for both formal and informal health teaching, as well as for opportunities for follow-up teaching with individuals.
- Promoting health through advocacy, the FCN represents the individual, family and congregation within the health care system and the community at large.
- The advocate, coordinator, and referral roles may all be simultaneously engaged to promote health by helping individuals and families navigate through systems, institutions, and agencies to access health care and by building connections when service gaps occur.

Health promotion and prevention program planning are extremely important to the practice of faith community nursing. In addition to the roles the FCN functions in to promote health in the faith community, additional tools are required to address the faith community's needs, which are varied and often extensive. The Scope and Standards of Practice for faith community nursing should be used to guide FCN practice.

Health promotion involves **teaching people about healthy behaviors**. The following list includes potential topics organized by age groups.

Infants and Children
- immunization guidelines
- bullying
- bicycle safety
- sex education classes
- sleep hygiene
- good touch and bad touch
- swimming safety
- self-esteem classes
- conflict resolution
- dental health
- first aid and CPR classes
- spiritual practices for health and healing

Adults
- prenatal care and childbirth
- fitness
- weight management
- advance directives
- relaxation and fitness
- conflict resolution
- marriage seminars
- parenting classes
- stress management
- first aid and CPR classes
- healthy cooking on a budget
- color your plate class (nutrition)
- disaster preparedness
- retirement planning
- spiritual practices for health and healing

Seniors
- advance directives
- importance of immunization for pneumonia and influenza
- finding health information on the Internet
- healthy cooking for one and two
- fitness
- spiritual practices for health and healing

In planning health promotion programs the FCN needs to be aware of **national and local resources**. In addition to resources that can be found in the *Accessing Resources* module, the following agencies have a primary focus on health promotion.

The American Public Health Association (APHA)
The mission of The American Public Health Association (APHA, www.apha.org) is to improve the health of the public and achieve equity in health status. APHA champions the health of all people and all communities. APHA strengthens the profession of public

health, shares the latest research and information, promotes best practices, and advocates for public health issues and policies grounded in research. This is the only organization that combines a perspective of more than 140 years, a broad-based member community, and the ability to influence federal policy to improve the public's health. APHA emphasizes the following areas:

- community
- science and evidence-based decision-making
- health equity
- disease prevention and wellness
- real progress in improving health

Centers for Disease Control and Prevention (CDC)

CDC (http://www.cdc.gov/healthyliving/) is one of the major operating components of the US Department of Health and Human Services. CDC's mission is to collaborate to create the expertise, information and tools that people and communities need to protect their health through health promotion; prevention of disease, injury and disability; and preparedness for new health threats. Whether diseases start at home or abroad, are chronic or acute, curable or preventable, human error or deliberate attack, CDC fights disease and supports communities and citizens to do the same.

As a health protection agency, CDC saves lives and protects people from health threats. To accomplish their mission, CDC conducts critical science and provides health information that protects against expensive and dangerous health threats, and responds when these arise. CDC provides tools and resources in the following areas.

- data and statistics
- health and safety features
- diseases and conditions features
- public health library and information center
- publications

Healthy People 2020

Healthy People 2020 (www.healthypeople.gov) is a 10-year agenda for improving the health in the US. This initiative is the result of a multiyear process that reflects input from a diverse group of individuals and organizations. The website contains information, clinical recommendations, and intervention strategies on a wide range of health topics. Healthy People 2020 works toward the following goals.

- Identify nationwide health improvement priorities.
- Increase public awareness and understanding of the determinants of health, disease, and disability and the opportunities for progress.
- Provide measurable objectives and goals that are applicable at the national, state and local levels.

- Engage multiple sectors to take actions to strengthen policies and improve practices that are driven by the best available evidence and knowledge.
- Identify critical research, evaluation, and data collection needs.

The overarching goals of Healthy People 2020 include the following.
- Attain high quality, longer lives free of preventable disease, disability, injury, and premature death.
- Achieve health equity, eliminate disparities, and improve the health of all groups.
- Create social and physical environments that promote good health for all.
- Promote quality of life, healthy development, and healthy behaviors across all life stages.

Four foundational health measures serve as indicators of progress towards achieving these goals.
- general health status
- health-related quality of life and well-being
- determinants of health
- disparities

Healthy People 2020 is organized into 39 established topic areas with objectives and these evolving new topics.
- adolescent health
- blood disorders and blood safety
- dementias, including Alzheimer's disease
- early and middle childhood
- genomics
- global health
- health care-associated infections
- health-related quality of life and well-being
- lesbian, gay, bisexual and transgender health
- older adults
- preparedness
- sleep health

Medline Plus
Medline Plus (http://www.nlm.nih.gov/medlineplus/aboutmedlineplus.html) is the US National Institutes of Health website for patients and their families and friends. Produced by the National Library of Medicine, it offers reliable, up-to-date information about diseases, conditions, wellness issues, drugs and supplements, and latest treatments. The site also features medical videos, illustrations, and links to the latest research.

World Health Organization (WHO, www.who.int/en/) is the directing and coordinating authority for health within the United Nations system and is responsible to provide leadership on global health matters, shape the health research agenda, set norms and standards, articulate evidence-based policy option,

Critical Thinking

How does the FCN demonstrate accountability for health promotion offerings?

How can an FCN include spiritual care when initiating health promotion activities?

provide technical support to countries and monitor and assess health trends. In the twenty-first century, health is a shared responsibility involving equitable access to essential care and collective defense against transnational threats.

OUTCOME 4

Use selected professional standards as a guide for developing health promotion programs.

Faith Community Nursing: Scope and Standards of Practice (2nd ed., 2012) delineates the practice of faith community nursing through specific standards that provide direction for professional nursing practice and a framework for evaluation of the practice.

FCNs may use a selection of these standards to develop a health promotion project for members of the faith community. The list of actions or activities offered with each standard is neither exhaustive nor complete. The following content is presented using the nursing process, which includes assessment, diagnoses, planning and evaluation.

Assessment

Standard 1: Assessment

Standard 1 says, "The faith community nurse collects comprehensive data pertinent to the health care consumer's wholistic health or the situation." Related to health promotion, this nursing step may include these actions or activities.

- Individual health risk appraisals can be brief self-assessment surveys (objective and subjective questions, biometric measurements and lifestyle questions).
- A comprehensive health risk appraisal includes biometric measurements, lab values, lifestyle questionnaire, used to determine personal strengths and health risks.
- A health needs assessment of the community at large will provide context for ministry within the faith community.
- A suggestion box helps develop information pertinent to FCN interventions and follow-up.
- Often, just knowing someone is listening will get people thinking differently and motivate them to verbalize needs and wishes.

Diagnoses

Standard 2: Diagnoses

Several standards apply to this step of the nursing process. Standard 2 says, "The faith community nurse analyzes the assessment data to determine the diagnoses or issues." Related to health promotion, **diagnoses** may include the following actions.

- Identify strengths, health risks, and issues to be addressed.
- Expect the assessments to provide the information for nursing diagnoses in order to prioritize and move forward in planning.

- Examining the individual or the groups within a congregation, and establishing their priorities or interests, provides a place to start.
- Determining the issues and building platforms for individuals and groups in the congregational setting helps the progress in planning for health awareness.
  - Comprehensive health risk appraisal tools: results should include national standards for health comparison and recommendations for improvement.
  - Self-assessment tools may be used for personalizing risks and interests and serve as the basis for planning short-term and year-long strategic health initiatives. Objective and subjective findings, biometric measurements and labs, and lifestyle questionnaires provide possible program content.
  - Community health needs assessment includes identification of environmental and social health determinants and helps identify best practices.

Standard 3 says, "The faith community nurse identifies expected outcomes for a plan individualized to the healthcare consumer or the situation." Related to health promotion, **outcomes identification** may include these activities.

Standard 3:
Outcomes Identification

- Discuss expectations with individuals, family and congregants involved. Clarification of outcomes improves participation and saves time and resources.
- Data from the assessment should be included in the discussion to clarify personal interpretation and understanding of issues.
- Discussion should help all parties decide if expectations, time requirements, and resources available are realistic and "doable." Planning should not progress until agreement is reached.
- Group goals must be identified and assessed to determine how they will support or hinder the expected outcome.
- Individual goals should be addressed and treated as delicately as group goals for the same reasons.
- Data collected related to health issues being addressed should include physical, mental, emotional and spiritual health.
- Open discussions of desired outcome and actions required to achieve each goal is essential.
- Projecting milestones to reach at certain points on a timeline is an element of expected outcome planning. What will be accomplished in three months, six months, and one year?
- Outline steps that need to be accomplished in order to reach the expected outcome.
- Cooperation of the pastor and other ministry leaders in planning for long-term projects can affect success. Remarks from the pulpit and respected leaders in the congregation about your project are often beneficial. Awareness of other

ministry initiatives will help avoid conflict and duplication of efforts.

- Distinguish health promotion from disease management in the outcomes and be specific as to either or both when identifying expected outcomes.

Planning

Several standards apply to the planning step of the nursing process.

Standard 4: Planning

Standard 4 says, "The faith community nurse develops a plan that prescribes strategies and alternatives to attain expected outcomes." Related to health promotion, **planning** includes these actions and questions.

- Identify the strategies to reach established goals and targeted priorities, such as weight loss, daily exercise and strength training, risk factor improvement, medication management, chronic disease management.
- During the planning process include the time to promote, present, and practice the elements of change.
- Review the organization's calendar for suitable times.
- Decide which, if any, pre-project training should take place. Are there refresher information presentations that will enhance or ensure the lifestyle change will be successful?
- Will you use experts to teach? How will you identify and contact them?
- Are any members of the congregation prepared and willing to work with you?
- Which community agencies or institutions will you work with?
- What will be the cost in time, for the team and monetarily?
- What data will you collect to measure your effort—attendance, number of men or women attending, elements of change achieved, and so on?

Standard 5: Implementation

Standard 5 says, "The faith community nurse implements the identified plan." Related to health promotion, **implementation** may include these actions.

- Create partnerships with individuals, families and congregational organizations to begin the plan in a safe, realistic and timely manner.
- Involve health cabinet or health ministry team members with tasks such as these.
  - Prepare room, sign in or register attendees, copy and distribute handouts, set up audio-visual equipment.
  - Develop a plan B in the event of equipment failures.
  - Assist with program presentations and data collections.

Standard 5B:
Health Teaching and
Health Promotion

Standard 5B says, "The faith community nurse employs strategies to promote wholistic health, wellness, and a safe environment." **Health teaching and health promotion** include these actions.

- Determine best practice material for presentation or speaker expertise.
- Select types of programs to present to accomplish outcomes, such as raising awareness or lifestyle change.
- Review program content prior to presentation for values clarification points.
- Include spiritual formation and progress as part of implementation.
- Track progress and collect data carefully.
- Expect goal revisions throughout course or term.
- Assure confidentiality of all procedures.

Standard 5C says, "The faith community nurse provides **consultation** to facilitate understanding and influence the specified plan of care, enhance the abilities of others, and effect change." Related to health promotion, consultation includes these actions.

Standard 5C: Consultation

- Seek guidance from the spiritual leader or other faith community leaders to ensure spiritual dimensions of health promotion are covered.
- Involve individuals, families and the faith community in decision-making regarding their goals and expectations.
- Offer recommendations.

Evaluation

Several standards apply to the evaluation step of the nursing process.

Standard 6 says, "The faith community nurse evaluates progress toward attainment of outcomes." The health committee or health ministry team and all participants in programming should be included in **evaluation** of efforts, lessons learned, what worked and what did not work, and so on. Related to health promotion, evaluation includes these points.

Standard 6: Evaluation

- components of the project
  - quality of speakers or presenters
  - module content
  - offering time—was it practical and effective?
  - resources (handouts, referrals, sources)—were they effective and economical?
  - results of data collection
  - individuals succeeding in personal goals
  - group achievement of goals
  - progress toward personal goal attainment
  - spiritual development through process of change (subjective is assumed)
- other necessary activities
  - celebration of successes
  - certificates of completion for all participants
  - gifts for special achievement, such as perfect attendance and positive attitude

Standard 7: Ethics

Standard 7 says, "The faith community nurse practices ethically." In relation to health promotion, **ethics** includes these points.

- The role of the FCN is to bring the results of the efforts into light for review at the local church level, for publication within denominations, and for state and national organizations.
- Results of evaluations are used to review for planning and future implementation.
- The cost-benefit ratios of the project as part of the overall theme for yearly implementation is evaluated in regard to:
  - number of successes
  - number of challenges and unsuccessful elements
- Aggregate data are shared with leadership, affiliated groups, and partners.

Standard 8: Education

Standard 8 says, "The faith community nurse attains knowledge and competence that reflect current nursing practice." Related to health promotion, **education** includes these points.

- The FCN uses the results to guide personal nursing practice.
- The FCN may need additional course preparation or continuing education to enhance teaching skills.
- A resource library for reference and ongoing health behavior information should be available for the congregation that includes such references as:
  - books, magazines and peer-reviewed journals
  - programs and courses
  - newsletters
  - online resources

Standard 13: Collaboration

Standard 13 says, "The faith community nurse collaborates with the healthcare consumer, family, and others in the conduct of nursing practice." Related to health promotion, **collaboration** includes these activities.

- The first collaboration the FCN makes is with participants during the assessment.
- Another important collaboration is with the spiritual leader and faith community leadership.
- During and after the planning stage, the FCN reaches out to other faith communities, professional organizations, state and local health departments to secure speakers, experts, materials and services to support the program being developed.
- The FCN works harmoniously with these organizations in resolving conflict and promoting trust.
- The FCN documents individual contributions and submits data for inclusion in the larger plan.

OUTCOME 5

Use health promotion and health teaching methods appropriate to the situation and the health care consumer's values, beliefs, health practices, developmental level, learning needs, readiness and ability to learn, language preference, spirituality, culture, and socioeconomic status.

Health promotion depends heavily on individuals, families, and groups such as faith communities having accurate, timely information in order to make decisions. Often the FCN can use resources within the faith community or from the broader community to provide information and supporting materials. There may also be times when the FCN has to construct original plans and present that information.

Preparing for Teaching and Learning

The information that follows is a brief introduction to teaching and learning, with an emphasis on adult learners who often comprise the target audience for health teaching and other health promotion activities.

Characteristics of Adult Learners

- Adult learners are self-directed and seek out learning activities to enhance their own knowledge and to meet their particular needs.
- Adult learners want to draw on their rich personal and professional experiences.
- Adults learn best when the information presented is contextual and relevant.
- Adults want to be able to apply new information and skills immediately.
- Sharing information with fellow participants is valued.
- While some adults may have a preference for material presented visually or auditorily, many adults are kinesthetic learners. They learn best when material is presented in a see, hear and *touch* format.
- Adult learning is most effective and enjoyable for the participant when it is interactive.
- When a learning activity builds in time for reflection during the learning process, the participant's application and retention of the material is enhanced.

Active Learning

When developing live educational activities to be presented to a small or large group, approximately 50 percent of the planning should be on content and 50 percent on the delivery of the material. Incorporating active learning strategies is a wise decision. When participants of any age are involved in their learning, rather than being passive observers, they are more

Critical Thinking

Does society have more responsibility for health than individuals? Explain your answer.

How can collaboration facilitate effectiveness of health promotion activities?

likely to master the information or concepts presented, apply them to their practice, and retain the information presented.

Active learning is a planned series of actions or events to invite the participant to process, interact and share experiences as part of the educational process. The interactive components support the goal and the educational objectives of the learning activity. When active learning strategies are used, the participant is reading, talking, writing, describing, touching, interacting, listening, and reflecting on the information and the materials presented.

- Active learning promotes problem solving, critical thinking, manipulation of materials, analysis, synthesis, and evaluation of the information.
- Active learning focuses on the desired outcome for the participant as a result of the learning activity.
- Active learning builds upon what we know from research regarding adult learning preferences and styles.

Learning Styles

Every person uses a mix of learning styles to process information. Knowing the learning styles of a person can assist the FCN in developing materials and presentations for that person. Numerous learning style inventories are available online. The recognized learning styles include the following.

- visual (spatial)—using pictures, images, and spatial understanding.
- aural (auditory-musical)—using sound and music
- verbal (linguistic)—using words, both in speech and writing
- physical (kinesthetic)—using your body, hands, and sense of touch
- logical (mathematical)—using logic, reasoning, and systems
- social (interpersonal)—learning in groups or with other people
- solitary (intrapersonal)—working alone and using self-study

Factors Affecting Learning

The importance of creating a learning environment is to accommodate learners so that they feel welcome, safe, and ready to take on learning tasks.

- Learners must perceive the learning environment as a safe place to share experiences and develop new ideas.
- FCNs can do this by setting a tone of mutual respect the very first day among everyone in the session.
- Ask participants to give examples of their good and bad past experiences related to sharing in classes. Sometimes experience is the best teacher!

The FCN should be the first to arrive in order to use the **welcoming approach**. Greet learners by name as they enter the room. Handshakes are good; hugs, if appropriate to the group, may also be exchanged.

A second important part of the learning environment for adult learners is **trust**.

- Creating a relationship of mutual trust between the facilitator and learner is imperative.
- Basic trust in relationships among adult learners requires openness, honesty and sensitivity.
- Trust leads to development of interpersonal communication skills, confidence, and desire to learn more.
- FCNs play a major role here. FCNs need to describe expectations and responsibilities of participants during the session as well as their own commitments and responsibilities to the participants. Discuss attendance, promptness, emergency contact numbers, successful completion of the project, and when and how to make suggestions, request changes, and express dissatisfaction.

Carefully consider the **physical environment** of the learning session.

- Control heating and ventilation for the comfort of participants.
- Lighting is an important consideration for the adult learner. Keep in mind visual acuity diminishes with age.
- Acoustics are an additional consideration for adult learners. Can everyone hear the discussion and comments?
- Information regarding restrooms, exits, breaks, lounges and public areas is important to discuss during the first meeting.
- Seating arrangements should foster communication. Use round large tables if the group is small or sit in a circle without tables. This formation gives the group a feeling of intimacy. If the room is large and rectangular tables are used place them in a *U* shape. This enables people to see each other face to face, and demonstrations can be performed in the *U* so everyone has a good sight line.

Make sure **equipment** used to support and enhance the learning session is properly functioning and in good repair.

- Facilitators should make certain they know how to operate the equipment even if there is a technical assistant with you. Practice before the session; do "a dry run" to refine your technique.
- Equipment should be set up and ready before participants arrive.
- Supplies should be accessible prior to class. Whenever possible have an extra set of handouts available.

Learning Objectives

The construction of a plan for teaching and learning usually begins with an assessment of the learners' needs or gap in their knowledge that prevents them from being or doing something. Often adult learners can provide this information through self-assessment.

HELPFUL RESOURCE

An example of self-assessment is completion of the wellness wheel in the Model for Healthy Living included in the Learning Activities.

A **learning objective or outcome** is a statement of what learners ought to be able to do as a consequence of instruction.
- What learners should be able to do at the end of a learning period that they could not do beforehand (Mager, 1997).
- " ... A description of a performance you want learners to be able to exhibit before you consider them competent. An objective describes an intended result of instruction, rather than the process of instruction itself" (Mager, 1997).
- " ... relatively specific statements about what learners should be able to do following instruction" (Gallagher and Smith, 1989).
- The **emphasis is on the learners** and what they should know or behaviors they should exhibit.

The **purpose of objectives** includes benefits for both instructor and learners.
- Guidance for instructor
  - selecting teaching and learning strategies
  - developing content
  - planning learner activities
  - determining evaluation techniques

- Guidance for learners
  - focus attention on what is important
  - know what to expect during the class

Strong objectives or outcomes include the **three domains of learning**.
- cognitive (knowing)
- psychomotor (doing)
- affective (feeling)

Precede your objectives with the statement: "At the conclusion of this activity, the learner will be able to ... "
- Start with a measurable verb, something you can see the learner do that indicates he or she has learned.
- Use Bloom's Taxonomy for action verbs such as: cite, discuss, demonstrate, analyze, formulate, evaluate.
- Avoid less measurable verbs such as *understand, know, learn, appreciate, familiarize.*
- When stating what the learner will be able to do at the conclusion of the activity focus on only one knowledge or behavior per objective: " ... the procedure for performing CPR."

HELPFUL RESOURCE

See Appendix C for action verbs in the three domains of learning.

Examples of Objectives
At the conclusion of the activity, the learner will be able to:
- interpret nutritional content listed on food labels
- demonstrate three relaxation exercises
- describe three risk factors of obesity

The **content of a health promotion** project depends on the intersection of several factors.
- needs identified by the target learners

- determination by the FCN of what the learner needs to know in order to change behavior
- institutional constraints placed on the FCN

Learning objectives that are correctly written direct the selection of what is to be included in the content.

- Objectives stated in measurable, observable terms, derived from stated needs in the assessment and that include three domains of learning lead to teaching plans tailored to the target learners.
- Institutional constraints imposed by the sponsor or funder of the project may limit time and money spent on the project.
- The FCN may have to adjust the amount and type of educational materials used in order to remain within these constraints.
- Knowledge of resources for free and low cost materials is invaluable for the FCN.

Teaching Strategies

A variety of strategies should be planned in order to accommodate differences in learning styles. Eliciting participation, questions, and even attention from a sea of faces in a **large class or lecture hall** can be a difficult task. Instructors often seek ways to make large classes feel smaller or more targeted.

Service learning is a pedagogy that combines classroom instruction, meaningful service in the community, and personal reflection.

In **case-based teaching and problem-based learning**, learners develop skills in analytical thinking and reflective judgment by reading and discussing complex, real-life scenarios. The FCN must practice how to use cases in teaching and provide case studies for health promotion that are relevant to the social sciences and other disciplines.

Discussion-based teaching helps students apply abstract ideas and think critically about what they learn.

- Studies show that discussions build learners' problem-solving skills more effectively than do lectures.
- However, fostering productive discussions can be difficult for even the most experienced instructors.
- The FCN must prepare for discussions by asking questions that promote discussion, getting students to talk, and handling common problems that arise during discussions.

Experiential learning and field work is the process whereby students "learn by doing" and by reflecting on the experience. Experiential learning activities can include, but are not limited to, hands-on laboratory experiments, practica, field exercises, and studio performances.

Cooperative learning, which uses group work and teamwork, involves having students work together to maximize their own and one another's learning. The FCN will benefit from reading about cooperative learning, designing effective small group activities, and taking courses that include guidance for creating and sustaining effective student learning groups.

Online teaching, ranging from hybrid courses that offer a combination of in-person and online instruction, to fully online experiences and distance learning, is increasingly common at many higher education institutions (www.crlt.umich.edu/tstrategies/tsot retrieved November 27, 2013).

Older, more common teaching strategies include these approaches.
- debates
- role-playing
- panels and seminars
- brainstorming
- problem solving
- structured controversy
- interviewing

The **evaluation** of the program focuses on content and process.
- content—learner needs are met; reflects objectives
  - post-instruction assessment
  - demonstration
  - observation of behavior change
  - satisfaction questionnaires
- process—educational effectiveness
  - appropriateness of materials
  - effectiveness of guest speakers and presenters
  - environment conducive to learning
  - peer observation

Critical Thinking

How is care of the spirit reflected in health promotion?

What skills does the FCN need to deliver effective health promotion programs?

Standards of Professional Performance for Faith Community Nursing

Standard 5B. Health Teaching and Health Promotion

The faith community nurse employs strategies to promote wholistic health, wellness, and a safe environment.

COMPETENCIES

The faith community nurse:

- Provides health teaching for individuals or groups that addresses such topics as healthy lifestyles, risk-reducing behavior, developmental needs, activities of daily living, preventive self-care, and spiritual practices for health and healing.
- Uses health promotion and health teaching methods appropriate to the situation and the healthcare consumer's values, beliefs, health practices, developmental level, learning needs, readiness and ability to learn, language preference, spirituality, culture, and socioeconomic status.
- Seeks ongoing opportunities for feedback and evaluation of the effectiveness of the strategies used.
- Uses information technologies to communicate health promotion and disease prevention information to the healthcare consumer in a variety of settings.
- Provides healthcare consumers with information about intended effects and potential adverse effects of proposed therapies.
- Teaches activities that strengthen the body-mind-spirit connection, such as meditation, prayer, and guided imagery.
- Evaluates health information resources for use in faith community nursing for accuracy, readability, and comprehensibility by healthcare consumers, and compatibility with the healthcare consumers' spiritual beliefs and practices.

Learning Activities

Definition of Health Critique

Instructions:
1. Complete the discussion of definitions of *health* in Outcome 1 of the Content Outline.
2. Ask participants to list the major concepts from their personal definitions on the board or flip chart.
3. Ask them to create a new list of major concepts based on the discussion they just heard.
4. After all concepts are on the list ask students to rank the concepts from most to least importance. Assure them that all concepts are important but they must force themselves to make a choice.

Questions:
1. What were the reasons for your ranking of concepts?
2. What would be your second choice ranking and why?
3. In what ways did the discussion influence your understanding of the definition of health?

Case Studies Related to Health Promotion Program Planning

Instructions:
1. Assign the participants to small groups and assign one or more case studies to each group.
2. Encourage the participants to discuss the case selected by using the questions provided.
3. Reconvene the entire group and have the small groups share their observations.

CASE 1
Tea and Toast

Calinda is an FCN working in a faith community serving a large senior population. Over the past two years, she has received a number of requests for comprehensive nutrition information, from both seniors and caregivers in the community. In her efforts to respond to these requests, Calinda notices that there are very few nutrition education resources focusing on older adults. She is committed to developing an educational resource to meet this information deficit. At the same time, she realizes that nutrition education for seniors in her community needs to be part of a broader comprehensive health promotion initiative. This will help the seniors avoid the "tea and toast" syndrome—eating nutritionally deficient and unbalanced meals—and support independence among older adults living in the community. Calinda decides that a comprehensive health promotion initiative is in order.

1. What practical advice could you give Calinda in order to ensure that her plans around a comprehensive health promotion initiative incorporate each of the key health promotion features discussed in this module?

2. List three to five community agencies Calinda should invite to be on her planning team.

3. How does this scenario relate to your own experience with addressing health issues in your faith community and community at large?

CASE 2
Baby and Beyond

Allison is an FCN working for a mega faith community in a large city. Her challenge is to provide educational opportunities for expectant and new mothers to ensure that they have the knowledge and skills necessary to give their children a healthy start in life. Her faith community does outreach work in the neighborhood nearby. Many of these parents are considered at-risk because they face barriers to good health such as low income, social isolation, and limited employment skills.

Allison collaborates with a program that offers pre- and post-natal classes for parents and caregivers. Through this program, she works closely with a group of outreach workers who are community parents living in the area.

Participants meet every week. The session opens with a short prayer and scripture reading. Participants are given the opportunity to silently reflect on the spiritual influence they felt during the week, and some members speak their feelings. At the end of each class, participants identify the topics they want addressed at the next session. In response to their information needs, Allison covers topics such as the birthing process, breastfeeding, healthy eating during and after pregnancy, smoking cessation, drug and alcohol addiction, healthy child development, making baby food, and parenting skills. To ensure that participants have adequate resources to meet their nutritional needs, food and milk vouchers are provided. Participants are reimbursed for their transportation costs to and from the classes. The program also provides access to child care so participants can attend the classes.

While the women were satisfied with the classes, there was a growing concern that other important health issues in the community were not being addressed. Over time, discussions held during the classes focused on other barriers to health faced by participants and their families, such as a lack of recreation facilities for young children and a shortage of affordable day care spaces. While many of the women expressed their need to get a job and support their families once their children were old enough, they were concerned that barriers such as a lack of proficiency in English and a lack of job training programs in the community would limit their ability to do so.

In response to the needs expressed by participants, Allison contacted several community service agencies in the neighborhood. The people with whom Allison spoke shared her concerns about the issues raised by the participants in her class. Allison collaborated with the other agencies to organize a community-wide forum at the auditorium of one of the local public schools. This event resulted in the formation of an inter-sectorial committee made up of agency representatives and community residents.

Over the next two years, the committee pursued the following activities in response to the needs and priorities identified by community members.

- One of the partner agencies provided parents with access to computers so they could develop résumés and upgrade their computer skills.
- Another partner agency started several English as a Second Language classes.
- A successful proposal for funding allowed a local day care center to offer free half-day play days twice a week for children ages two to four years.

- Residents successfully lobbied the city to clean and upgrade playground facilities in two community parks.
- The committee applied for, and received, a community services grant to offer a summer camp for preschool children.
- The local library expanded its storytelling program to include local language stories every week.
- During the summer, the committee organized monthly barbecues as a fun social event for community residents.
- Allison's church set up an education and support group for new fathers.

Discuss this case study in terms of:
- wholistic view of health
- focus on participatory approach
- focus on determinants of health; building on strengths and assets
- use of multiple strategies

Case Study Instructor Notes

This case incorporates the key features of health promotion practice, including:

- **Wholistic view of health** that goes beyond the physical health status of new and expectant mothers and children to encompass the social and mental dimensions of health and well-being.
- A **focus on participatory approaches** that entails the direct involvement of community members in planning and implementing activities in response to their shared health concerns.
- A **focus on the determinants of health** through activities addressing the social, economic and environmental factors contributing to health such as employment, recreation, social support, literacy skills, healthy child development and access to child care.
- **Building on existing strengths** and assets by making use of existing community resources and facilities wherever possible and building on the capacity of community residents.
- Using **multiple, complementary strategies**, including health education, self-help/mutual aid, organizational change, community mobilization, and advocacy.

Model for Healthy Living

Instructions:
1. Print copies of the Model for Healthy Living Assessment Wheel from the Church Health Center website.
2. Read together the following article, "What Is Integrated Health?" and the explanation of the Model for Healthy Living.
3. Explain how the Church Heath Center's Model for Healthy Living as a model of integrated health can be used as a self-assessment strategy.
4. Give each student a copy of the wheel. Read the descriptions for each part of the wheel; allow participants time to think about the descriptions before marking their wheels.

What Is Integrated Health?

Christianity is a faith tradition filled with body imagery but has produced an institution disinterested in the embodied existence of its believers. We Christians like our spirituality clean and unencumbered by the realities of bodily experience. The flip side of this attitude is equally disturbing, and can be found among many health care professionals who pay little attention to the role that spirituality can play in the maintenance of optimum human health. So we divide the various aspects of our lived experience and assign them to the appropriate professionals when necessary. To the physicians go our bodies; to the ministers, our souls. And never the twain shall meet.

The apostle Paul knew firsthand how stifling a house divided like this can be. The church in Corinth was notorious for the way it parceled out the gifts of the spirit into separate spheres. It took the patience of a teacher like Paul to remind them that a truly healthy community functions less like a machine, with its various parts working independently of each other, and more like an organism. "The church is the body of Christ," he said, "... don't treat it like a cadaver." We find harmony in our diverse capacities by the invigorating and unifying Spirit of our Redeemer.

Despite two thousand years of reflection on the importance of this insight, the church—and Western society—finds itself committing some of the same mistakes that were made in Corinth. Health has come to be defined as the *absence* of disease, when in fact the Shalom that God wills for the world is more concerned with the *presence* of vitality, of well-being and wholeness. For this

reason, Christians need now more than ever to work toward a new vision of integrated health. If we have learned anything from Paul it is this: we do not stand alone, but are instead communal creatures. Our lives are marked by interdependence. At the individual level, we are body, mind, and spirit. Optimum human health can only be achieved when all three of these are brought into harmony with each other. At the social and ecological level, we are members of many networks whose vitality is equally important to us. From an integrated health perspective, my well-being is a function of the communities of which I am a part. What good is a clean bill of health if I bring it home to a violent relationship, or to a poverty-stricken home, or to an environmentally contaminated neighborhood?

I wish that Christianity had a spiritual discipline like yoga. Perhaps we can work on creating one, and with the weight of tradition behind us. The real affront to God lies not in exploring the practices of another world religion, but rather in living as if our spirituality has nothing to do with the body that God so consistently affirms throughout scripture. While society encourages us to place the various aspects of our lived experience in little cubbyholes, the real insight of Christian spirituality is that all of this is of a piece—integrated—and should be celebrated as such. "And there are varieties of activities, but it is the same God who activates all of them in everyone" (1 Corinthians 12:6).

This article appeared in Church Health Reader *(2013). Daniel G. Deffenbaugh is professor of philosophy and religion at Hastings College in Hastings, Nebraska, and author of* Learning the Language of the Fields.

The Model for Healthy Living

Many of us separate out the various parts of life, yet true healthy living means that all aspects of our lives are in balance.

The Model for Healthy Living is a tool designed to help us consider the interconnectedness of key areas of life and to help improve the health and wellness of individuals and communities. It was developed on-site at Church Health Center Wellness in Memphis, Tennessee, as a way of aiding the Center's patients and clients to consider life as a whole. Work habits can affect nutrition; emotions can impact physical health; our relationships with family and friends might influence our faith life. Living healthy lives doesn't just mean that you see the doctor regularly. Rather, every aspect of the model—your faith life, movement, medical health, work, emotions, nutrition, and family and friends—contributes to a life filled with love, joy, and most important, a stronger connection with God.

Faith Life—*Building a relationship with God, your neighbor, and self*

We have moved a universe away from seeing faith as an important part of health, and it's time to bring the two back together. Faith traditions vary widely, but at the core, a faith life helps us build a relationship with God, our neighbors, and ourselves. This affirms that we are body-and-spirit beings created and loved by God. Even if you don't consider yourself "religious," you can explore a richer faith life and enjoy the benefits this experience will bring to your overall wellness.

Emotional—*Managing stress and understanding your feelings to better care for yourself*

It's pretty easy to turn to unhealthy habits in response to stress in our lives. For many people, that habit—whether food, mindless television, excessive spending, alcohol, or something else—makes us momentarily feel better even though we know it's bad in the long term. Through understanding your feelings and emotional needs, you can make changes to take better care of yourself and manage stress in healthier ways.

Work—*Appreciating your skills, talents, and gifts*

We were made to work, and the value of work is intrinsic. You can appreciate the skills, talents, and gifts you bring to your work situation, whatever it is. You can find meaning for your life through your job or volunteer commitments.

Medical—*Partnering with your health professional to manage your health*

You are the expert in your own health care. Your doctor is your partner. Yes, doctors have education, training, and experience you don't have, but you know yourself better than any doctor ever will. When it comes to your medical care, you bring something important to the conversation. You can build a partnership with your health care provider that lets you participate in managing your medical care.

Movement—*Discovering ways to enjoy physical activity*

We were created to move. When you consider the way the parts of the body are hinged together, rotate, and reach in every direction, it's easy to see that God means for us to move. It is part of how we celebrate our body-and-spirit connection to God. No matter what your physical activity level is now, you can discover ways to enjoy movement.

Nutrition—*Making smart food choices and developing healthy eating habits*

Good nutrition builds strong bodies that can lead to being whole people better connected to God. What you eat matters. Whatever your eating habits are now, you can increase your understanding of how food affects your overall well-being, learn to make smart food choices, and develop healthy eating habits.

Friends and Family—*Giving and receiving support through relationships*

God, Jesus, and Holy Spirit were the very first relationship. Even God exists in community. Coping with life is sometimes hard, but friends and family make it easier. You can both give and receive support through the relationships in your life.

Visit www.chreader.org for more information on the Church Health Center's Model for Healthy Living

Model for Healthy Living

Assessment Wheel

Circle the number on the wheel that best describes your satisfaction in each of these areas in your life or the life of your church (1- unsatisfied, 10- completely satisfied). Connect the circles. What areas would you like to improve?

Faith Life
Building a relationship with God, your neighbors, and yourself.

1   2   3   4   5   6   7   8   9   10

Movement
Discovering ways to enjoy physical activity.

1   2   3   4   5   6   7   8   9   10

Medical
Partnering with your health care provider to manage your medical care.

1   2   3   4   5   6   7   8   9   10

Work
Appreciating your skills, talents, and gifts.

1   2   3   4   5   6   7   8   9   10

Emotional
Managing stress and understanding your feelings to better care for yourself.

1   2   3   4   5   6   7   8   9   10

Nutrition
Making smart food choices and developing healthy eating habits.

1   2   3   4   5   6   7   8   9   10

Family & Friends
Giving and receiving support through relationships.

1   2   3   4   5   6   7   8   9   10

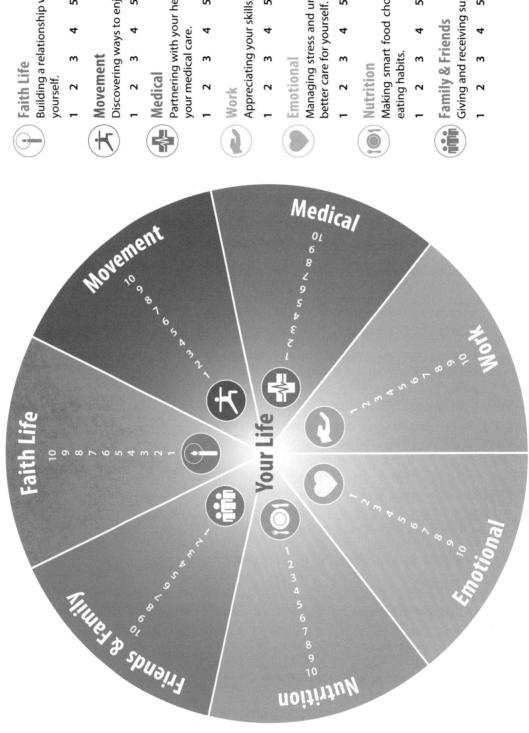

Evaluation of a Health Promotion Program

Instructions:

1. If participants are involved with a community-based health promotion action, they may evaluate that initiative.

2. If participants have access to the Internet, refer them to the Community Tool Box website.

3. Access the Community Tool Box website, http://ctb.ku.edu/en, and select "learn a skill"; then, select "toolkits"; then select "3 Analyzing Problems and Goals."

4. Select the tab "Outline" and read the outline thoroughly. Study the outline for the process of analyzing problems and goals. Use the outlined process to evaluate the situation selected in the next step.

5. Then select "Examples," choose one of the six situations and answer the questions in the outline about the example you chose.

Questions:

1. What additional questions do you have?

2. What is your opinion of the activity? Prepare a report of your evaluation to share with the class.

3. Watch the PowerPoint slides on the site. You may want to use them in your class presentation.

Expanded Learning Activities

Instructions:

1. Ask participants to write a personal definition of health. This could be assigned as a pre-class activity.

2. As a pre-class activity, ask participants to read *Faith Community Nursing: Scope and Standards of Practice* (2nd ed., 2012).

3. Use the information in Appendix A to explore health beliefs of diverse faith traditions. Discuss how important it is for the FCN to have awareness of health beliefs in various faith traditions.

4. Guided by the content in Outcome 3 of the Content Outline, ask participants to evaluate the following objectives, and then practice writing objectives for their own ministries.

   • Study the effects of a time management course on the practice of nursing in the US.

   • Be aware of the incidence of recidivism at Mercy Hospital during the summer of 2012.

   • Design a decision-making flow chart for registered nurse delegation to non-licensed personnel.

References

Required Textbook

American Nurses Association and Health Ministries Association. (2012). *Faith community nursing: Scope and standards of practice* (2nd ed.). Silver Spring, MD: Nursesbooks.org.

References

Bartholomew, L. K., Parcel, G. S., Kok, G., & Gottlieb, N. H., Fernandez, M. E. (2011). *Planning health promotion programs: An intervention mapping approach* (3rd ed.). San Francisco, CA: Jossey-Bass.

Brown, J., Kazi, L., Spitz, P., Gertman, P., Fires, J., & Meehan, R. (1984). The dimensions of health outcomes: A cross-validated examination of health status measurement. *American Journal of Public Health, 74*, 159–161.

Carlson, J. (2003). *Basic concepts in complementary therapies and wellness.* Upper Saddle River, NJ: Prentice Hall.

Church Health Center (2013). The model for healthy living. *Church Health Reader, 3(1)*, 8.

Deffenbaugh, D. (2013). What is integrated health? *Church Health Reader, 3*(1), 9.

DiClemente, C. C., Prochaska, J. O., Fairhurst, S. K., Velicer, W. F., Velasquez, M. M., & Rossi, J. S. (1991). The process of smoking cessation: An analysis of precontemplation, contemplation, and preparation stages of change. *Journal of Consulting and Clinical Psychology, 59*(2), 295–304.

Fagan, D., Kiger A., van Teijlingen, E. (2013). A survey of faith leaders concerning health promotion and the level of healthy living activities occurring in faith communities in Scotland. *Global Health Promotion*, June 1, 2012 (1), 27–36. doi: 10.1177/1757975910383927.

Gallagher, R. & Smith, D. (1989). Formulation of teaching/learning objectives useful for the development and assessment of lessons, courses, and programs. *Journal of Cancer Education, 4*(4), 231–234. doi: 10.1080/0885819 8909528016.

Goldsmith, S. (1972). The status of health indicators. *Health Service Reports, 87*, 212–220

Hickman, J. S. (2011). *Fast facts for the faith community nurse: Implementing FCN/parish nursing in a nutshell.* New York, N.Y.: Springer Publishing Company.

King, I. M. (1981). *A theory for nursing: Systems, concepts, process.* New York: Wiley.

Levin, J. (2014). Faith-based initiatives in health promotion: History, challenges, and current partnerships. *American Journal of Health Promotion, 28*(3), 139–41. doi:10.4278/ ajhp.130403-CIT-149.

Mager, R. (1997). *Preparing instructional objectives: A critical tool in the development of effective instruction* (3rd ed.). Atlanta, GA: CEP Press.

McNamara, J. W. (2014). *Stronger together: Starting a health team in your congregation.* Memphis, TN: Church Health Center.

Naumann, J. F., & Finn, R. W. (2010). *Principles of Catholic social teaching and health care reform: A joint pastoral statement.* http://www.catholic.net/index.php?option=dedest aca&id=3787. Retrieved November 2013.

Odulana, A. A., Kim, M. M., Isler M. R., Green, M. A., Taylor, Y. J., Howard, D. L., Godley, P. A. & Corbie-Smith, G. (2014). Examining characteristics of congregation members willing to attend health promotion in African American churches. *Health Promotion Practice, 15*(1), 125–133.

Parsons, T. (1951). *The social system.* New York: The Free Press.

Pender N. J. (1987). *Health promotion in nursing practice* (2nd ed.). Norwalk: Appleton & Lange.

Pender, N., Murdaugh, C., & Parsons, M. (2011). *Health promotion in nursing practice* (6th ed.). Boston, MA: Pearson Publishing Company.

Prochaska, J. O. & Prochaska, J. M. (2008). Termination at each stage of change. In M. O'Donnell (Ed.). *A Clinician's Guide to the Termination of Psychotherapy.* New York, NY: Brunner-Routledge, Taylor & Francis.

Raingruber, B. (2014). *Contemporary health promotion in nursing practice.* Burlington, MA: Jones & Bartlett Learning.

Rosenstock, I. (1974). Historical origins of the health belief model. *Health Education Behavior 2*(4), 328–335.

Thompson, P. (2010). Clergy knowledge and attitudes concerning faith community nursing: Toward a three-dimensional scale. *Public Health Nursing, 27*(1), 71–78. doi: 10.1111/j.1525-1446.2009.00828.x. PMID:20055970. [PubMed - indexed for MEDLINE] retrieved August 2013.

Tountas, Y., (2009). The historical origins of the basic concepts of health promotion and education: The role of ancient Greek philosophy and medicine. *Oxford Journals Medicine, 24*(2), 185–192. http://heapro.oxfordjournals.org/content/24/2/185.full. Retrieved September 2013.

Online Resources:

American Public Health Association: http://www.apha.org/

Centers for Disease Control and Prevention: http://www.cdc.gov/healthyliving/

Church Health Reader: www.chreader.org

Community Tool Box: http://ctb.ku.edu/en/

Health Belief Model: http://www.utwente.nl/cw theorieen overzicht/theory%20clusters/health%20communication/health_belief_model/

Healthy People: www.healthypeople.gov

International Council of Nurses, Health Information for Patients and Consumers: http://www.icn.ch/matters_healthpromo.htm

MAP-IT 5-step guide to implementing Healthy People 2020 in a community: http://www.healthypeople.gov/2020/implement/mapit.aspx

Office of Disease Prevention and Health Promotion: http://odphp.osophs.dhhs.gov/

Pender Health Promotion Model Manual: http://deepblue.lib.umich.edu/bitstream/handle/2027.42/85350/health_promotion_manual_rev_5-2011.pdf?sequence=1

Precede–Proceed Model: www.lgreen.net

United States Army Public Health Command: http://phc.amedd.army.mil/Pages/default.aspx

White House Office of Faith-based and Neighborhood Partnerships: http://www.whitehouse.gov/administration/eop/ofbnp

World Health Organization, Health Topics: http://www.who.int/topics/health_promotion/en/

Wrap-Up and Evaluation

Measuring Competency

This chart can be used to assess the individual outcomes in this module.
- A copy of this chart is attached to the Participant Module, so that each participant can complete this short evaluation.
- Have participants read each outcome and then place an X in the box that best matches their opinion about the objective being met.
- Encourage each participant to write a short reflection about this module in the space provided at the bottom of this chart.
- Use this data to make any necessary changes.

Outcome	Not Met	Somewhat Met	Met
1. Use knowledge of various definitions of health to compose a personal definition of health.			
2. Compare and contrast health promotion and disease prevention.			
3. Provide health teaching for individuals or groups that addresses such topics as healthy lifestyles, risk-reducing behaviors, developmental needs, activities of daily living, preventive self-care, and spiritual practices for health and healing.			
4. Use selected professional standards as a guide for developing health promotion programs.			
5. Use health promotion and health teaching methods appropriate to the situation and the health care consumer's values, beliefs, health practices, developmental level, learning needs, readiness and ability to learn, language preference, spirituality, culture, and socioeconomic status.			
Reflection: *In one paragraph, write a reflection on this module.*			

Appendix A

Health Belief Model

One of the first theories of health behavior (Rosenstock, 1974) identified four basic tenets.

1. People must realize and believe that they are at personal risk of disease or a life-threatening condition. The work of health promotion must personalize the risk. This moves beyond reading about statistical risk for the general public: i.e. "1 in 8 women are at risk of breast cancer."

2. People must understand the risk they face has consequences that could damage or shorten their life if not addressed.

3. People must be brought to understand that the remedy to reduce the risk of becoming ill or manage the illness is through lifestyle changes, available tests, or treatments.

4. People must believe that the benefits of illness prevention outweigh the costs of the changes to their life or treatments they will encounter.

Any health education program or individual encounter must include these concepts in order to engage the individual in important thought processes which lead to active involvement in managing his or her health. This health belief approach links to the Transtheoretical Model developed by Prochaska and DiClemente from their work with smoking cessation, and most recently with weight loss.

Transtheoretical Model

This model has six basic stages describing personal engagement for change.

Stage 1: Precontemplation
In this stage, "It isn't that they can't see the solution. It is that they can't see the problem" (G. K. Chesterton).

- People at this stage usually have no intention of changing their behavior, and typically deny having a problem.
- Others surrounding the person see clearly there is a problem, but the individual is in a state of denial, and resistant to change.
- He or she lacks information about his or her condition, and there is comfort in the state of ignorant bliss.
- Often, these individuals don't want to hear about their problems and will not be attending any programs the church or corporate program has to offer.

Stage 2: Contemplation
- During this stage, people with a problem begin thinking about it and begin thinking about changing their circumstance.
- People in this stage may read about the issue they face and want to discuss it.
- They may not be ready for acting on their thinking at this point.

- Many remain at this stage for lengthy periods of time, knowing they should change but being unable to take the steps necessary to begin the process.
- Often at this stage, people substitute thinking about change for the action they need to take.
- Moving people through this stage is an important feature of health ministry.
- People must be brought to understand the solution to the problem.
- As this focus shift is made, they can begin to visualize the future differently.
- That desire motivates movement and action.

Stage 3: Preparation
- This stage is identified by those who are "preparing" to make a change within the next month.
- They are thinking through the life changes necessary to begin to change. This can be as simple as thinking through what is necessary to attend a class:
  - The class is held on Thursday evening.
  - The time is from 6 PM to 8 PM.
  - They need to pick up the children, drop them off at home, think through the preplanning for meals, and have a babysitter lined up.

- The time it takes to drive to the class from home to arrive on time.
- Do they need to have another person pick up the children and take them home?
- Will the congregation simplify these issues by providing meal and babysitting service during the class?
- These are all considerations experienced by the individual, and the possible intervention to move the person forward in the desire to change.

Stage 4: Action

- The action phase is where the individuals are actively engaged in modifying their behavior.
- They are attending the course, moving forward with their decisions, making the change they determined to make.
- The individual who enters this phase without having addressed the earlier stages soon may encounter barriers which he or she hasn't worked through.
- When this occurs, often the individual will attend a few classes and then drop out.
- In congregations, we often place 90 percent of our efforts around holding class events, and have spent minimal time in working through the various stages for personal development needed for successful change.
- When this lack of preparation occurs, we often see a class with a beginning participation of 40, and at the end of the classes, we have only 11 still attending.
- At any given time, an estimate of only about 12–15 percent of the population is ready for the Action stage.
- Each class offered must address the issues of the earlier stages in order to assist those attending to work through the necessary stages in order to meet their goals.

- Classes that do not address these often have severe dropout rates.

Stage 5: Maintenance

- During the maintenance phase, all the issues of behavior change will be tested.
- Can the gains made during the class be sustained?
- A good test of time for maintenance is six months.
- Depending on the issue being changed, maintenance may last a lifetime. During this phase the individual is constantly applying knowledge to practice, encountering challenges, meeting them successfully (or not), and having backup systems in place so that as they encounter lapses in behavior they are prepared to begin again and continue.

Stage 6: Termination

- Prochaska & Prochaska (2008) state this as the ultimate goal.
- The behavior of the past is no longer a temptation or a threat for the future.
- Some in the field of health science say that people never terminate from the decisions, and are always affirming their choices and learning to choose each day.
- It is critical to remember that as people progress through the stages, lapses and relapses may occur.
- Provision and coaching must remain, with supportive relationships so that those who relapse are able to regain their place and begin again within a warm and loving environment.
- Progress for health behavior change is not a linear progression, but often moves forward and back—"Two steps forward, one step back, three steps forward."

Appendix B

Why Health and Faith?

Through the ages, health and healing have been important components of the world's religions, stressing attention to health, care for the sick, and positive behavioral choices. Norman Shealy, in his book entitled *Sacred Healing: The Curing Power of Energy and Spirituality*, cites teachings that exemplify how various religions view health.

Baha'i: *"All healing comes from God."*

Buddhism: *"To keep the body in good health is a duty ... otherwise we shall not be able to keep our mind strong and clear."*

Christianity: *"The prayer of faith shall heal the sick, and the Lord shall raise him up."*

Confucianism: *"High mysterious heaven hath fullest power to heal and bind."*

Hinduism: *"Enricher, Healer of disease, be a good friend to us!"*

Islam: *"The Lord of the worlds created me ... and when I am sick, He healeth me."*

Jainism: *"All living beings owe their present state of health to their own karma."*

Judaism: *"O Lord, my God, I cried to Thee for help and Thou hast healed me."*

Shinto: *"Foster a spirit that regards both good and evil as blessings, and the body spontaneously becomes healthy."*

Sikhism: *"God is Creator of all, the remover of sickness, the giver of health."*

Taoism: *"Pursue a middle course. Thus will you keep a healthy body and a healthy mind."*

Zoroastrianism: *"Love endows the sick body of man with firmness and health."*

As integral and vital elements of every community, faith communities are a fundamental part of the lives of millions of people. They are the places we go first for guidance, the people we seek first for support. And they make up the very core of many individuals' systems of belief—and behavior.

It comes as no surprise that the World Health Organization (1998) defines health not merely as the absence of disease or infirmity, but as a dynamic state of complete physical, mental, social, and spiritual well-being.

Adapted from C. Norman Shealy. (2001). Sacred Healing: The Curing Power of Energy and Spirituality. Rockport, MA: Element Books, Ltd.

Appendix C
Action Verbs for Writing Objectives

Affective Domain			
Category or level	**Behavior descriptions**	**Examples of experience, or demonstration and evidence to be measured**	**Key words (verbs which describe the activity to be trained or measured at each level)**
Receiving	Open to experience, willing to hear	Listen to teacher or trainer, take interest in session or learning experience, take notes, turn up, make time for learning experience, participate passively	Ask, listen, focus, attend, take part, discuss, acknowledge, hear, be open to, retain, follow, concentrate, read, do, feel
Responding	React and participate actively	Participate actively in group discussion, active participation in activity, interest in outcomes, enthusiasm for action, question and probe ideas, suggest interpretation	React, respond, seek clarification, interpret, clarify, provide other references and examples, contribute, question, present, cite, become animated or excited, help team, write, perform
Valuing	Attach values and express personal opinions	Decide worth and relevance of ideas, experiences; accept or commit to particular stance or action	Argue, challenge, debate, refute, confront, justify, persuade, criticize
Organizing or Conceptualizing Values	Reconcile internal conflicts; develop value system	Qualify and quantify personal views, state personal position and reasons, state beliefs	Build, develop, formulate, defend, modify, relate, prioritize, reconcile, contrast, arrange, compare
Internalizing or Characterizing Values	Adopt belief system and philosophy	Self-reliant; behave consistently with personal value set	Act, display, influence, solve, practice

Based on Krathwohl, D. R., Bloom, B. S. and Masia, B. B. (1964). Taxonomy of educational objectives, Book II. Affective domain. New York, NY. David McKay Company, Inc.

Psychomotor Domain			
Category or level	**Behavior Descriptions**	**Examples of activity or demonstration and evidence to be measured**	**Key words (verbs which describe the activity to be trained or measured at each level)**
Imitation	Copy action of another; observe and replicate	Watch teacher or trainer and repeat action, process or activity	Copy, follow, replicate, repeat, adhere, attempt, reproduce, organize, sketch, duplicate
Manipulation	Reproduce activity from instruction or memory	Carry out task from written or verbal instruction	Re-create, build, perform, execute, implement, acquire, conduct, operate
Precision	Execute skill reliably, independent of help, activity is quick, smooth, and accurate	Perform a task or activity with expertise and to high quality without assistance or instruction; able to demonstrate an activity to other learners	Demonstrate, complete, show, perfect, calibrate, control, achieve, accomplish, master, refine
Articulation	Adapt and integrate expertise to satisfy a new context or task	Relate and combine associated activities to develop methods to meet varying, novel requirements	Solve, adapt, combine, coordinate, revise, integrate, adapt, develop, formulate, modify, master
Naturalization	Instinctive, effortless, unconscious mastery of activity and related skills at strategic level	Define aim, approach and strategy for use of activities to meet strategic need	Construct, compose, create, design, specify, manage, invent, project-manage, originate

Based on R. H. Dave's version of the Psychomotor Domain (Developing and Writing Behavioral Objectives, 1970. The theory was first presented at a Berlin conference 1967; hence you may see Dave's model attributed to 1967 or 1970). *Adapted from: http://www.businessballs.com/bloomstaxonomyoflearningdomains.htm*

Cognitive Domain			
Category or level	Behavior descriptions	Examples of activity to be trained, or demonstration and evidence to be measured	Key words (verbs which describe the activity to be trained or measured at each level)
Knowledge	Recall or recognize information	Multiple-choice test, recount facts or statistics, recall a process, rules, definitions; quote law or procedure	Arrange, define, describe, label, list, memorize, recognize, relate, reproduce, select, state
Comprehension	Understand meaning, restate data in one's own words, interpret, extrapolate, translate	Explain or interpret meaning from a given scenario or statement; suggest treatment, reaction, or solution to given problem; create examples or metaphors	Explain, reiterate, reword, critique, classify, summarize, illustrate, translate, review, report, discuss, rewrite, estimate, interpret, theorize, paraphrase, reference, give example
Application	Use or apply knowledge, put theory into practice, use knowledge in response to real circumstances	Put a theory into practical effect, demonstrate, solve a problem, manage an activity	Use, apply, discover, manage, execute, solve, produce, implement, construct, change, prepare, conduct, perform, react, respond, role-play
Analysis	Interpret elements, organizational principles, structure, construction, internal relationships; quality, reliability of individual components	Identify constituent parts and functions of a process or concept, or deconstruct a methodology or process, making qualitative assessment of elements, relationships, values and effects; measure requirements or needs	Analyze, break down, catalogue, compare, quantify, measure, test, examine, experiment, relate, graph, diagram, plot, extrapolate, value, divide
Synthesis (create/build)	Develop new unique structures, systems, models, approaches, ideas; creative thinking, operations	Develop plans or procedures; design solutions; integrate methods, resources, ideas, parts; create teams or new approaches; write protocols or contingencies	Develop, plan, build, create, design, organize, revise, formulate, propose, establish, assemble, integrate, re-arrange, modify

Cognitive Domain			
Evaluation	Assess effectiveness of whole concepts, in relation to values, outputs, efficacy, viability; critical thinking, strategic comparison and review; judgment relating to external criteria	Review strategic options or plans in terms of efficacy, return on investment or cost-effectiveness, practicability; assess sustainability; perform a SWOT (strengths, weaknesses, opportunities, and threats) analysis in relation to alternatives; produce a financial justification for a proposition or venture; calculate the effects of a plan or strategy; perform a detailed and costed risk analysis with recommendations and justifications	Review, justify, assess, present a case for, defend, report on, investigate, direct, appraise, argue, project-manage

Based on Bloom's Taxonomy.

Unit III: Wholistic Health

Behavioral Health

and Faith Community Nursing

Behavioral Health
and Faith Community Nursing

Introduction

Learning Outcomes

Upon completion of this module, the participant will be able to:

1. Identify signs and symptoms of mental illness and spiritual implications.
2. Identify barriers to effective ministering to the behavioral health of the faith community.
3. Make appropriate referrals, based on assessment, to behavioral health resources.
4. Create a plan to transform/ enhance the current environment of the faith community to an environment that is recognized as caring by those needing behavioral health services.

Description

This module addresses the role of the faith community nurse (FCN) in providing behavioral health care in the faith community. It also illustrates how the faith community can minister effectively to the mentally ill.

In 1979 behavioral health emerged promoting individual responsibility in the maintenance of health and prevention of illness. Mental health is the psychological state of someone who holistically functions at a satisfactory level. The outcome of a mental health diagnosis cannot change by changing your behavior (for instance, schizophrenia). It is possible, however, to control it with medicine. In contrast, *behavioral health* is a state of mental and emotional being or choices and actions that affect wellness (SAMHSA, 2011). It is an aspect of identity that can be changed. Perhaps the term behavioral health is less stigmatized than *mental health* because a kinder, gentler name opens more doors for people.

Hours: 2

Research

Recently, there is evidence of increasing research on faith and mental illness. A study published in the *Psychiatric Review* stated that religious coping improves outcomes for people being treated for severe psychiatric illness (Rosmarin, et al., 2013). Baylor researchers concluded in their study that many churches have turned a blind eye to the needs of the mentally ill and their families (Rogers, et al., 2012). There is a movement among churches in the US to develop programs to change their culture and remove barriers to care of the mentally ill.

Faith Tradition

The early church's care of people with mental illness was positive until mental illness became associated with demons and evil spirits. During the 1980s, psychiatric wards removed religious influence from the treatment of mental illness. More recent studies recommend that therapists change their attitudes from considering religious beliefs harmful to treatment.

In non-Western cultures, where the predominant religions are Judaism, Islam, Buddhism, and Hinduism, mental health care also had a religious framework (Koenig, 2005). However, professional counseling and psychotherapy is not used as often by Muslim patients as by patients in Western culture. Attempts to integrate indigenous knowledge from religious practices in Islam have resulted in increased awareness about their effectiveness and value. One of the most basic and mandatory acts in Islamic tenets is obligatory prayer five times daily. Sayeed and Prakash (2013) suggest that this act of worship alone can provide solutions to most psychological and somatic problems in humans.

Reflection

"Do not fear, for I am with you, do not be afraid, for I am your God; I will strengthen you, I will help you, I will uphold you with my victorious right hand."
—Isaiah 41:10

"In God I trust; I am not afraid. What can a mere mortal do to me?"
—Psalm 56:11

Key Terms

Behavioral health: a state of mental and emotional being or choices and actions that affect wellness (Substance Abuse Mental Health Services Administration, 2011)

Caring environment: a faith community environment that is recognized by the mentally ill as accepting, sympathetic, and well-informed

Mental health: a state of well-being in which the individual realizes his or her own abilities, can cope with the normal stresses of life, can work productively and fruitfully, and is able to make a contribution to his or her community (World Health Organization, 2013)

Model of Friendship: acceptance and friendship; a powerful deterrent to the internalization of the stigma of mental illness by the mentally ill

Multicultural faith community: a faith community comprised of many cultures, such as the deaf, people from other countries, people from distinct regions or heritage, etc.

Role of the faith community: being involved in the compassionate care of the mentally ill and advocating to change the stigma surrounding mental illness

Serious mental illness: illness that causes serious functional impairments that substantially interfere with life activities

Silence in the congregation: the way most congregations and families of the mentally ill react to mental illness in the congregation

Stigma: a mark of disgrace associated with a particular circumstance, quality, or person; persists due to lack of knowledge, portrayal of people with mental illness by the media, and fear

HELPFUL RESOURCE

See Appendix H for "Daily Prayer for People Living with Mental Illness," a spiritual exercise for persons with mental illness.

Behavioral Health
and Faith Community Nursing

Content Outline

OUTCOME 1
Identify signs and symptoms of mental illness and spiritual implications.

Mental and Behavioral Health Definitions

The World Health Organization (WHO) defines **mental health** as "a state of well-being in which the individual realizes his or her own abilities, can cope with the normal stresses of life, can work productively and fruitfully, and is able to make a contribution to his or her community." Cultural differences, subjective assessments, and competing professional theories all affect how mental health is defined.

Behavioral health is a state of mental and emotional being or choices and actions that affect wellness (WHO, 2013).

In 2012, the National Survey On Drug Use and Health (NSDUH) estimated that there are 96 million adults age 18 or older in the United States with **serious mental illness** that cause serious functional impairments interfering with major life activities. This represents 4.1 percent of the US adult population (www.nimh.nih.gov/statistics).

Serious mental illness is defined in the NSDUH survey as:
- mental, behavioral, or emotional disorder (excludes developmental and substance disorders)
- diagnosable currently or within the past year
- of sufficient duration to meet diagnostic criteria specified within the 4th edition of the *Diagnostic and Statistical Manual of Mental Disorders (DSM IV)*
- resulting in serious functional impairment which substantially interferes with or limits one or more major life activities (NSDUH, 2012)

Signs and Symptoms of Mental Illness in Adults

The American Psychiatric Association (APA), 2013 identifies these signs and symptoms associated with the most prevalent disorders.

Major Depression
- loss of interest in favorite activities
- depressed mood for longer than two weeks
- threatening to kill himself or herself; talking or writing about death, dying or suicide
- feeling hopeless or overwhelmed or helpless
- withdrawing from social network and family
- difficulty with sleep (too much, too little)

Schizophrenia
- delusions
- hallucinations
- lack of concentration, difficulty remembering, inability to plan
- loss of motivation involving self-care
- blunted emotions
- social withdrawal

Bipolar Disorder
There are two subtypes of bipolar disorder.
- bipolar I (mania then depression)
- bipolar II (depression, then hypomania)

Depression in bipolar has some or all of the symptoms of major depression. **Mania episodes** will have some of the following symptoms:
- increased energy and over-activity
- elevated mood: feels high, full of energy, invincible
- long periods of not sleeping
- irritability
- rapid thinking and speech
- lack of inhibitions: spends money recklessly, very sexually active, disregards risks
- grandiose delusions: superhero, person of great superiority
- lack of insight: doesn't realize manic behavior is unreasonable and a sign of illness

Anxiety Disorder—excessive and unrealistic worry over a period of at least six months
- restlessness
- fatigue
- difficulty concentrating
- irritability or explosive anger
- muscle tension
- sleep disturbances
- personality changes, such as becoming less social
- includes phobic disorders (fear of certain objects, situations)
- panic attacks (intense periods of fear or feelings of doom developing over a very short time frame up to 10 minutes)

Post-traumatic stress disorder (PTSD) is anxiety caused by the exposure to either death or near-death circumstances or to events that threaten one's own or another person's physical

---

MENTAL ILLNESSES

The Diagnostic and Statistical Manual of Mental Disorders—5 (5th edition, 2013) lists many mental illnesses. These are the most prevalent diagnoses.

In adults:
- *major depression*
- *schizophrenia*
- *bipolar disorder*
- *anxiety disorder*
- *borderline personality disorder*
- *antisocial personality disorder*

In children:
- *attention deficit hyperactivity disorder*
- *depression*
- *behavioral disorders*

Substance-induced disorders affect adults, adolescents and children.

well-being. The traumatic event is re-experienced with fear or feelings of helplessness or horror and may appear in dreams or thoughts.

Borderline Personality Disorder—a pervasive pattern of instability of interpersonal relationships, self-image and affects, and marked impulsivity beginning by early adulthood
- frantic efforts to avoid real or imagined abandonment
- a pattern of unstable and intense interpersonal relationships characterized by alternating between extremes of idealization and devaluation
- identity disturbance: markedly and persistently unstable self-image or sense of self
- impulsivity in at least two areas that are potentially self-damaging (e.g., spending, sex, substance abuse, reckless driving, binge eating)
- recurrent suicidal behavior, gestures, threats, or self-mutilating behavior
- affective (mood) instability
- chronic feelings of emptiness
- inappropriate, intense anger or difficulty controlling anger (e.g., frequent displays of temper, constant anger, recurrent physical fights)
- transient, stress-related paranoid ideation or severe dissociative symptoms

Antisocial Personality Disorder—condition in which a person has a long-term pattern of manipulating, exploiting, or violating the rights of others, behaviors which often are criminal in nature
- acts witty and charming
- is good at flattery and manipulating others' emotions
- breaks the law repeatedly
- disregards the safety of self and others
- has problems with substance abuse
- lies, steals and fights often
- doesn't show remorse or guilt for actions
- often angry and arrogant

Signs and Symptoms of Mental Illness in Children

Major Depression—many children display the same symptoms as adults, such as sadness and low mood
- primary symptoms revolve around sadness, a feeling of hopelessness and mood changes
- complaints of physical illnesses such as recurring stomachaches that do not respond to treatment
- thoughts of death and suicide

Attention Deficit Hyperactivity Disorder (ADHD)—children show signs of inattention, hyperactivity, or impulsivity in specific ways

HELPFUL RESOURCE

The Toolkit for Community Conversations About Mental Health, *from the Substance Abuse and Mental Health Services Administration, is designed to support communities interested in holding conversations about mental health. Access this helpful tool at http://content. govdelivery.com/accounts/ USSAMHSA/bulletins/84b053.*

- are in constant motion
- squirm and fidget
- do not seem to listen
- have difficulty playing quietly
- often talk incessantly
- interrupt or intrude on others
- do not finish tasks
- easily distracted

Behavior Disorders—involve a pattern of behavior that is hostile, aggressive and disruptive for a period of more than six months and is not developmentally age-appropriate
- harming or threatening themselves, others, or their pets
- damaging or destroying property
- lying or stealing
- not doing well in school, skipping school
- early smoking, drinking, or drug use
- early sexual activity
- frequent arguments and tantrums
- hostility toward authority figures

Substance-Induced Disorders in Adults or Children

- alcohol-related disorders
- cannabis-related disorder
- hallucinogen-related disorders
- opioid-related disorders
- sedative- and hypnotic-related disorders
- anxiolytic-related disorders
- stimulant-related disorders
- other disorders listed in *DSM—5* (2013)

These disorders share some common symptoms such as:
- substance is usually taken in larger amounts than intended
- increased activity to obtain the substance
- recurrent results in failure to fulfill major role at work, home or school
- social, occupational, and recreational activities are given up or reduced due to substance use
- recurrent substance use in situations that are considered risky
- sleep difficulty or restlessness is present with some substances
- nervousness, anxiety, irritability, anger and in some aggression (APA, 2013)

Implications of Mental Illness on Spirituality

Spirituality and faith beliefs may be impacted by the signs and symptoms of mental illness in the following ways.
- Isolation, withdrawal from family and community promotes feelings of being alone and abandoned.

KEY TERM

Stigma *is a mark of disgrace associated with a particular circumstance, quality, or person. Stigma about mental illness persists due to lack of knowledge, portrayal of people with mental illlness by the media, and fear.*

- Illness promotes negative attitudes toward God as individuals become more frustrated with the emotional pain they experience. Many people rely on God to relieve their pain and may experience a growing distance in their relationship with God if their prayers are unanswered (Koenig, 2005).
- **Stigma**, a mark of disgrace associated with a particular circumstance, quality, or person with mental illness, leads to feelings of shame adding to the pain of emotional illness and disengagement with the church community.
- Hallucinations and delusions which are present in the psychotic mental illnesses may lead mentally ill individuals to believe that God is talking to them and they may interpret biblical readings erroneously (Simpson, 2013).

OUTCOME 2

Identify barriers to effective ministering to the behavioral health of the faith community.

History of the Church's Care for People with Mental Illness

Understanding the issues that form barriers to ministering to people with mental illness requires first understanding the **history of the church's involvement in the care of people with mental illness.**

- The relationship between religion and mental illness has not always been a positive relationship.
- People with mental illness were believed by religious leaders, especially in the Western cultures, to be possessed by demons or evil spirits.
- The concern about demons and evil spirits led to fears that mental illness was contagious. This in turn led to confinement, exorcism, or death (Koenig, 2005).
- In spite of these concerns, history shows that major religious traditions throughout the world have been at the forefront of providing care for the mentally ill and emotionally vulnerable (Koenig, 2005).
- Many of the breakthroughs in caring for people with mental illness have been championed by members of religious organizations crusading for change (Koenig, 2005).
- Congregations turn a blind eye to mental illness, which in turn leads many families to leave the faith community (Rogers, et al., 2011).
- Families of people with mental illness would like for the church community to provide assistance with the issues of their family member.
- Data indicates that the faith community overlooks the needs of the mentally ill. "The data give the impression that mental illness, while prevalent within a congregation, is also nearly invisible" (Stanford, 2011).

Critical Thinking

What have you seen happen spiritually to people living with mental illness as a result of their disease?

Barriers to Effective Ministry

Amy Simpson (2013) calls mental illness the **"no-casserole" disease.** She reports that families dealing with mental illness watch the congregation delivering casseroles and offering support and help to the physically ill while the mentally ill suffer in silence.

Silence in the congregation and from the families affected by mental illness seems to be the main barrier to church involvement. Unfortunately, this is the way most congregations and families of the mentally ill react to mental illness in the congregation. Families are silent due to the stigma that still exists, and congregations are silent in many instances due to lack of knowledge of the signs of mental illness. The portrayal in the news media regarding the mental illness of perpetrators of many of the mass shootings may also cause the congregation to be hesitant in becoming involved with the mentally ill.

Other barriers in the faith community include
- resistance within mental health services to involve faith communities
- lack of knowledge and training regarding behavioral health in faith communities
- lack of financial resources in faith communities to become more active in behavioral health (Koenig, 2005)

HELPFUL RESOURCE
See Appendix A, History of Mental Health Care and the Church in Western Cultures.

KEY TERM
Silence in the congregation is the way most congregations and families of the mentally ill react to mental illness.

Critical Thinking
What barriers in the faith community have you seen interfere with ministering to people living with mental illness?

OUTCOME 3
Make appropriate referrals, based on assessment, to behavioral health resources.

Appropriate Assessment

The **goals of the assessment** of a faith community member who has presented with signs and symptoms of mental illness are:
- to keep the person safe
- to refer to the appropriate level of care

An appropriate assessment includes the following (Kitchner, et al., 2009):
1. **Assess for threat of harm to self or others.**
- Do not be afraid to ask the question "Are you thinking of hurting yourself or others?"
- If the answer is yes, do not leave the person alone. (See Appendix B for appropriate questions if the answer is yes.)
2. **Listen non-judgmentally.** Use empathetic listening skills—open-ended questions, clarification, restating, an open and inviting presence, listening to tone of voice and nonverbal clues, and avoid giving unhelpful advice, such as "Pull yourself together."
3. **Give reassurance and information.**
- Do not make promises you cannot keep.

- If a person is hallucinating or delusional, he or she may not be able to understand any information. This can be offered when the person is in touch with reality.
- Reassure with statements validating the person's feelings such as "I know you believe the visions are real. I will help keep you safe."
- Assist in contacting the individual's therapist or contact the therapist directly if the person is a not able to do so due to mental state.

4. **Encourage appropriate professional help.**
For those experiencing **suicidal or homicidal ideations**, appropriate referrals include:
- If the person has a therapist, assist in contacting the therapist.
- Accompany the person to the local hospital emergency room for evaluation.
- File a Mental Detention Order with the local sheriff department if you cannot persuade the person to go to the ER.

For those experiencing **panic attacks, fear of dying, or extreme distress:**
- Monitor physical symptoms as well as mental and emotional symptoms.
- A person experiencing a panic attack may think he or she is having a heart attack, especially if this is the first panic attack.
- In this case, a person having chest pain would be referred to the emergency room, or call 911.
- If the individual has had panic attacks previously, ask him or her what has worked to relieve the attack and provide assistance.

For those experiencing symptoms suspected to be **signs of substance abuse:**
- Try to get the individual to a safe place.
- Do not argue if he or she shows signs of inebriation. This is one argument you will not win.
- Do not let the person drive or engage in any activity that will cause harm to themselves or others.
- Contact Alcoholics or Narcotics Anonymous as a resource.
- If unable to manage the situation or the person becomes aggressive, keep yourself and others safe by isolating the person if at all possible.
- Contact law enforcement for assistance and describe the situation, including the substance being used if it is known.

For those experiencing **exacerbation of their mental illness without aggression:**
- Encourage the person to seek counseling.
- Provide local resources and help make an appointment.

For those who are **aggressive**:
- **Keep yourself safe. *Take all threats seriously.***

- **De-escalate the situation.**
  - Stay calm.
  - Use a calm tone of voice.
  - Use nonthreatening language.
  - Allow the person to pace if needed.
  - Do not involve law enforcement unless absolutely necessary as the situation may escalate; if you involve law enforcement, be sure to fully describe the behavior you are observing.
  - Sometimes passing the person off to another member of the health team or the spiritual leader may help de-escalate the situation if the person is directing anger toward you personally.

Cultural Considerations

A **multicultural faith community** is comprised of many cultures, such as the deaf, people from other countries, people from distinct regions or heritage, etc. In a multicultural faith community, it is appropriate to ask the faith community member the following questions, which allow the faith community member a feeling of control about the referral.

- What would you like for your provider (psychiatrist, psychologist, social worker, or therapist) who is taking care of you to know about your religious or spiritual beliefs and practices?
- What forms of healing are respected in your religion?
- Is there a spiritual leader or healer you would find helpful to you while you are receiving care? (This material is based on the copyrighted work of NKI CECC and is used with its permission. *A Pastoral Education Workbook: responding to the needs of a multicultural faith community* can be obtained from NKI CECC at http://cecc.rfmh.org)

Cultural questions that will be helpful in assessing the needs of the faith community member include:

- What do you call your complaint or condition?
- What do you think caused this?
- What do you think will happen because of this condition?
- When you think about getting a diagnosis and treatment from a mental health professional, how will this affect your life? (This material based on the copyrighted work of NKI CECC and is used with its permission. *A Pastoral Education Workbook: responding to the needs of a multicultural faith community* can be obtained from NKI CECC at http://cecc. rfmh.org)

Obtain consent to share this information with the therapist.

HELPFUL RESOURCE
See Appendix C for a sample referral list to compile and keep on hand.

KEY TERM
A **multicultural faith community** *is comprised of many cultures, such as the deaf, people from other countries, people from distinct regions or heritage, etc.*

Critical Thinking
What behavioral health resources are available in a faith community and the external community to support a person with mental illness in an exacerbation of disease?

KEY TERM

The **role of the faith community** *is to be involved in the compassionate care of the mentally ill and advocate to change the stigma surrounding mental illness.*

KEY TERM

A **caring environment** *is a faith community recognized by the mentally ill as accepting, sympathetic and well-informed.*

KEY TERM

Model of Friendship—Acceptance and friendship are powerful deterrents to the internalization of the stigma of mental illness by the mentally ill.

HELPFUL RESOURCE

The full description of the Creating Caring Faith Communities model can be found at http://www.mentalhealthministries.net/resources/caring_congregations_model.html

HELPFUL RESOURCE

See Appendix D for a Communities of Compassion and Justice Action Plan.

OUTCOME 4

Create a plan to transform/enhance the current environment of the faith community to an environment that is recognized as caring by those needing behavioral health services.

Families with family members suffering from mental illness would like to experience an accepting, sympathetic, and well-informed community. They believe that in this type of community, they would be in a situation to express their feelings and share their experiences in a nonthreatening environment without fear of rejection or condemnation (Swinton, 2000).

The role of the faith community today is twofold (Lambert and Lambert, 2008):

- one of being involved in the compassionate care of the mentally ill
- one of advocacy to change the stigma surrounding mental illness

Rather than being a place where stigma around mental illness persists, the faith community can be a **caring environment** recognized by the mentally ill as accepting, sympathetic and well-informed. Several models have met with success in changing the culture of faith communities to one that provides resources, support, and acceptance.

Model of Friendship (Swinton 2000). Acceptance and friendship are powerful deterrents to the internalization of the stigma of mental illness by the mentally ill.

- This type of friendship is modeled on the relationships of Jesus: unconditional acceptance (John 4:5-30) and solidarity with the poor and the marginalized (Matthew 9:10).
- Swinton's basic model for the church is one of education about friendship as Jesus demonstrated, seeking out information regarding the needs for advocacy and empowerment of the mentally ill, formulating a plan for church involvement, and developing relationships with other agencies that are working in the community.

Creating Caring Faith Communities (Mental Health Ministries, 2013) has created a five-step program. This model includes education of the faith community regarding mental illness, commitment to the intentional care and support of those with mental illness, welcoming those with mental illness as full members of the faith community, support, and advocacy.

Communities of Compassion and Justice is a model proposed by the Commission on Mental Illness and Faith Fellowship for People with Mental Illness, Archdiocese of Chicago (2008). This model also focuses on education of the faith community, along with identification of the justice issues and the church's response. The model outlines a specific plan to assist in adopting this model for the church's care of those with mental illness.

Pathways to Promise offers a tool kit for mental health ministries that includes national resources, monthly activities focusing on mental health issues, and suggestions for how to be welcoming to those who suffer from mental illness. It includes tools needed to start and maintain a ministry focusing on people with mental illness. This model includes education, community, hospitality, service and advocacy.

HELPFUL RESOURCE

See examples of this program in Appendix E. The tool kit can be downloaded at www. pathways2promise.org.

Critical Thinking

Can a non-behavioral health professional adequately assess a mental health issue for correct referral? Explain your answer.

Standards of Professional Performance for Faith Community Nursing

It is to be expected that all standards of care will apply to FCN practice. In connection with behavioral health, the FCN will be heavily involved in the assessment of the client and the church culture, education and advocacy to reduce stigma, appropriate referral, and resource utilization.

Standard 1. Assessment

The faith community nurse collects comprehensive data pertinent to the healthcare consumer's wholistic health or the situation.

COMPETENCIES

The faith community nurse:

- Collects wholistic data including but not limited to physical, functional, psychosocial, emotional, cognitive, sexual, cultural, age-related, environmental, economic, and spiritual or transpersonal assessments in a systematic and ongoing process, while honoring the uniqueness of the person and placing a particular emphasis on spiritual beliefs and practices.
- Elicits the healthcare consumer's values, preferences, expressed needs, and knowledge of the healthcare situation.
- Involves the healthcare consumer, family, group, spiritual leader, other healthcare providers, and others, as appropriate, in wholistic data collection.
- Identifies barriers (e.g., psychosocial, literacy, financial, cultural) to effective communication and makes appropriate adaptations.
- Recognizes the impact of personal attitudes, values, and beliefs.
- Assesses family dynamics and impact on healthcare consumer health and wellness.
- Prioritizes data collection activities based on the healthcare consumer's immediate condition, or the anticipated needs of the health care consumer or situation.
- Uses appropriate evidence-based assessment techniques and instruments in collecting pertinent data as a basis for wholistic care.

- Synthesizes available data, information, and knowledge relevant to the situation to identify patterns and variances in individuals, families, groups, or the faith community as a whole.
- Applies ethical, legal, and privacy guidelines and policies to the collection, maintenance, uses, and dissemination of data and information.
- Recognizes healthcare consumers as the authority on their own health by honoring their care preferences.
- Documents relevant data in a retrievable format that is both confidential and secure.

Standard 5A.
Coordination of Care

The faith community nurse coordinates care delivery.

COMPETENCIES

The faith community nurse:

- Coordinates implementation of a wholistic plan of care.
- Coordinates the health care of individuals across the life span using principles of interprofessional models of care delivery and case management.
- Organizes the components of the plan.
- Manages a healthcare consumer's care in order to maximize independence and quality of life.
- Assists the healthcare consumer to identify options for alternative care.
- Communicates with the healthcare consumer, family, and system during transitions in care.
- Advocates for the delivery of dignified and humane care by the interprofessional team.
- Documents the coordination of care.

Standard 8. Education

The faith community nurse attains knowledge and competence that reflect current nursing practice.

COMPETENCIES

The faith community nurse:
- Participates in ongoing educational activities related to appropriate knowledge bases, professional issues, and spiritual care.
- Demonstrates a commitment to lifelong learning through self-reflection and inquiry to address learning and personal growth needs.
- Seeks experiences that reflect current practice to maintain knowledge, skills, abilities, and judgment in clinical practice or role performance for faith community nursing.
- Acquires knowledge and skills appropriate to the role, population, specialty of faith community nursing, setting, or situation.
- Seeks formal and independent learning experience to develop and maintain clinical, professional, and theological skills and knowledge.
- Identifies learning needs based on nursing knowledge, the various roles the nurse may assume, and the changing needs of the population.
- Participates in formal or informal consultation to address issues in nursing practice as an application of education and knowledge base.
- Shares educational findings, experiences, and ideas with peers.
- Contributes to a work environment conducive to the education of healthcare professionals.
- Maintains professional records that provide evidence of competence and lifelong learning.

Standard 15. Resources Utilization

The faith community nurse utilizes appropriate resources to plan and provide nursing services that are safe, effective, and financially responsible.

COMPETENCIES

The faith community nurse:
- Assesses individual healthcare consumer care needs and resources available to achieve desired outcomes.
- Identifies healthcare consumer care needs, potential for harm, complexity of the task, and desired outcome when considering resource allocation.
- Delegates elements of care to appropriate healthcare workers in accordance with any applicable legal or policy parameters or principles.
- Identifies the evidence when evaluating resources.
- Advocates for resources, including technology, that enhance nursing practice.
- Modifies practice when necessary to promote a positive interface between healthcare consumers, care providers, and technology.
- Assists the healthcare consumer and family in identifying and securing appropriate and available resources to address health and spiritually related needs across the healthcare continuum.
- Assists the healthcare consumer and family in factoring costs, risks, and benefits in decisions about treatment and care.
- Develops innovative solutions and applies strategies to obtain appropriate resources for faith community nursing care.

Learning Activities

Quiz on Mental Illness

Instructions:
1. Before beginning the lecture on mental illness, instruct participants to turn to Appendix G and fill out the *Quiz on Mental Illness.*
2. Score the quiz before beginning the lecture.

Question:
At the conclusion, ask the participants how they scored on the quiz and if there were any surprising answers.

Barriers to Behavioral Health

Instructions:
Break into small groups. Give each group a piece of paper from the flip chart and a marker. Instruct the groups to discuss and record the barriers present in their individual faith communities to minister to people with mental illness. Identify the most common barrier and develop a plan to address that barrier (10 minutes). Instruct each group to identify a group member to present their plan to the large group (5 minutes).

Quick Look at Mental Health Disorders

Instructions:
1. Break into small working groups. Make sure each group has at least one laptop or tablet to access the Internet.
2. Direct groups to go to http://www.nimh.nih.gov, the website of the National Institute of Mental Health.
3. Assign each group a different disorder listed under the button labeled "Health Topics."
4. Ask each group to prepare a brief synopsis of findings to the large group.

Question:
What surprised you most about the disorder you investigated?

Case Studies

Break into small groups. Give each group a piece of paper from the flip chart and a marker. Assign each group either Case Study 1 or Case Study 2. Ask them to assess the symptoms presented by the faith community member and identify the appropriate referral. Record the symptoms and the referral on the paper provided (8 minutes). Instruct each group to identify someone to present their findings to the large group (5 minutes). Select a group that has Case Study 1 to present their findings, and then ask the other groups who have Case Study 1 if they have anything different to add. Do the same with Case Study 2.

CASE 1

On Wednesday evening at church, a congregant approaches you and asks you to talk with her about getting a doctor's appointment. She tells you that she is feeling hopeless and helpless, has no interest in doing her crafts, and is sleeping all the time. She is not sure what is the matter with her and doesn't know who to consult.

What do these complaints suggest to you? What questions and actions would your assessment include?

Questions:
1. What symptoms is the faith community member presenting?
2. What is the appropriate referral?

CASE 2

On Sunday morning you are taking blood pressures. While taking Mr. Zane's blood pressure, you notice that he is continually cocking his head and looking around. You also observe that he is disheveled with body odor. When you talk with him about his condition, he is slow to answer as if you have interrupted a conversation he is having.

What do these observations suggest to you about Mr. Zane? What questions and actions would your assessment include?

Questions:
1. What symptoms is the faith community member presenting?
2. What is the appropriate referral?

Faith Community Behavioral Health Assessment

At the conclusion of the course content lecture, ask the participants to complete an assessment of their faith community in Appendix F (5 minutes). When they have completed their assessment, instruct them to use this assessment to develop a plan to remove one identified barrier as a starting point for moving their faith communities to being places of caring for the mentally ill.

References

Required Textbook

American Nurses Association and Health Ministries Association (2012). *Scope and standards of practice: Faith community nursing* (2nd ed.). Silver Spring, MD: Nursesbooks.org.

References

American Psychiatric Association. (2013). *Desk reference to the diagnostic criteria from DSM–5*. Arlington, VA: American Psychiatric Association.

Baylor study finds church congregations blind to mental illness. (2011, June 22). *Baylor University Media Communications*. Retrieved from http://www.baylor.edu/mediacommunications/news.php?action=story&story=95800

Kitchener, B. A., Jorm, A. F., and Kelly, C. M., Maryland Department of Health and Mental Hygiene, Missouri Department of Mental Health, and National Council for Community Behavioral Healthcare. (2009). *Mental health first aid USA*. http://www.mentalhealthfirstaid.org/cs/about/. Retrieved June 10, 2014.

Koenig, H. (2005). *Faith & mental health: Religious resources for healing*. West Conshohocken: Templeton Foundation Press.

Koenig, H. (2010). Spiritual and mental health. *International Journal of Applied Psychoanalytic Studies, 7*(2), 2622-2634.

Lambert, T. & Lambert, R. (2008). *Mental illness and faith community outreach*. (Revised). Retrieved June 10, 2014 from http://www.ministry.org/booklet.pdf

Mental Health Ministries. (2012). *Creating caring congregations*. Retrieved from http://www.mentalhealthministries.net/resources/dvds/creating_caring_congregations_dvd.html

Mental Health Ministry, A toolkit for congregations. (2009). Pathways to Promise. Retrieved from http://www.pathways2promise.org

National survey on drug use and health (NSDUH, 2012). Retrieved from http://www.nimh.nih.gov/statistics

A pastoral education workbook: Responding to the mental health needs of multicultural faith communities. (2011). New York State Office of Mental Health: The Nathan Kline Institute for Psychiatric Research & Center of Excellence in Culturally Competent Mental Health. Retrieved June 10, 2014 from http://ssrdqst.rfmh.org/cecc/sites/ssrdqst.rfmh.org.cecc/UserFiles/mentalhealthclergyguide101711A.pdf

Rogers, E.B., Stanford, M. & Garland, D. R. (2012). The effects of mental illness on families within faith communities, *Mental Health, Religion & Culture, 15*:3, 301–313. http://dx.doi.org/10.1080/13674676.2011.573474

Rosmarin, D., Begda, J., Ongier, P., Pargament, K., Bjorgivensson, T., (2013). Faith and healing: Religious coping improves outcomes for people being treated for severe psychiatric illness. *Psychiatric Research, 210*(1). 182–187.

Sayeed, S. & Prakash, A. (January 2013). The Islamic prayer (Salah/Namaaz) and yoga togetherness in mental health. *Indian Journal of Psychiatry, 55*(2), 224–230.

Scheinholtz, M., Substance Abuse and Mental Health Services Administration. (2013). Overview of behavioral health for aging information and referral/assistance professionals. Retrieved from http://www.nasuad.org/documentation/l_R/call_notes/1-9-13%20Behavioral%20Health%20Overview.pdf

Simpson, A. (2013). *Troubled minds: Mental illness and the church's mission*. Downers Grove, IL: InterVarsity Press.

Swinton, J. (2001). *Resurrecting the person: Friendship and the care of people with mental health problems*. South Nashville, TN: Abingdon Press.

Additional References

Anaebere, A., & DeLillly, C. (2012). Faith community nursing: Supporting mental health during life transitions. Issues in *Mental Health Nursing, 33*(5), 337–339. doi:10.3109/01612840.2011.631164

Corrigan, P. W. (2011). Best practices: Strategic stigma change (SSC): Five principles for social marketing campaigns to reduce stigma. *Psychiatric Services, 62*, 824–826. http://dx.doi.org/10.1176/appi.ps.62.8.824

Franklin, C. & Rowena, F. (Eds.) (2011). *The church leader's counseling resource book*, Oxford: Oxford University Press.

Haugk, K. (2000). *When and how to use mental health resources: A guide for Stephen Ministers, Stephen Leaders, and church staff*. St. Louis: Stephen Ministries.

Huguelet, P. & Koenig, H. (Eds.) (2009). *Religion and spirituality in psychiatry*. Cambridge: Cambridge University Press.

Johnson, E. (Ed.) (2010). *Psychology & Christianity: Five views* (2nd ed.) Downers Grove, IL: InterVarsity Press.

Koenig, H. (Ed.). (1998). *Handbook of religion and mental health*. San Diego: Academic Press.

Koenig, H. (2008). *Medicine, religion, and health: Where science and spirituality meet*. West Conshohocken: Templeton Foundation Press.

Leroy, J., Rippentrop, R., Sayer, N., Sierra-Swiech, R., & Skrocki, R. (2013). *Best practices in connecting faith communities to mental health resources*.

Marshak, L. & Prezant, F., (2007). *Married with special-needs children: A couples' guide to keeping connected*. Bethesda, MD: Woodbine House.

Mindful of grace: Mental illness and the church. (2012). *Church Health Reader, 4*(2).

Reinert, K., & Koenig, H. (2013). Re-examining definitions of spirituality in nursing research. *Journal of Advanced Nursing, 69*(12), 2622–2634.

Scheinholtz, M. (2013). Substance Abuse and Mental Health Services: Overview of behavioral health for aging information and referral/assistance professionals training. Teleconference January 9, 2013. Retrieved from http://www.nasuad.org/documentation/l_R/call_notes/1-9-13%20Behavioral%20Health%20Overview.pdf.

Stanford, M. (2012) Mindful of grace: Viewing mental illness through the eyes of faith. *Church Health Reader, 2*(4), 8–10.

Substance Abuse and Mental Health Services Administration (2003). Core competencies for clergy and other pastoral ministers in addressing alcohol and drug dependence and the impact on family. *Substance abuse and family: Defining the role of the faith community*. Report of an Expert Consensus Panel Meeting Feb. 26–27, 2013. Retrieved from http://store.samhsa.gov/product/Core-Competencies-for-Clergy-and-Other-Pastoral-Ministers-In-Addressing-Alcohol-and-Drug-Dependence-and-the-Impact-on-Family-Members/PHD1060

Substance Abuse and Mental Health Services Administration. (2014). Community conversations about mental health. Retrieved from http://beta.samhsa.gov/community-conversations

Taylor, R., Ellison, C., Chatters, L., Levin, J., & Lincoln, K. (2000). Mental health services in faith communities: The role of clergy in black churches. *Social Work, 45*(1), 73–87.

Warnock, A. (2013, May 24). How can faith communities and society better respond to mental illness? Retrieved from http://www.patheos.com/blogs/adrianwarnock/2013/05/how-can-faith-communities-and-society-better-respond-to-mental-illness/

Zwier, J., & Visser, W. (2012). *Let's talk: Breaking the silence around mental illness in our communities of faith.* Faith and Hope Ministries. Retrieved from http://faithand hopeministries.net/bible-studies-c144.php

Online Resources

Alcoholics Anonymous: www.alcoholics-anonymous.org/

Association of Professional Chaplains, Schaumburg, IL: http://professionalchaplains.org

Autism Society of America: http://www.autism-society.org/

Centers for Disease Control and Prevention: http://cdc.gov

Mental Health First Aid: http://www.mentalhealthfirstaid.org/cs/

Narcotics Anonymous: www.na.org/

National Alliance on Mental Illness. http://www.nami.org

National Institute of Mental Health: http://www.nimh.nih.gov

National Suicide Prevention Lifeline: https://www.suicide preventionlifeline.org/

Substance Abuse and Mental Health Services Administration: http://www.samhsa.gov/index.aspx

World Health Organization: http://www.who.int/en/

Wrap-Up and Evaluation

Measuring Competency

This chart can be used to assess the individual outcomes in this module.
- A copy of this chart is attached to the Participant Module, so that each participant can complete this short evaluation.
- Have participants read each outcome and then place an X in the box that best matches their opinion about the objective being met.
- Encourage each participant to write a short reflection about this module in the space provided at the bottom of this chart.
- Use this data to make any necessary changes.

Outcome	Not Met	Somewhat Met	Met
1. Identify signs and symptoms of mental illness and spiritual implications.			
2. Identify barriers to effective ministering to the behavioral health of the faith community.			
3. Make appropriate referrals, based on assessment, to behavioral health resources.			
4. Create a plan to transform/enhance the current environment of the faith community to an environment that is recognized as caring by those needing behavioral health services.			
Reflection: *In one paragraph, write a reflection on this module.*			

Appendix A

History of Mental Health Care and the Church in the Western Cultures

Pre-Middle Ages
- 5th century BC: severe mental illness was understood to be caused by a psychological condition. Mental illness was called the sacred disease. Care for the mentally ill was considered to be the responsibility of the family. If no family was available, the town might assign a caregiver or put the person in jail.
- 250 AD: the Christian church developed an outreach program for the mentally ill.
- 344–372 AD: several hostels were set up in Antioch, a poor house was built in Sebasteia, and the first great hospital, the Basileias, was built. These establishments took care of both the physically and mentally ill.
- Middle of 4th century AD: some mental illnesses were thought to be the result of demonic possession.

Middle Ages (500–1500 AD)
- 5th century: records of church helping the mentally ill.
- 6th century: Christian church-run monasteries cared for the mentally ill.
- 1225–1230: Bartholomaeus, a Franciscan monk and professor of theology, wrote an encyclopedia that dealt with the natural causes of mental illness as opposed to the prevailing theory that mental illness was caused by supernatural causes (Koenig, 2005).
- 1247: the first psychiatric hospital was built in London, the Priory of St. Mary of Bethlehem.
- 1409: Spain built a religious sponsored hospital to care specifically for the mentally ill.
- 1487: with the publication of *Malleus Maleficarum*, which describes the diagnosis and treatment of those demonically possessed, the church became involved in the persecution of the mentally ill, as well as witches and sorcerers. (Koenig, 2005).
- 1547: St. Mary's was torn down and replaced by Bethlem Hospital, commonly called "Bedlam."
- 1676: a new Bethlem Hospital was built and often frequented by tourists who came to observe and be entertained by patients.
- Historians disagree on how extensive the persecution of the mentally ill was during this time.

Renaissance and Reformation (mid-1300s–1800s)
- Ideas about mental illness did not change much.
- As the scientific revolution evolved, references to demons as the cause of mental illness began to subside.

Age of Reason and Enlightenment
- Followed after the Reformation era.
- Religious beliefs were not tolerated as well as in previous eras.
- Appearance of nonsupernatural and nonreligious explanations for mental illness began as the medical community sought scientific explanations for causes of mental illnesses.
- Abuse became less common in the hospitals.
- 1793: in France, a new approach which focused on compassion and less use of restraints was successful.
- 1796: the York Retreat was established in England using a treatment protocol of intelligent and humane care. The goal was one of self-control and restoration. Eventually this protocol was adopted throughout England (Koenig, 2005).

Origins of American Psychiatry
- Greatly influenced by the treatment protocols in England.
- Quakers brought moral treatment in the early 1800s (Koenig 2005).
- 1813: Friends Hospital established in Philadelphia.
- Treatment was a mix of science and religion.
- Mid-1800s: Dorothea Dix became the champion for humane care of the mentally ill in America (Koenig 2005). She also influenced the care offered in England and Scotland for the mentally ill.

Modern Times
- Heavily influenced the decline of religion's input into psychiatry and led to an almost complete separation of the two (Koenig 2005).
- 1980: a number of psychiatric hospitals and psychiatric treatment settings had completely removed any evidence of religious influence on treatment.
- Spirituality is increasingly being examined as a factor in mental health. Recent studies have found that spirituality may serve as a psychological and social resource for coping with the negative impact of traumatic stress on mental health (Reinert & Koenig, 2013).

Appendix B

Questions for Suicide Assessment

Once risk of suicide has been determined, address these questions to determine appropriate referral.
- Do you have a plan? Please describe your plan.
- Do you have access to the things you need to accomplish your plan?
- Have any members of your family committed suicide? What was your relationship to the person who committed suicide? Did you observe this action or find the family member after suicide had occurred?

The degree of danger increases with a positive answer to these questions.
- The more detailed the plan the more danger of suicide occurring.
- Accessibility to lethal weapons increases the probability of a suicide attempt.
- High risk of suicide occurs when a family member has committed suicide.
- Finding a family member after suicide also carries high risk.

If there are positive responses to the above assessment, involve a behavioral health professional. Do not leave your congregant alone until a mental health evaluation can be done at your local mental health center or emergency room or a Medical Detention Order (MDO) has been obtained, if necessary, and the congregant has been moved by law enforcement for evaluation.

Appendix C

Quick Reference Resource List
Mental Health Ministry Local Resources

Organization or Professional	Contact Information
Pastoral Counselor	
Licensed Behavioral Health Providers	
Chemical Dependency Counselors	
Alcoholics Anonymous	
Narcotics Anonymous	
Psychiatrists	
Community Mental Health Center	
Suicide Crisis Hotline	
Emergency Room	
Local Behavioral Health Unit	
National Alliance on Mental Health	
Mental Health Chaplain	

Appendix D
Communities of Compassion and Justice Action Plan

Once the faith community leadership has studied the issues of compassion and justice around mental and behavioral health themes, effective outreach can begin in a variety of ways. It is important that persons with mental illness feel welcomed and supported within the faith community. As people of faith, we do this by loving unconditionally. Faith communities should be places of nonjudgmental love for their members experiencing mental illness and for those who have a family member with mental illness. Then parishioners can feel safe to acknowledge their needs and overcome their fears of rejection. A faith community can establish that reputation with persons who have a mental illness and their families in a variety of ways.

1. **People with mental illness and their families will often come to a clergy person and faith community leaders first when symptoms of the illness strike.**
   It is important for clergy and leaders to listen with compassion and to know when to refer people to mental health professionals rather than attempt to solve psychological problems themselves or dismiss the problem. It is also important to know where in the community one can refer people for competent professional help and services. This can be done by forming relationships with mental health professionals and agencies. And it is equally important to stay in touch with the person and/or their family after a referral as major mental illness can cause a crisis of faith. People with mental illness and their families need the ongoing support of the faith community as well as professional help. The faith community can make a real difference in people's lives when it reaches out and continues to support individuals and families affected by mental illness.

2. **Incorporate into intercessory prayer at worship services specific prayers for those suffering with schizophrenia, manic depression, anxiety disorders.**
   This lets the faith community know that the community prays and cares for people with mental illness. Do not identify names or information that could compromise confidentiality of members who may suffer from mental health disorders. Rather, the purpose is to model publicly the safety of talking about these topics in the faith community. The prayer sends the welcoming message to those who suffer with mental illness and to their family members that their community supports them.

3. **Preach on the subject of mental and behavioral health.**
   Include references to persons with mental illness and their issues in homilies about social justice, caring for the poor, discrimination, and compassionate outreach to others. Avoid words or phrases in all sermons and communications that add to stigmatizing those who have mental illness.

4. **Let faith community members know that their leaders or ministers want to visit people with mental illness when they are hospitalized.**
   A hospitalization for mental illness is a traumatic time for the person and their family. It is an important time for ministerial presence. As for any major disease, the individual and family will have questions about God, faith, and "why me?" Ministerial presence and support will help them to understand and accept that this disease of the brain is not a punishment from God and not due to lack of faith.

5. **Give the peace and justice ministry teams the opportunity to get involved in the systemic problems that affect persons with mental illness.**
   At least half of the prison population suffers with mental illness and at least one-third of the homeless population suffers with mental illness. The high recidivism rate among prisoners and the issues of capital punishment and mental illness raise serious questions about the legal system's ability to deal with mental illness. The failure of the mental health system to meet the basic needs of persons with mental illness and their families is a moral issue for us as a very wealthy country that has the means to provide not only basic services but much more. The community mental health system throughout the country continues to be underfunded and provides inadequate or incomplete services for persons with mental illness and their families. Mental health workers are generally the poorest paid. Programs for persons with mental illness are the last to receive budget increases and the first to receive budget cuts. This is morally unconscionable.

6. **Advocacy is needed with the political leaders and the legislative process.**
   Since much of the problem with obtaining adequate care comes from the lack of funding for existing programs and decent wages for healthcare workers, state legislators who pass laws and control the budget are key to improving the system. Faith communities can write letters and/ or advocate directly with their elected officials to bring about justice to these inequities. Mental illness and the legislative process is a faith community issue since it deals with justice and compassion for people in need. The faith community can speak powerfully about doing what is right and just.

7. **Housing and jobs are critical to the recovery process and to the dignity of the individual.**
   Many people in faith communities own businesses or housing or work in the real estate industry. Faith communities can encourage members to help find jobs and places to live for persons with mental illness.

8. **Publicize the issues in the church bulletin or newsletter through a series of short articles.**
   It is important to have a series of articles rather than one or two. A series of *short* articles, preferably more than five, keeps the information readable by not giving too much to digest at one time. It also keeps the issues in the minds of people rather than a one-time exposure soon forgotten like yesterday's news. A series also gives a chance to explain the facts, the moral implications, and what faith communities can do.

9. **Healing prayer and services, such as Sacrament of Anointing of the Sick, for illnesses should include mental illnesses.**
   This gives a sign to the community that all forms of illnesses are included in the faith community's care and concern. Faith communities have to be particularly sensitive in this area as there is a history of misguided prayer in the past. Mental illness is not demon possession or God specifically giving us a cross to bear or God's lack of love for us. It is a disease like any other disease. The healing prayer should reflect the biological nature of the illness just like any other disease. We should pray for a healing and continue with sound medical practices.

10. **Many organizations and groups within the faith community are looking for speakers and topics for their meetings.**
    The topic of mental illness should be encouraged as subject matter for one of their meetings. Speakers could be from the medical community, mental health field, or advocacy groups. It is important to check out ahead of time what the speakers have to say on the subject, as there is a lot of misinformation about mental illness. A few good resources for information and speakers include the Chicago Archdiocesan Commission on Mental Illness, the National Catholic Partnership on Disability, The National Alliance for the Mentally Ill, the American Psychiatric Association, and the Mental Health Association.

11. **Peer-to-peer ministry is an important outreach for persons suffering with major mental illness.**
People with mental illness often do not have a circle of friends that care for them. An important element to recovery and healing is a caring community. The peer is not a professional but is a person who is caring and able to be a good listener. Peer-to-peer program information is available through NAMI.

12. **Network within your vicariate or with other faith communities in the area, and have an annual liturgical celebration of the lives of persons with a mental illness, their families, and mental health workers/professionals.**
This gathering should be celebratory and positive with a gathering after the liturgy to share fellowship and conversation.

13. **Host speakers, workshops, and educational events for families of persons with a mental illness.**
NAMI groups can help organize these gatherings. Families in crisis need spiritual guidance and advice. The long-term nature of serious mental illnesses means the family also needs long-term spiritual guidance. NAMI has an excellent "Family to Family" program that assists families with education and networking.

14. **Promote the dignity of the individual.**
God loves us each as we are. Use "people first language," including phrases such as "people with a mental illness" rather than "the mentally ill." No one wants to be known as a disease.

Adapted from Commission on Mental Illness and Faith Fellowship for People with Mental Illness, Archdiocese of Chicago (2008).

Appendix E

Pathways to Promise Program and Toolkit

Pathways to Promise (www.pathways2promise.org) is an interfaith technical assistance and resource center that offers liturgical and educational materials, program models, and networking information to promote a caring ministry with people with mental illness and their families. These resources are used by people at all levels of faith group structures from local faith communities to regional and national staff.

The website includes information on "Three Steps to a Mental Health Ministry" for developing the capacity of faith communities to support recovery and wellness.

Pathways to Promise offers help for building a mental health ministry in a faith community setting and suggestions for working with others in the local community.

Some resources included are:
- "Companionship: A Ministry of Presence"
- a description of a Local Mental Health Training Cooperative
- a survey instrument to help you identify mental health concerns in your faith community
- a pdf of the **Mental Health Ministry Toolkit**

The Mental Health Ministry Toolkit is a great resource for many ideas and simple ways to increase awareness of mental health issues and support for these persons and families in any faith community. Even small actions, such as messages in bulletins, an usher's greeting, or larger efforts, such as services and prayers to be more inclusive of these members, can help us all reach out to those suffering from the isolating and stigmatizing effects of these illnesses.

Pathways to Promise materials are user-friendly for FCNs and health ministry teams.

Appendix F
Faith Community Health Assessment

Yes = 2   Maybe = 1   No = 0

Enter your faith community's score in the space beside each question. Then add the numbers to find the total score.

____ 1. Does your faith community support a health ministry?

____ 2. Does your spiritual leader give sermons regarding the faith community's care of the vulnerable?

____ 3. Does your faith community have a process in place to greet new people when they visit?

____ 4. Do you think that you can safely disclose your feelings in your faith community and your confidentiality will be honored?

____ 5. Is your faith community open to members sharing their pain?

____ 6. Does your faith community survey the members regarding their experience as a member of the faith community and give them an opportunity to provide their feedback?

____ 7. Is your faith community one that listens, processes, and aids in problem solving or one that tells you what to do, directs the process without your input, and is judgmental?

____ 8. Is your faith community environment one that encourages members to feel like they can be themselves and be honest about their feelings, pain, or situation?

Score_____ /16

This survey can be helpful in surveying the faith community's opinion of the church culture. It can also be used by the health ministry team to develop a plan for changing or enhancing the culture to be one of caring and support for the mentally ill.

Appendix G
Quiz on Mental Illness

1. Mental illness only affects people in poverty.	Y	N
2. Many of the homeless have a form of mental illness.	Y	N
3. People with mental illness are violent.	Y	N
4. Only non-Christians experience mental illness.	Y	N
5. Mental illness results because people are sinful or evil.	Y	N
6. There is no effective treatment for mental illness.	Y	N
7. People will avoid the subject of mental illness due to fear of the mentally ill.	Y	N
8. Medication is a useful form of treatment for mental illness.	Y	N
9. Many view mental illness as weakness.	Y	N
10. Most faith communities are open and welcoming to the mentally ill.	Y	N

ANSWERS:
1.N; 2.Y; 3.N; 4.N; 5.N; 6.N; 7.Y; 8.Y; 9.Y; 10.N.

Appendix H

Daily Prayer for People Living with Mental Illness

Each Day

I will recall that I am a child of God. I am one who is created out of love. I am chosen, good, holy, and have purpose ... a task to perform here on Earth before I return to the Father. I deserve to be treated as a person who has value and dignity.

I will look this day for what my illness is teaching me about the mystery of God and life.

I will not allow the stigma of mental illness to defeat me this day. I will choose to have power over stigma by detaching myself from the stigma.

I will talk to someone today who will encourage me to see my goodness and holiness as a child of God. Maybe we will share a prayer together for one another.

I will look for humor and reasons to laugh and be happy. Quiet joy will be my goal.

I will read a passage from Scripture or something from a book of devotion, inspiration or spiritual reading that will encourage me to trust and hope in the power and love of God.

I will seek twenty minutes of solitude, silence, or prayer this day. If my mind won't quiet down, if my thoughts keep racing, I will offer that as my prayer to God. If necessary and helpful, I will listen to soothing instrumental music or inspirational/religious music to quiet me and remind me that God is present.

I will walk outdoors marveling at a sunrise, a sunset, the song of a bird, the soothing colors of nature, the serenity of green grass, a blue sky, the softness of the pastel colored blossoms of springtime, and the peaceful waters of a river, lake or stream that ripple and flow. I will remind myself that everything in nature is a reflection of the Creator and pleases the Creator just as it is, and so do I just as I am.

I will delight in the knowledge that we are each created different, because it is in our differences we make a more powerful and beautiful whole. We each reflect a different aspect of the mystery of life and God. Individually and together we are a masterpiece!

In God is my hope and my joy. I will give honor, glory and praise to God, knowing and trusting what God has in store for me. We do not seek or like suffering but our suffering can make us strong in many ways and more compassionate and loving to others, our brothers and sisters in the Lord.

Knowing for sure that although I long for God, God's longing for me is even greater, I will rest in that knowledge this day.

Adapted from Lambert, T. & Lambert, R. (2008). Mental illness and faith community outreach. From a workshop on spirituality by Rita Sebastian Lambert.

Unit III: Wholistic Health

Transforming Life Issues

Family Violence

Transforming Life Issues
Family Violence
Introduction

Learning Outcomes

Upon completion of this module, the participant will be able to:

1. Recognize family violence and the five forms of abuse.
2. Describe the incidence, prevalence, and risk factors of family violence.
3. Assess intimate partner abuse, child, and elder abuse.
4. Assist the vulnerable in the context of faith traditions, spiritual interventions, and faith community nursing Scope and Standards of Practice.

Description

This module provides an overview of issues pertaining to family violence. Besides defining and describing family violence, it includes information addressing the incidence, prevalence, and risk factors. The module will also describe the methods to assess and respond to those who are victims of abuse. Participants will discuss the faith community nurse's role of employing faith community nursing Scope and Standards of Practice that promote wholistic health, wellness, and a safe environment.

Hours: 2

Research

Family violence is a globally widespread issue that transcends all socioeconomic communities and population groups, has no religious boundaries, and has both immediate and lifelong health consequences. Much of the scholarship in this area includes qualitative studies with populations who face increased vulnerability to interpersonal trauma. Research in this area covers the life span from childhood to later adulthood and encompasses both domestic and international studies. One of the protective factors emerging in the literature is religious coping. Religious coping, spirituality, and faith-based approaches to trauma recovery include endorsement of beliefs, engagement in behaviors, and access to support from faith communities. Spirituality and positive religious coping have been associated with decreased psychological distress, a finding established with survivors of child abuse, sexual violence, intimate partner violence, community violence, and war (Bryant-Davis and Wong, 2013).

Faith Tradition

Many faith communities (Christian denominations, Jewish, Islamic and others) voice concern about family violence. Unfortunately, many victims of family violence find it difficult to seek help from their faith communities as domestic issues may be accompanied by denial, shame, and guilt. Some faith communities offer guidance and prevention training, whereas others may choose to ignore the issue. Although religious families may be considered sacred, many individuals are victimized and live in unsafe households consumed by silence related to concerns bound in their personal beliefs and religious ideology (Casey, 2014). Advocates for trauma survivors are encouraged to attend to the faith traditions and beliefs of persons confronting the potential devastation of traumatic events (Bryant-Davis and Wong, 2013). Faith community nurses are in an excellent position to be involved with other professionals in providing an interprofessional approach to education, prevention, evaluating, and coordinating services (Humphreys and Campbell, 2010).

Key Terms

Economic abuse: the attempt to make the victim financially dependent upon the abuser as a means to have total control over all financial resources. This may include holding any funds received through public assistance or social security, forbidding employment, requiring intense financial accountability, and withholding information on expenses that could overextend the family's financial capabilities

Emotional abuse: the attempt or act of undermining a person's self-worth, which may include constant criticism, belittling the victim's abilities and competency, insults and manipulating the victim's feelings and emotions to induce guilt

Family violence: the pattern of violent and coercive behavior directed by someone toward a partner, sibling, child or elder

Physical abuse: the infliction or attempt to harm someone by physical force, which may include behaviors such as hitting, shoving, kicking, burning, punching or restraining

Psychological abuse: threatening a partner or another person by instilling fear, which may include threats of physical harm to self, the victim or others through blackmail, harassment, property destruction, and stalking

Sexual abuse: coercing or forcing someone into sexual contact without consent, which may include rape, forcing prostitution, or sodomy

Reflection

Gracious God, you created us and gave us the breath of life. In gratitude, we want to live in your enduring love and trust. We ask that you be with those who suffer from oppression. We pray for those who suffer in silence and are fearful to utter a word and be misunderstood. Surround them with your care and protect them by your love. Heal their pain of suffering and give them strength. Bind up the wounds of abuse and permit the vulnerable to walk in peace, clarity of mind, and the joy of your blessings. Empower them so that they may give love with confidence and dignity. Amen.

Prayer used by permission of Chaplain Anne Gifford, FCN, DEdMin.

Using the Church Health Center's Model for Healthy Living, explore the interconnectedness in the context of how family violence and abuse affects one's life (Appendix A).

Transforming Life Issues
Family Violence
Content Outline

KEY TERM

Understanding these five key forms of **family violence** *is essential to responding to victims.*
- **physical abuse**
- **sexual abuse**
- **psychological abuse**
- **emotional abuse**
- **economic abuse**

OUTCOME 1

Recognize family violence and the five forms of abuse.

Family violence is the pattern of violent and coercive behavior directed by someone toward a partner, sibling, child or elder.
- **Physical abuse** is the infliction or attempt to harm someone by physical force. It may include behaviors such as hitting, shoving, kicking, burning, punching, or restraining.
- **Sexual abuse** is coercing or forcing someone into sexual contact without consent. It may include rape, forcing prostitution, or sodomy.
- **Psychological abuse** is threatening a partner or another person by instilling fear. It may include threats of physical harm to self, victim or others through blackmail, harassment, property destruction, and stalking.
- **Emotional abuse** is the attempt or act of undermining a person's self-worth. It may include constant criticism, belittling the victims' abilities and competency, insults, manipulating the victim's feelings and emotions to induce guilt.
- **Economic abuse** is the attempt to make the victim financially dependent upon the abuser as a means to have total control over all financial resources. This may include holding any funds received through public assistance or social security, forbidding employment, requiring intense financial accountability, and withholding information on expenses that could overextend the family's financial capabilities.

OUTCOME 2

Describe the incidence, prevalence, and risk factors of family violence.

Family violence impacts many population groups.
- Family violence affects everyone, regardless of sexual orientation.
- Family violence affects all racial, ethnic, religious, and socioeconomic groups.

- Family violence is a community problem, but it is rarely talked about.
- Domestic violence is the leading cause of injury to women.
- Men are also affected by domestic violence.
- There is no specific type of abused woman. All types of women are vulnerable.

Violence is usually a **recurrent phenomenon that escalates** in severity and frequency over time. The highest risk for serious injury or death from violence in an intimate relationship is at the point of separation or at the time when the decision to separate is made.

Drug or alcohol abuse is a contributing factor.
- Drug or alcohol abuse may occur simultaneously with family violence.
- Eliminating drugs or alcohol does not necessarily eliminate the abuse.
- Substance abuse is no excuse for family violence.

Who is the abuser or perpetrator?
- There is an increasing awareness that women are also abusers of men.
- In about half of the reported cases of domestic violence, both male and female are active combatants.
- Nearly two-thirds of women who report being raped, physically assaulted, or stalked were victimized by a current or former husband, partner, boyfriend, or date.
- Intimate partners perpetrate the majority of all violent crimes against women, while men are more likely to be victimized by strangers.
- Abusers are often extremely jealous, possessive, controlling. They may experience rage at the possibility of being abandoned and would rather kill their partners than let them leave the relationship.
- Reports suggest that the single most common element among violent adult abusers is having been **neglected or abused in childhood.**

Children and Minors as Victims

It is important to emphasize that **children are the victims and are never to blame** for maltreatment. A number of characteristics of an individual child may increase the likelihood of being maltreated.
- being either under four years old or an adolescent
- being unwanted, or failing to fulfill the expectations of parents
- having special needs, crying persistently or having abnormal physical appearance

There are four main categories of maltreatment of children and minors.

> **Critical Thinking**
> *What is the faith community's responsibility toward victims of family violence?*

1. Neglect of meeting the basic needs—food, shelter, clothing, health care, protection
2. Physical—hitting, shaking, burning, forceful restraint, extreme spanking
3. Sexual—incest, rape, sodomy, exhibitionism, pornography, attempted or actual fondling
4. Emotional—attacks on child or adolescent's self-esteem and sense of self; verbal threats or name calling; belittling statements

In armed conflict and refugee settings, girls are particularly vulnerable to sexual violence, exploitation and abuse by combatants, security forces, members of their communities, aid workers and others.

Caregivers Who May Abuse
Most child abuse occurs within families. Parents and relatives who were abused themselves are most often the perpetrators. Characteristics of a parent or caregiver that may increase the risk of child maltreatment include the following.
- difficulty bonding with a newborn
- not nurturing the child
- having been maltreated as children themselves
- lacking awareness of child development or having unrealistic expectations
- misusing alcohol or drugs, including during pregnancy
- being involved in criminal activity
- experiencing financial difficulties

Family Characteristics That May Contribute to Abuse
Characteristics of relationships within families or among intimate partners, friends and peers that may increase the risk of child maltreatment include the following.
- physical, developmental or mental health problems of a family member
- family breakdown or violence between other family members
- isolation or lack of a support network
- lack of support from the extended family in child-rearing

Community Risk Factors
Characteristics of communities and societies that may increase the risk of child maltreatment include the following.
- gender and social inequality
- lack of adequate housing or services
- high levels of unemployment or poverty
- easy availability of alcohol or drugs
- inadequate policies and programs to prevent child maltreatment, child pornography, child prostitution and child labor (World Health Organization, 2014).

Consequences of Child Maltreatment
Child maltreatment causes suffering to children and families and can have **long-term consequences**.

Research by Shaley et al. (2013) found that 10-year-olds who experienced violence had significant biological aging changes in DNA. Maltreatment causes stress that is associated with disruption in early brain development. Extreme stress can impair the development of the nervous and immune systems. Consequently, as adults, maltreated children are at increased risk for behavioral, physical and mental health problems.

- perpetrating or being a victim of violence
- depression
- smoking
- obesity
- high-risk sexual behaviors
- unintended pregnancy
- alcohol and drug misuse

Preventive Approaches

Preventing child maltreatment requires a multifaceted approach. Effective programs that support parents and teach positive parenting skills may include:

- Visits by nurses to parents and children in their homes to provide support, education, and information.
- Parent education, usually delivered in groups, to improve child-rearing skills, increase knowledge of child development, and encourage positive child management strategies.
- Multiple interventions, which typically include support and education of parents, preschool education, and childcare (World Health Organization, 2014).

Elders as Victims

Elder maltreatment is a single or repeated act, or lack of appropriate action, occurring within any relationship where there is an expectation of trust, which causes harm or distress to an older person. This type of violence constitutes a violation of human rights and includes:

- physical, sexual, psychological, emotional; financial and material abuse
- abandonment
- neglect
- serious loss of dignity and respect

Elder maltreatment can lead to physical injuries, ranging from minor scratches and bruises to broken bones and head injuries leading to lasting disabilities.

- It may also cause serious, sometimes long-lasting, psychological consequences, including depression and anxiety.
- For older people, the consequences of maltreatment can be especially serious because their bones are more brittle and convalescence is longer.
- Even relatively minor injuries can cause serious and permanent damage, or even death.

Neglect is the most common form of elder maltreatment in domestic settings followed by physical abuse and financial or material exploitation.

- Many elders live away from their children and may depend on friends and their faith community family for support.
- Most victims suffer from some sort of disability which requires assistance.
- The elderly are often isolated. One common factor is migration of young couples, leaving elderly parents alone, in societies where older people were traditionally cared for by their offspring.
- Financial exploitation is a common form of elder abuse.
- Family members are the most frequent abusers of the elderly.
- A shared living situation is a risk factor for elder maltreatment.

It is not yet clear whether spouses or adult children of older people are more likely to perpetrate abuse.

- An abuser's dependency on the older person (often financial) also increases the risk of abuse.
- In some cases, a long history of poor family relationships may worsen as a result of stress and frustration as the older person becomes more dependent.
- Finally, as more women enter the workforce and have less spare time, caring for older people becomes a greater burden, increasing the risk of abuse (World Health Organization, 2011).

Impact of Violence on the Family

Violence or the threat of violence increases the risk for behavioral and emotional problems and impairment of vocational, social, and academic functioning. Exposure to family violence is associated with increased rates of:

- suicide
- homicide
- conduct disorder
- depression
- post-traumatic stress disorder
- alcohol and drug abuse
- impaired self-esteem
- feelings of helplessness and hopelessness

Recent research (Koeppel and Bouffard, 2014) found that children who are exposed to intimate partner violence are more likely to grow up to experience partner violence themselves.

Critical Thinking
Why is it important for FCNs to understand how to care for victims of family violence?

OUTCOME 3
Assess intimate partner abuse, child, and elder abuse.

Laws for reporting family violence vary from state to state.

- Most federal and state laws address reporting family violence.
- Nursing Practice Acts require reporting of abuse, neglect, or exploitation.

If abuse is present, the victim frequently is kept isolated from any social network and activities.
- The victim has restricted access to health providers and services.
- The victim has personality changes or is excessively private.
- The victim frequently is nervous, anxious and easily upset.
- The victim's partner has excessive control of victim's activities and involvement with others.
- The partner speaks for and makes victim's decisions.
- The partner insults or ridicules victim in public.
- The victim has unexplained injuries or minimizes visible injuries.
  - attributes injuries to 'an accident.'
  - may wear long sleeves in warm weather, sunglasses indoors, or heavy makeup.

Possible indicators of child abuse or neglect include the following.
- hygiene and appearance
  - consistently dirty, hungry or inappropriately dressed
  - lacks appropriate medical care
  - bruises or welts on body or face
  - burns, fractures, or lacerations
  - human bite marks
  - burning or itching in genital area
- social
  - no supervision for extended periods of time is evident
  - frequently absent from school
  - wary of physical contact with adults
  - fearful of parents
  - shy or aggressive of peers
  - inappropriate sexualized behavior
- behavioral
  - "acts out" or withdraws from others
  - begs or steals food
  - threatens or attempts suicide

Possible indicators of elder abuse include the following. When visiting the setting in which an individual lives, make observations of the individual and the living environment.
- Observe for malnutrition or dehydration, poor personal hygiene, dirty clothes and bedding.
- Recognize if the person appears to be over- or under-medicated or is untreated for physical health problems.
- Look for evidence of multiple injuries, burns or bruises that are in various stages of healing.
- Consider whether the caretaker appears to be openly hostile or the elder is unwilling to discuss his or her injuries in the presence of the caretaker.
- Watch for whether the elder acts fearful of caretaker but appears eager to please caretaker.

> ## Critical Thinking
> *Discuss how the FCN can respond to intimate partner, elder, and child abuse.*

OUTCOME 4

Assist the vulnerable in the context of faith traditions, spiritual interventions, and faith community nursing Scope and Standards of Practice.

Statistics show that more people go to spiritual leaders (clergy, FCNs, chaplains, spiritual directors) than any other helping professional for assistance with personal problems. The prepared FCN can play a critical role.

The FCN can begin with simple **self-assessment** about readiness to become involved with family violence issues and consider how to be better prepared.

1. If I have had a personal experience with family violence, have I sufficiently dealt with and healed from my own victimization so that I can care for others?
2. What is my current attitude about family violence?
3. Am I qualified to work with victims and perpetrators of family violence?
4. Do I need training about family violence and ways to deal with it?
5. Have I realistically evaluated and admitted my limitations?
6. What resources can I access to assist victims of family violence?

The following list suggests actions FCNs can take to **help the faith community engage** with issues of family violence.

1. Be cognizant of religious teachings of faith communities.
2. Become aware of the legal concerns on abuse regarding assault, battery, and neglect.
3. Attend additional training offered by your denomination, faith, or organizations who work with family violence.
4. Educate your spiritual leaders, faith community, and larger community about family violence with sermons, articles, programs, and prayers.
5. Encourage age-appropriate curriculum on healthy relationships and bully prevention in children's classes and youth groups.
6. Invite local family violence organizations, law enforcement, and emergency medical services (EMS) to partner with your faith community to raise awareness and care for victims.
7. Post contact information for local services and national family violence hotlines in bathrooms and other places where it will not be obvious who is receiving or reading the materials.
8. Explore the resources available through your denomination or religious affiliation.
9. Practice a safe sanctuary policy including background checks and screening volunteers and staff members.
10. Always have more than one adult involved with youth activities and classes.
11. Encourage the faith community to offer parenting classes and support for single parents.

Be ready to **respond to suspicious incidents** of family violence and abuse.

1. Speak with the victim alone.
    - Ask if the victim would like to share his or her story with you.
    - Ask open-ended questions in a nonjudgmental manner.
    - Listen; don't ask for detailed descriptions of the violence.
    - Believe what the victim says until proven otherwise.
    - Maintain confidentiality.
    - Do not minimize or take ownership of the situation.
    - Reassure the victim that feelings of fear, shame, isolation, guilt, confusion, hopelessness, and powerlessness are normal.
2. Assist the victim to assess personal strengths and support systems.
3. Offer and strongly encourage seeking help from medical or mental health care providers.
    - Refer the victim to a trained specialist who can help develop an escape plan.
    - Present information and options, but insist that the victim make his or her own decisions.
4. Support the victim's decisions even when you disagree.
5. Remember that reporting suspected abuse is required by law.

Safety is always the top priority.
- Never take a victim into your own home as it may create a potential risk of a dangerous situation for all parties.
- Never attempt to confront a batterer as it may escalate the violence.
- Never blame the victim for the abuse or his or her attempt to justify the abuser's actions.
- Never give in to the temptation to "rescue" the victim by taking ownership of his or her problems.
- Never use clichés such as "It's God's will" or "All things work together for good."

Critical Thinking
What are some self-assessment issues that the FCN should consider before working with victims of family violence?

Standards of Professional Performance for Faith Community Nursing

Standard 1. Assessment

The faith community nurse collects comprehensive data pertinent to the healthcare consumer's wholistic health or the situation.

COMPETENCIES

The faith community nurse:

- Collects wholistic data including but not limited to physical, functional, psychosocial, emotional, cognitive, sexual, cultural, age-related, environmental, economic, and spiritual or transpersonal assessments in a systematic and ongoing process, while honoring the uniqueness of the person and placing a particular emphasis on spiritual beliefs and practices.
- Assesses family dynamics and impact on healthcare consumer health and wellness.
- Applies legal, ethical, and privacy guidelines and policies to the collection, maintenance, uses, and dissemination of data and information.

Standard 5B. Health Teaching and Health Promotion

The faith community nurse employs strategies to promote wholistic health, wellness, and a safe environment.

COMPETENCIES

The faith community nurse:

- Provides health teaching for individuals or groups that addresses such topics as healthy lifestyles, risk-reducing behaviors, developmental needs, activities of daily living, preventive self-care, and spiritual practices for health and healing.

Standard 7. Ethics

The faith community nurse practices ethically.

COMPETENCIES

The faith community nurse:

- Takes appropriate action regarding instances of illegal, unethical, or inappropriate behavior that can endanger or jeopardize the best interests of the healthcare consumer or situation.

Standard 9. Evidence-Based Practice and Research

The faith community nurse integrates evidence and research findings into practice.

COMPETENCIES

The faith community nurse:

- Utilizes current evidence-based nursing knowledge, including research findings, to guide practice.

Standard 15. Resource Utilization

The faith community nurse utilizes appropriate resources to plan and provide nursing services that are safe, effective and financially responsible.

COMPETENCIES

The faith community nurse:

- Identifies healthcare consumer care needs, potential for harm, complexity of the task, and desired outcome when considering resource allocation.

Learning Activities

Faith Traditions and Family Violence

Instructions:
1. Ask participants to form small groups.
2. Assign each group a section of the following faith tradition material from Christianity, Islam and Judaism. Discuss how the content relates to family violence and the faith community.
3. Have each group write key points on a flip chart or white board.
4. Ask each group to share key points with all participants.

Question:
What similarities and differences do you see in these passages?

The LORD lives! Blessed be my rock,
and exalted be the God of my salvation,
the God who gave me vengeance
and subdued peoples under me;
who delivered me from my enemies;
indeed, you exalted me above my adversaries;
you delivered me from the violent.
For this I will extol you, O LORD, among the nations,
and sing praises to your name.
—Psalm 18:46–49

O mankind! reverence your Guardian-Lord, who created you from a single person, created, of like nature, His mate, and from them twain scattered (like seeds) countless men and women; reverence Allah, through whom ye demand your mutual (rights), and (reverence) the wombs (That bore you): for Allah ever watches over you.
And do not give the weak-minded your property, which Allah has made a means of sustenance for you, but provide for them with it and clothe them and speak to them words of appropriate kindness.
—The Qur'an 4:1, 4:5 (Yusuf Ali translation)

And among His Signs is this, that He created for you mates from among yourselves, that ye may dwell in tranquility with them, and He has put love and mercy between your (hearts): verily in that are Signs for those who reflect.
—The Qur'an 30:21 (Yusuf Ali translation)

Judaism has always recognized dignity to all human beings: just as God cares. Victims of abuse draw comfort, encouragement, and support from their Judaism. *Pikuah Nefesh*, saving a life, is commanded of Jews even if the life is one's own; therefore Jewish battered women are instructed to count themselves in. Comfort is offered by God, "I will give you peace in the land and you will lie down, and no one will make you afraid" (Leviticus 26:6).
—Toby Meyer, *Jewish Perspectives in Domestic Violence.*

Understanding the Cycle of Violence

Instructions:
1. Distribute copies of Dr. Walker's model of the cycle of violence (Appendix B).
2. Allow time for participants to read the material.
3. Discuss how the FCN should respond to an observation of a suspicious incident in each phase of Dr. Walker's cycle.

Question:
In what ways do you think you can better prepare yourself to respond to a suspicion of family violence?

Guest Speaker

Instructions:
1. Invite representatives from area women's shelters, child advocate organizations, adult protective services, and other local organizations that work with family violence, abuse, and neglect to share their criteria for services and accessing information.
2. It is also helpful to invite representatives from organizations who work with abusers.
3. Be sure to give clear expectation about topics, format, and length of presentation.

Question:
After hearing from guest speakers on family violence topics, what aspects of the subject do you feel you need to understand better?

Expanded Learning Activities

Instructions:

1. Watch and discuss an online video or DVD.

   - Elder Justice Now Campaign. (2010). *An Age for Justice: Confronting Elder Abuse in America* [16 minute Video webcast. Free]. Retrieved November 23, 2013 from http://www.youtube.com/watch?v=-eaJXBj87to.

   - Faith Trust Institute. (2009). *Broken vows: Religious perspectives on domestic violence* [60 minutes DVD and Study Guide. $89.00] Available from www.faithtrustinstitute.org.

   - Faith Trust Institute. (2009). *Domestic violence: What churches can do*, [20 minute video/DVD. $31.00]. Available from Faith Trust Institute www.faithtrustinstitute.org.

   - Faith Trust Institute. (2004). *Hear Their Cries: Religious Response to Child Abuse.* [48 minute video/DVD. $70.00]. An award-winning video on the role of clergy and lay leaders in ending child abuse is a critical resource. Available at: http://www.faithtrustinstitute.org.

   - Lewkowicz, Sara Naomi (Time Lightbox). (2013). *A Portrait of Domestic Violence* [6.5-minute video webcast]. Retrieved November 23, 2013 from http://lightbox.time.com/2013/03/25/video-a-portrait-of-domestic-violence/

   - TED: Ideas Worth Spreading. (2012). *Leslie Morgan Steiner: Why domestic violence victims don't leave* [16 minute video webcast. Free]. Retrieved November 23, 2013 from http://www.ted.com/talks/leslie_morgan_steiner_why_domestic_violence_victims_don_t_leave.

2. Lead a group discussion on FCN collaboration.

   In a large group, discuss the following questions.

   - Describe your faith community's family violence education program.

   - How is your faith community reaching out to the family violence concerns of the community (support/assists in community education, battered women's shelter, etc.)?

   - Discuss ways the different faith communities might collectively collaborate and coordinate to present a community family violence awareness program.

References

Required Textbook

American Nurses Association and Health Ministries Association. (2012). *Scope and standards of practice: Faith community nursing* (2nd ed.). Silver Spring, MD: Nursesbooks.org.

References

Bryant-Davis. T. & Wong, E. (2013). Faith to move mountains: Religious coping, spirituality, and interpersonal trauma recovery. *American Psychologist 68*(8), 675–684.

Casey, K. (2014). Jesus loves me this I know: 'cause my mother told me so! ... being a child of religion and violence. *Feminist Theology: The Journal of the Britain & Ireland School of Feminist Theology, 22*(2), 123–132.

Humphreys, J., & Campbell, J. (2010). *Family violence and nursing practice* (2nd ed). New York, NY: Springer Publishing Company.

Koeppel, M., & Bouffard, L. (February 2014). *The consequences of intimate partner violence victimization by sexual orientation.* Sam Houston University: College of Criminal Justice Crime Victims' Institute.

Shalev, I., Moffitt, T., Sugden, K. Williams, B. Houts, R. Danese, A., Mill, J., Arseneault, L., Caspi, A. (2013). Exposure to violence during childhood is associated with telomere erosion from 5 to 10 years of age: A longitudinal study. *Molecular Psychiatry, 32*, 576–581.

World Health Organization. (2011). Elder maltreatment: Fact sheet N°357. August 2011 Retrieved June 4, 2014from http://www.who.int/mediacentre/factsheets/fs357/en/

World Health Organization. (2014). Child maltreatment: Fact sheet N°150. Updated January 2014 Retrieved June 4, 2014 from http://www.who.int/mediacentre/factsheets/fs150/en/

Additional References

Alkhateeb, M., & Abugideiri, S. (2007). *Change from within: Diverse perspectives on domestic violence in Muslim communities.* USA: Peaceful Families Project.

Anderson, J. (2007). *Woman submit! Christians and domestic violence.* Auburndale, FL: One Way Cafe Press.

Branson, B., & Silva, P. (2007). *Violence among us: Ministry to families in crisis.* Valley Forge, PA: Judson Press.

Capaldi, D. M., Knoble, N. B., Shortt, J.W., & Kim, H. K. (2012). A systematic review of risk factors for intimate partner violence. *Partner Abuse, 3*(2), 231–280.

Cook, P. (2009). *Abused men: The hidden side of domestic violence.* Westport, CT: Praeger Publishers.

Duke University. (2012, April 24). Violence puts wear and tear on kids' DNA. *Science Daily.* Retrieved June 6, 2014, from www.sciencedaily.com/releases/2012/04/120424095946.htm.

Ephesians 525 Ministries. (2014). *Help! There's an abused woman in my church: How to spot her and what to do—A guide for pastors and other Christians.*

Fortune, M. (1995). *Keeping the faith: Guidance for Christian women facing abuse.* San Francisco, CA: Harper Collins.

Gellert, G. (2002). *Confronting violence: Answers to questions about the epidemic destroying America's homes and communities.* Washington DC: American Public Health Association.

Hollies, L. (2006). *Inner healing for broken vessels: A domestic violence survival guide.* Cleveland, OH: Pilgrim Press.

Kaufman, C. (2003). *Sins of omission: The Jewish community's reaction to domestic violence.* Boulder, CO: Westview Press.

Kramer, Alice & Nosbursch, Jane. (2012). Safe mom, safe baby. *The Journal of Perinatal and Neonatal Nursing, Oct/Dec 2012,* 307–316.

MacDonnel, K. Watson. (2012). The combined and independent impact of witnessed interparental violence and child maltreatment. *Partner Abuse, 3*(3), 358–378.

Mindlin, Jessica & Brandl, Bonnie. (2013) Rural domestic and sexual abuse program advocates: Making a difference in the lives of older survivors of abuse. *National Clearinghouse on Abuse in Later Life* [pdf document]. Retrieved June 6, 2014 from http://ncall.us/content/rural

Mosqueda, Laura & Dong, XinQi. (Aug 3, 2011). Elder abuse and self-neglect. *Journal of American Medical Association, 306*(5), 532–539.

Myers, T. (2009). *Jewish perspectives in domestic violence* [paper published online]. Retrieved June 6, 2014 from http://www.ncdsv.org/images/Myers_JewishPerspectivesinDV_2009.pdf

O'Brien, K. (2013). Lifting the domestic violence cloak of silence: Resilient Australian women's reflected memories of their childhood experiences of witnessing domestic violence. *Journal of Family Violence, 28*(1), 95–108.

Sam Houston State University. (2013, October 30). Study explores intimate partner violence across generations. *ScienceDaily.* Retrieved June 6, 2014 from www.sciencedaily.com/releases/2013/10/131030093140.htm

Santovena, E., Lambert, T., & Hamel, J. (2013). Partner abuse worldwide. *Partner Abuse, 4*(1).

Schrager, Sarina. (2012). *Family violence: what health care providers need to know.* Sudbury, MA: Jones and Bartlett Learning.

Shwayder, Maya. (Nov, 2013) A same-sex domestic violence epidemic is silent. *The Atlantic.* Retrieved November 6, 2013 from http://www.theatlantic.com/health/archive/2013/11/a-same-sex-domestic-violence-epidemic-is-silent/281131/

Simmons, Barbara & Baxter, Jennifer Scotese. (2010). Intimate partner violence in older women. *Home Healthcare Nurse, 28*(2), 82–89.

Steiner, Leslie Morgan. (2010). *Crazy love.* New York, NY: St. Martin's Griffin.

Sturge-Apple, M. L., Skibo, M. A., & Davies, P. T. (2012). Impact of parental conflict and emotional abuse on children and families. *Partner Abuse, 3*(3), 379–400.

US Department of Justice, Bureau of Justice Statistics. (2013). Intimate partner violence: Attributes of victimization 1993–2011. Retrieved June 4, 2014 from http://www.bjs.gov/index.cfm?ty=pbdetail&iid=4801

Walker, L. (1979). *The battered woman.* New York: Harper and Row.

Walls, J. (2005). *The glass castle.* New York: Scribner.

Zarif, Marjan. (2010). Feeling shame: Insights on intimate partner violence. *Journal of Christian Nursing, 8*(1), 40–45.

Online Resources

Catalano, Shannan. Intimate partner violence: Attributes of victimization, 1993–2011. *Bureau of Justice Statistics.* Retrieved June 6, 2014 from http://www.bjs.gov/index.cfm?ty=pbdetail&iid=4801

CDC releases data on interpersonal and sexual violence by sexual orientation. *Centers for Disease Control and Prevention.* Retrieved November 23, 2013 from http://www.cdc.gov/media/releases/2013/p0125_NISVS.html

Chamberlain, L. (2008, March). A prevention primer for domestic violence: Terminology, tools, and the public health approach. *VAWnet.* Retrieved November 9, 2013 from http://www.vawnet.org/summary.php?doc_id=1313&find_type=web_desc_AR

National Clearinghouse on Abuse in Later Life. *Mandatory reporting of elder abuse.* Retrieved November 23, 2013 from http://ncall.us/content/mr

Rituals for healing from trauma and abuse. *Ritualwell: tradition and innovation.* Retrieved June 23, 2014 from www.ritualwell.org/categories/63

Safe-at-last's survival guide for victims of family violence & domestic abuse. *Safe-at-last hubpages.* Retrieved November 1, 2013 from http://safe-at-last.hubpages.com/hub/Domestic-Violence-OK-So-its-Abuse-What-Now

Safe Havens Interfaith Partnership Against Domestic Violence and the National Clearinghouse on Abuse in Later Life. (2013). Partnering to address faith and safety: A guide for faith leaders and domestic and sexual violence service providers to assist older victims of abuse [pdf document]. Retrieved November 23, 2013 from http://www.ncall.us/content/eafaith-toolkit

DVD/Videos

Centers for Disease Control and Prevention (CDC-TV). (2008). *Breaking the Silence—Stop the Violence* [5-minute video webcast]. Retrieved November 23, 2013 from http://www.cdc.gov/CDCTV/BreakTheSilence.

Elder Justice Now Campaign (2010). *An age for justice: Confronting elder abuse in America* [16-minute video webcast. Free]. Retrieved June 6, 2014 from http://www.youtube.com/watch?v=-eaJXBj87to

Faith Trust Institute (2004). *Hear their cries: Religious response to child abuse* [48 minute video/DVD. $70.00]. Available from http://www.faithtrustinstitute.org

Faith Trust Institute (2009). *Broken vows: Religious perspectives on domestic violence* [60-minute DVD and study guide. $89.00]. Available from www.faithtrustinstitute.org.

Faith Trust Institute (2009). *Domestic violence: What churches can do,* [20-minute video on DVD. $31.00]. Available from www.faithtrustinstitute.org

Faith Trust Institute (2010). *Hear their cries,* [2.33-minute video. Free]. Retrieved on November 15, 2013 from http://www.youtube.com/watch?v=YjkjqrfV71g

Lewkowicz, Sara Naomi (Time Lightbox). (2013). *A Portrait of Domestic Violence* [6.5-minute video webcast]. Retrieved November 23, 2013 from http://lightbox.time.com/2013/03/25/video-a-portrait-of-domestic-violence/

TED: Ideas Worth Spreading (2012) *Leslie Morgan Steiner: Why domestic violence victims don't leave* [16-minute video webcast. Free]. Retrieved June 6, 2014 from http://www.ted.com/talks/leslie_morgan_steiner_why_domestic_violence_victims_don_t_leave

Resources by phone

In the US: call the National Domestic Violence Hotline at 1-800-799-7233 (SAFE).

In the UK: call Women's Aid at 0808 2000 247.

In Australia: call 1800RESPECT (1 800 737 732).

Wrap-Up and Evaluation

Measuring Competency

This chart can be used to assess the individual outcomes in this module.
- A copy of this chart is attached to the Participant Module, so that each participant can complete this short evaluation.
- Have participants read each outcome and then place an X in the box that best matches their opinion about the objective being met.
- Encourage each participant to write a short reflection about this module in the space provided at the bottom of this chart.
- Use this data to make any necessary changes.

Outcome	Not Met	Somewhat Met	Met
1. Recognize family violence and the five forms of abuse.			
2. Describe the incidence, prevalence, and risk factors of family violence.			
3. Assess intimate partner abuse, child, and elder abuse.			
4. Assist the vulnerable in the context of faith traditions, spiritual interventions, and faith community nursing Scope & Standards of Practice			
Reflection: *In one paragraph, write a reflection on this module.*			

Appendix A

The Church Health Center
Model for Healthy Living

Using the Church Health Center's Model for Healthy Living, explore the interconnectedness in the context of how family violence and abuse affects one's life.

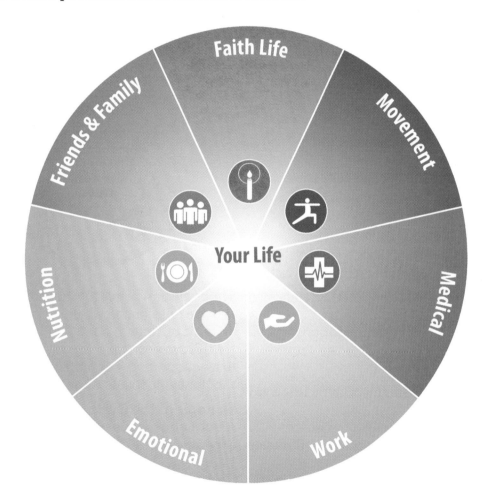

Faith Life
Building a relationship with God, neighbors and yourself.

Movement
Discovering ways to enjoy physical activity.

Medical
Partnership with your health care provider to manage your medical care.

Work
Appreciating your skills, talents and gifts.

Emotional
Managing stress and understanding your feelings to better care for yourself.

Nutrition
Making smart food choices and developing healthy eating habits.

Family & Friends
Giving and receiving support through relationships.

Appendix B

Cycle of Violence

Many organizations and websites with missions to assist battered women have descriptions of the cycle of violence. These descriptions have their root in the work of Dr. Lenore Walker, a clinical psychologist who pioneered studies of domestic violence and abused women. Her book, *The Battered Woman*, is a classic work in this field and provides a foundational understanding of four stages of the cycle that entraps women and other victims.

Stage 1: Tension Building
During this phase, the batterer uses increasingly abusive behaviors, such as name-calling, criticism, and public embarrassment. The victim responds with heightened anxiety.
- The abuser starts to get angry.
- Nonphysical abuse advances to minor battering.
- Communication breaks down.
- The victim feels the need to keep the abuser calm.
- Tension escalates.

Stage 2: Abuse
The batterer acts with an incident of physical, emotional or sexual violence against the victim.
- Physical forms of abuse are often accompanied by severe verbal abuse.
- The abuser establishes intimidation.
- The victim tends to minimize the abuse.

Stage 3: Honeymoon
The abuser feels remorse and acts lovingly toward the victim.
- The abuser gives gifts and compliments.
- The abuser promises the abuse will never happen again.
- This encourages the victim to remain in the relationship.
- The victim apologizes for provoking the violence.
- In some cases the abuser denies the abuse happened, causing self-doubt in the victim.

Stage 4: Calm
A period of calm and peace follows the apology.
- The abuser acts as if the abuse never happened.
- Promises made during the Honeymoon phase may be kept for a period of time.
- The victim hopes the abuse is over.

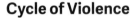

Cycle of Violence

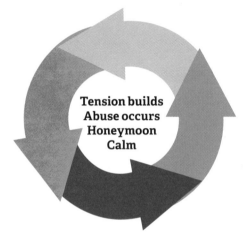

Tension builds
Abuse occurs
Honeymoon
Calm

The cycle can repeat hundreds of times in an abusive relationship. Each stage lasts a different amount of time in a particular relationship, so the full cycle can take anywhere from a few hours to a year or more to complete. As times goes on, the Honeymoon and Calm stages may disappear.

Example of the Cycle of Violence
A man abuses his wife. After he beats her, he experiences self-directed guilt. He says, "I'm sorry I hurt you." What he does not say is, "Because I might get caught." He then rationalizes his behavior by saying that his wife is having an affair with another man. He tells her, "If you weren't such a worthless woman, I wouldn't have hit you." He then acts contrite, reassuring her he will never hurt her again. Then he fantasizes and reflects on past abuse and how he will hurt her again. He plans to ask her to go to the store to pick up some groceries. What he does not tell her is that she has only a limited amount of time to do the shopping and get back home. When she is held up in traffic and is a few minutes late, he feel justified in hitting her and says, "You're having an affair with the store clerk." He has just set her up.

Appendix C

Could It Be Me?

Could it be me? You'll never know, because my door is so tightly closed.

I want to yell, I want to scream, "Could you, or would you, help me please?"

I'm so ashamed by what he did to me. I try to hide the marks so no one will see.

I know that one day I'm going tell him to stop, but I just didn't know how. Do I leave or not?

I have these three children I love so much, but how in the world will I care for the bunch?

Oh no, he is home. He's yelling my name. Should I go, should I hide, or now make my stand?

He's mad; he's angry in spite of my tears. I close my eyes, then feel pain once again as he nears.

I have learned not to make noise or to scream, for I've found when I do he just gets more angry.

I think now he's done. I stand up from the floor. I look in his eyes, and I cry, "Is there more?"

He leaves out the door and I reach for the phone. Who can I call before he comes home?

I gather my children and some of our things, but it's too late, for he's back, screaming my name.

Children crying, he's screaming, there's a gun he's been cleaning.

I feel pain, as I fall looking back to the door and see my children that I adore.

"I love you," I call, as I close my eyes. If only I would have had enough time.

Rebekah Seymour © 2005

Unit III: Wholistic Health
Transforming Life Issues
Loss, Suffering and Grief

Transforming Life Issues
Loss, Suffering and Grief
Introduction

Learning Outcomes

Upon completion of this module, the participant will be able to:

1. Define life issues and terms related to loss, suffering and grief.
2. Apply the basic tenets and theories related to suffering, grief and mourning in faith community nursing practice.
3. Engage in activities that support and facilitate the transition of life events for individuals in the faith community.
4. Apply the competencies of faith community nursing to professional development that supports working in the field of grief and loss.

Description

This module recognizes the significant life-altering events that transform people's lives as related to loss, suffering and grief. It discusses the basic tenets of suffering and grief, the tasks of mourning, and coping with loss. It addresses the roles of the faith community nurse (FCN) as a companion to the bereaved and as a faith community coordinator promoting wholistic health and wellness. The module culminates with a discussion of the personal feelings and attitudes that facilitate or interfere with the support of those who are suffering or dying and the bereaved.

Hours: 2

Research

The loss of something or someone, or the confrontation of a life-threatening and life-altering event is difficult. Dealing with a significant loss may challenge a person's sense of security and confidence. Grief is natural and may manifest with a range of emotions that includes sadness and depression, as well as anger, guilt, and fear (Neimeyer, 2012). For some, experiencing a loss can be life-transforming (Winokuer & Harris, 2012).

A review of the literature shows many professional treatment modalities to help one through a process of healing after loss. Neimeyer (2012) prefers a constructivist approach to grief with a professional counselor helping the client find meaning in life through narrative reframing. Shepherd and Shepherd (2013) find value in the process of sharing grief and bereavement through support groups, and several studies (Greenwood et al., 2013; Locock and Brown, 2010; Dyregrov et al., 2013) explore specific dimensions of support groups. Dominek et al. (2009), Softka et al. (2012), and Schotanus-Dijkstra et al. (2014) supported the use of computerized technology where participants can creatively tell their story through text-based communication.

In context, the FCN focuses on the spiritual health while helping clients who are suffering.

Faith Tradition

Granger Westberg's parish nurse model is grounded in the Judeo-Christian history of engaging both the spiritual and physical aspects of healing. Christians are instructed to help and serve one another, following the example of Christ (Galatians 6:2; 1 Thessalonians 5:11). Other faith traditions also focus on spiritual and physical aspects of healing. The tenet to care for individuals in need is applicable to all faith communities. They are committed to reaching out in compassion to relieve suffering and to giving comfort to people who are mourning.

The basic **message of Judaism** on death and Jewish mourning is to provide comfort by making a *shiva* call to provide meals and to sit *shiva* (seven days of mourning following a death).

In **Islamic literature**, effective spiritual care means to compassionately engage in *sohba*, a term that denotes uplifting comfort, encouragement, companionship and presence.

Key Terms

Anticipated loss: a loss that is expected, as with an impending death due to a terminal illness

Bereavement: period of mourning in a state of intense grief after a loss, especially after the death of a loved one

Countertransference: the conscious and unconscious feelings experienced by the clinician toward the patient

Grief: deep sadness or distress when a person experiences a loss

Mourning: symbolic social process and outward expression of grief and sorrow

Loss: the experience of not being able to keep or have access to something; having something taken away or destroyed

Prolonged grief disorder: a syndrome consisting of extended intense emotions and feelings following loss that persists and does not exhibit any signs of resolution

Stephen Ministers: church volunteers trained in the Stephen Ministries model to provide one-to-one care to people experiencing a difficult time in life, such as grief and loss

Suffering: experiencing physical, emotional, or spiritual anguish, pain or distress

Reflection

"A loss often produces suffering and grief. One can suffer a loss when they lose a possession or experience the separation from someone. How we deal with a loss can impact our sense of happiness or unhappiness."
—Norman Wright

"Healing means, first of all, the creation of an empty but friendly space where those who suffer can tell their story to someone who can listen with real attention."
—Henri Nouwen

"Bear one another's burdens, and in this way you will fulfill the law of Christ."
—Galatians 6:2

"Therefore, encourage one another and build up each other, as indeed you are doing."
—1 Thessalonians 5:11

Transforming Life Issues

Loss, Suffering and Grief

Content Outline

SOME TYPES OF LOSS

- Body image
- Pet
- Health
- Job
- Objects
- Safety
- Home
- Fertility
- Parent
- Stillbirth
- Colleague
- Sibling
- Dreams
- Finances
- Identity
- Relationship

KEY TERM

Loss *is the experience of not being able to keep or have access to something.*

KEY TERM

Anticipated loss *is an expected loss.*

OUTCOME 1

Define life issues and terms related to loss, suffering and grief.

To understand loss, one must understand life. Life is the process from birth to death. Life is terminal; it always has an end. Human life is not forever.

Loss is the experience of not being able to keep or have access to something; having something taken away or destroyed; losing something that is an emotional investment.

- Loss is an inevitable part of life.
- It is part of existence as a living, breathing human being.
- Loss is part of life's story, part of the journey of one's life path.
- Loss can make one feel disconnected from the outside world.
- Losses can vary as to the amount of pain that may be experienced.

Everyone experiences loss and grief in a distinct way. Dealing with a significant loss can be one of the most difficult times in a person's life. Paradoxically, sometimes loss can cause positive change and help someone move forward.

- The destabilizing feature of loss can initiate or promote self-reflection.
- One may make a life-changing decision or behavior change. This is especially true when the mourner shares his story and is validated and supported in the process.

Loss may be sudden. For instance, sudden or shocking losses may be events associated with a crime, accident, or suicide.

- Often there is no way one can prepare or prevent this loss.
- This kind of loss can challenge one's sense of security and confidence in life's predictability.

An **anticipated loss** is an expected loss, such as impending death due to a terminal illness. The benefit is having the opportunity to plan and prepare for the loss.

Suffering is part of the life process. L. M. Wright (2005) describes suffering as the state of "physical, emotional, or spiritual anguish, pain, or distress. Experiences of suffering can include:
- serious illness that alters one's life and relationships as one knew them
- the forced exclusion from everyday life
- the strain of trying to endure
- longing to love or be loved
- acute or chronic pain
- conflict, anguish, or interference with love in relationships."

Grief is the internal thoughts and feelings expressed after significant loss. It is the deep sadness or distress when a person experiences loss. Grief is a normal process, not a disease state.

Mourning is the external expression of sorrow that a person goes through to adapt to the loss or death of a person. It is an outward expression of the grief process when one may be dependent upon the support of others (Worden, 2009).

Bereavement describes the period of mourning and state of intense grief after a loss, especially the death of a loved one.
- During this time the person tries to adapt to the loss and find direction for life and search for meaning.
- Worden (2009) identified three basic assumptions that are challenged by the death of a loved one.
  - The world is a benevolent place.
  - The world makes sense.
  - The bereaved person is worthy.

OUTCOME 2

Apply the basic tenets and theories related to suffering, grief and mourning in faith community nursing practice.

Basic Tenets and Theories of Suffering

Loss and suffering may be congruent. Suffering is often associated with a loss because it may have an effect on an individual, one's relationship or one's place within the world.
- Suffering can be physical, psychological, social, cultural, developmental, or spiritual.
- Pain is usually associated with suffering, but suffering may occur in the absence of pain.
- Although suffering is not always synonymous with physical pain, it may be closely associated to psychological, social, and spiritual distress.

Suffering can be physiological, such as when there is a change in a person's physical well-being. It can be emotional, such as when a person feels diminished and broken. Suffering can also be related to spiritual distress in one's relationship with a higher being.

KEY TERM
Suffering *is the state of physical, emotional or spiritual anguish.*

KEY TERM
Grief *is the internal thoughts and feelings expressed after significant loss. It is the deep sadness or distress when a person experiences loss. Grief is a normal process, not a disease state.*

KEY TERM
Mourning *is the external expression of sorrow that a person goes through to adapt to the loss or death of a person. It is an outward expression of the grief process when one may be dependent upon the support of others (Worden, 2009).*

KEY TERM
Bereavement *is the period of mourning and state of intense grief after a loss.*

Critical Thinking
How have your personal losses affected your personal and spiritual growth?

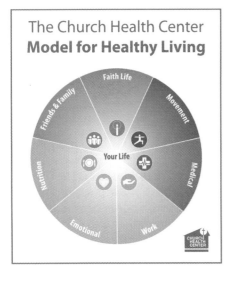

The Church Health Center
Model for Healthy Living

For the purpose of this module, the focus will be on the physical, emotional, and spiritual parts of the **Church Health Center's Model for Healthy Living**. This model addresses all aspects of keeping life in balance so that one may live a life of joy, love and connection with God.

Suffering is an intensely personal experience closely related with one's physical and mental well-being. The response to suffering may include a range of emotions such as sadness, anguish, fear, abandonment, despair, and others.

- Suffering people often feel helpless, voiceless, trapped and unable to escape their circumstances.
- Suffering can be deeply linked to one's awareness of mortality and may initiate fear.
- Suffering people may ask "why?" and seek to find meaning and answers for that which is unknowable.
- Suffering is often associated with separation from the world, leading to feelings of loneliness and yearning for connection. Some may struggle with distress about being dependent on others.

Suffering is often accompanied by spiritual distress.

- Regardless of religious or denominational affiliation, individuals experiencing illness or the threat of dying may express fear and a sense of hopelessness.
- When life is threatened and in time of vulnerability, one may experience a time of self-evaluation and reevaluate his/her relationship with a higher being.

KUBLER-ROSS'S FIVE STAGES OF GRIEF:

1. **Denial:** *a temporary defense that may be closely associated with the shock value of a diagnosis or event.*
2. **Anger:** *projecting resentment and intense frustration.*
3. **Bargaining:** *negotiating as a way to exchange or postpone the inevitable or something that has already happened.*
4. **Depression:** *realization of what will happen or has already happened and acknowledging the reality of the event.*
5. **Acceptance:** *the acknowledgement of coming to terms with the inevitable.*

Basic Tenets and Theories of Grief

Kubler-Ross's 1969 theory is the model most referenced. She depicted grief as a journey through five distinct stages with a final resolution. However, not all individuals manifest these characteristic stages as a progression from one stage to the next. Contemporary models portray grief as an ongoing process that does not end (Doka & Tucci, 2011). Therefore, the FCN needs to consider the stages as being fluid and fluctuating with the emotions of grief.

The Tasks of Mourning

Worden (2009) suggested four tasks of mourning as an active process.

1. **Accept the reality of the loss.** Loss is difficult; therefore, people need to get control of denial so they can begin to deal with their loss.
2. **Work through the pain of grief.** This process takes time as it involves feeling pain rather than ignoring or avoiding it.
3. **Adjust to an environment in which the deceased is missing.** Sometimes a loss involves taking on responsibilities, learning

new skills and assuming new roles. This phase may involve a person in reorganization of self and reintegration of the loss.

4. **Emotionally relocate the deceased and move on with life.** This may seem like a difficult task as one refocuses his or her life on others or possibly on another relationship. It is not betrayal of the deceased, but rather moving on and healing.

According to Worden (2009), coping with loss is not an isolated healing process. It is a continuing process that overlaps with activities of daily living and takes time. Worden describes a task-based model for coping with loss with tasks that integrate the physical, psychological, social, and spiritual.

Physical tasks relate to symptom management and meeting basic bodily needs. Attending to one's own routine physical needs is important in the healing process and maintaining a healthy life. See The Church Health Center Model of Healthy Living.

Psychological tasks are concerned with security, autonomy, and the value of living with dignity.

Social tasks are those related to sustaining interpersonal attachments and interacting with social systems.

Spiritual tasks are related to the effectiveness of a person's sources of spiritual energy to invigorate and to enrich life.

Sustaining hope is an individualistic view. It is dependent on a person's culture, history, environment, and condition. Hope should be grounded in reality and based on the person's faith and conviction about whether or not life is basically good and meaningful.

> ## Critical Thinking
>
> *In what ways have you witnessed the range of reactions to loss?*
>
> *In your experience, what helps or hinders a person moving through the necessary stages of grief?*

OUTCOME 3

Engage in activities that support and facilitate the transition of life events for individuals in the faith community.

Helping someone through the grief process may not heal the wounds of the loss, but it may help the person move forward by accelerating a natural healing process. A review of the literature shows that the FCN's communication skills and referrals to professional treatment modalities may help others through the healing process of loss. The FCN communicates effectively in a variety of formats in all areas of practice, in service through presence and companionship, to those who are suffering in loss, grief or bereavement. The FCN is committed to:

- Listening and to making supportive and caring comments.
- Serving as an advocate to help individuals regain control of events and cope with vulnerability and uncertainty.
- Serving as a compassionate voice with those who are struggling with health concerns and spirituality.
- Being culturally competent, respectful, and cognizant of the mourner's culture and spirituality.

Engaging on a Personal Level

The FCN engages the client at a personal level as a companion on another person's journey. Wolfelt (2012) describes companioning as:

- Being present to another person's pain; it is not about taking away the pain.
- Listening with the heart; not analyzing with the head.
- Bearing witness to the struggles of others; not judging or directing them.
- Walking alongside; not leading them.
- Discovering the gift of sacred silence and being quiet in the moment.
- Respecting disorder and confusion; not imposing order and logic.
- Learning from others; not teaching them.
- Having a curiosity, not being about expertise.
- Paying attention to the experiences that give life richness and meaning.

The FCN listens to the client's life journey as a story that represents who the person is and as a means to help the individual cope with a loss. Listening is an invitation to possibly help make sense of one's suffering. Sharing one's journey also helps to alleviate or diminish emotional, physical, and/or spiritual suffering.

The FCN as a Referral and Resource Agent

Since grief and loss typically interfere with the person's social and occupational functioning, the nurse may direct or provide the client with helpful and appropriate learning resources. These may include counseling, support groups, pamphlets, books, cognitive behavior material, and websites. In consideration of the client and the family, the FCN should offer self-help resources specific to the needs of the bereaved individual as each person's needs are unique to his or her loss.

Professional counseling may help the client through the grieving process. Neimeyer (2012) prefers a constructivist approach to grief by helping the client find meaning in life through **narrative reframing**.

- Reframing goes beyond the practice of listening. It is a way to help the client expound on their understanding of an event or problem. It can help a person create ways to respond to the issues.
- Neimeyer proposes that telling one's story may help one with the grief process by integrating the mourner with who they are in the world, and in relation to the deceased and one's self.

Support groups offer opportunities for shared stories, validation of feelings, psychosocial support, mutual understanding and compassion. Many lives are impacted with the diagnosis of a disease process, whether it is personal, or a family member or friend.

Shepherd & Shepherd (2013) find value in sharing grief and bereavement through support groups. Although each person's grief experience varies, there is still a sense of therapeutic unity in a caring environment when people share similar problems.

Research conducted by Locock and Brown (2010) found that support group participants valued a sense of camaraderie as members share and compare lives with others. Doing so helped them realize they were not alone and they actually ended up feeling better as they compared events and realized others were worse off than they were. Another study (Greenwood et al., 2013) revealed that both caregivers and peer volunteers benefited from support groups that gave the opportunity to make connections, talk freely about their emotions, share helpful information, and exchange advice.

Dyregrov (2013) conducted a qualitative study on support group dynamics. He found that participants valued an organized group meeting structure that included a defined purpose as well as possible effects and limitations. The participants also stressed the need for a screening process for assessing and assigning individuals to an appropriate therapeutic support group.

The FCN is an agent for topical support group services, referrals and resources.

- Offering the faith community a support ministry is a wholistic approach in helping patients, families and friends process through the stages of grief from the actual diagnosis of illness to learning to cope with illness.
- Groups give opportunity for individuals to tell their story, share information and exchange knowledge.
- The FCN might consider inviting guest speakers who have been professionally trained and have professional credentials. These outside speakers can provide objective and nonbiased information without endorsing personal biases, products or services.

Internet resources can provide help to people without access to counseling or support groups.

- Several studies have been conducted on the value of online resources as a support system for those without access to support groups.
- Softka, et al. (2012) suggests the use of computer technology where participants can creatively tell their story. Those with technological and social media access are able to seek help and healing through computerized tools to creatively tell their story through text-based communication and multimedia, including Skype. This was also found to be an effective tool for people who live in isolated or rural communities.
- Dominic et al, (2009) and Softka, et al. (2012) also stress the value of the Internet as a self-help tool for education and support.

The FCN uses the ANA nursing process to evaluate the client's progress and need for additional services. The FCN observes for

HELPFUL RESOURCE

Bereavement Ministry Program: A Comprehensive Guide for Churches *by J. Nelson and D. Aaker (Notre Dame, IN: Ava Maria Press, 2009) includes a guide for getting basic resources for adults, children, and teens; templates for letters to the bereaved at certain times after the loss; speaker evaluations and more.*

KEY TERM

Prolonged grief disorder *is a syndrome of extended intense emotions and feelings following loss that persist.*

Critical Thinking

How would you discern whether professional counseling, support groups, or online resources would be your first recommendation to a person experiencing loss?

symptoms of **prolonged grief disorder**, a syndrome consisting of extended intense emotions and feelings following loss that persists and does not exhibit any signs of resolution, or complicated grief, described as grief disorders that may be chronic, delayed, exaggerated, and mask grief reactions (Worden, 2009). Such concerns may require the services of professionals experienced in grief therapy.

The FCN is a communicator to faith community leadership by:
- Assisting with healing services and faith community cultural rituals.
- Providing community education and arranging workshops that focus on areas such as loss and grief, end-of-life, funeral planning, and Advance Directives.
- Working with the faith community's **Stephen Ministers**, who are church volunteers trained in the Stephen Ministries model to provide one-to-one care to people experiencing a difficult time in life, such as grief and loss.

OUTCOME 4

Apply the competencies of faith community nursing to professional development that supports working in the field of grief and loss.

The FCN has a professional duty and responsibility to adhere to the professional practice standards as addressed under Standard 14 of *Faith Community Nursing: Scope and Standards of Practice* (2012, 2nd ed.).

When providing care, the FCN must consider issues and concerns in relation to the client's chronological age as well as mental and physical development. The FCN engages in self-evaluation by identifying areas of strength and areas where professional development is needed. When the FCN recognizes that he or she is lacking in specific skills or knowledge, it is important to obtain appropriate knowledge and skills by attending educational workshop or seminar opportunities.

The professional and personal support and nurturing of the FCN is vital to the care the nurse provides to others. The FCN works with professional faith community leadership and mentoring nurses for knowledge sharing, guidance, and spiritual support. The leadership and mentors will work together to periodically conduct the FCN's formal review of practice actions, establish goals, and provide constructive feedback.

Reflective Learning

Competency is an ongoing process that integrates the FCN's knowledge, skills, abilities, and reflective learning. Gamino and Ritter (2012) discuss the value of having skilled and competent health care providers work with a client's problems related to loss and bereavement. It is important that health care workers be able to manage their own feelings of fear and disillusionment while giving comfort, hope and help to those who suffer with loss and grief.

The reflective learning process serves as a thoughtful personal self-assessment, analysis, and synthesis of identifying one's strengths and opportunities for improvement. In order to minister to another's grief and loss, the FCN must periodically recruit FCN peers, mentors, and faith community leaders.

The FCN engages in self-evaluation of practice and identifies areas of strength as well as areas in need of professional development. The FCN must also set goals and take action to achieve the goals identified during the evaluation process.

It is important that the FCN first reflect on personal losses and understand how he or she coped with those losses. This is essential to being able to truly empathize with other people's grief. This reflection can be accomplished in several ways.

- Explore previous experiences with loss and ways of coping.
- Periodically conduct a self-examination to determine if you are comfortable working with those who are suffering.
- Attend and participate in loss, grief, and bereavement conferences, workshops and seminars.
- Periodically confer with and seek informal peer and ministry leader's feedback on your practice and spiritual care.

Countertransference

The FCN should be aware of one's vulnerability to be circuitously influenced in the ethical practice of personal **countertransference**, which refers to the conscious and unconscious feelings experienced by the clinician toward the patient and family. Gamino and Ritter (2012) encourage the health care worker to develop a personal awareness and understanding of one's personal issues as a key to identifying the presence of countertransference.

- Recognize what directed the FCN to work in the field of loss and grief.
- Consider "Whose needs are being met?" Sharing one's own grief can be detrimental.
- Caregivers must have the courage to identify and confront the totality of their own responses in view of the patient's needs.
- Focus on listening skills and validate the patient's story of loss.
- Respect the patient's sacred space and their level of discomfort by not embedding one's own past experiences of grief.
- Avoid assuming burdens that are the responsibility of others.

KEY TERM
Countertransference *means feelings experienced by the clinician toward the patient and family.*

Critical Thinking
What methods or tools help you in the personal reflection process?

Standards of Professional Performance for Faith Community Nursing

Standard 11. Communication

The faith community nurse communicates effectively in a variety of formats in all areas of practice.

COMPETENCIES

The faith community nurse:

- Assesses communication format preferences of healthcare consumers, families, and colleagues.
- Assesses his or her own communication skills in encounters with healthcare consumers, families, and colleagues.
- Seeks continuous improvement of his or her communication and conflict-resolution skills.
- Conveys information to healthcare consumers, families, the interprofessional team, and others in communication formats that promote accuracy.
- Questions the rationale supporting routine approaches to care processes and decisions when they do not appear to be in the best interest of the healthcare consumer.
- Discloses observations or concerns related to hazards and errors in care or the practice environment to the appropriate level.
- Maintains communication with other providers to minimize risks associated with transfers and transition in care delivery.
- Contributes her or his own professional perspective in discussions with the interprofessional team.

Standard 14. Professional Practice Evaluation

The FCN evaluates his or her own nursing practice in relation to professional practice standards and guidelines, relevant statutes, rules, and regulations.

COMPETENCIES

The faith community nurse:

- Provides age-appropriate and developmentally appropriate care in a spiritually, culturally, and ethnically sensitive manner
- Engages in self-evaluation of practice regularly, identifying areas of strength as well as areas in which professional development would be beneficial.
- Obtains informal feedback regarding her or his own spiritual care and nursing practice from healthcare consumers, peers, spiritual leaders, health committee members, faith community volunteers, professional colleagues, and others.
- Participates in systematic formal review, as appropriate.
- Takes action to achieve goals identified during the evaluation process.
- Provides evidence for practice decisions and actions as part of the informal and formal evaluation processes.
- Interacts with peers and colleagues to enhance her or his own professional nursing practice or role performance.
- Provides peers with formal or informal constructive feedback regarding their practice or role performance.

Learning Activities

Compare and Contrast Videos

Instructions:
1. Watch the free four-minute video *The Grieving Process: Coping with Death* from Watchwellcast (http://www.youtube.com/watch?v=gsYL4PC0hyk) and the two-minute free video from PBS on Katie Couric's loss, *Born on a Sunny Day* (http://www.pbs.org/thisemotionallife/video/born-sunny-day).
2. Discuss the producer's approach to addressing grief in the first video.
3. Compare the second video to the first one.

Question:
What new insight did one of these videos provide to your understanding of approaching grief and loss?

The Pallium Project

Instructions:
1. Watch the free six-minute video *Talking About End of Life Care* from the Pallium Project (http://www.youtube.com/watch?v=Qo5mCB9gbfY).
2. Discuss the video's approach to talking about this difficult topic.

Question:
How might this video's content affect the next conversation you have about end-of-life care?

Loss Time Line

Instructions:
1. Before or during the module, ask participants to engage in a reflective self-assessment as a means to identifying personal vulnerability while caring for others and maintaining a professional therapeutic and ethical practice.
2. Have participants develop a personal time line for their lives, starting with birth and continuing through childhood and into adulthood.
3. Mark significant life events along the time line.
4. Identify experiences of loss.
5. Reflect on what helped or did not help during a time of bereavement.

Question:
Ask for volunteers to share their time lines and explain what promoted healing during times of loss.

Case Studies

Instructions:
1. Break the participants into small groups.
2. Assign each group one of the case studies below.
3. Have each group select a transcriber-reporter for the group.
4. Allow 15–20 minutes to discuss the case study and develop a plan of care. Have each group write the key points on a flip chart or white board.
5. Invite each small group to present their care plan and discuss the questions listed below the case study.

Question:
What insights did your group's discussion provide that you can practically apply in your practice?

CASE 1

An FCN is called to visit a faith community member who has been diagnosed with late stage breast cancer. The individual has refused hospice care. She has been discharged to home since her daughter is able to care for her. On one visit the FCN assesses the client's pain level, which is high; the client comments that she does not want pain medication. She believes that she must endure the pain to atone for her sins and that God will heal her.
- How would you respond to the individual's beliefs related to her illness and pain?
- What referral resources would you suggest?

Some considerations for Case #1
Following assessment of pain and spiritual beliefs, list the advantages of pain relief, such as: ease of burden on her daughter, increased ability to eat, comfort in moving around, and sleep that will improve the quality of her life. Discuss fear of addiction, if appropriate. For instance, if medication is needed to relieve pain, there is no reason to fear the possibility of addiction. Refer to the spiritual leader for counsel regarding remarks about "atone for her sins" and "God will heal her."

CASE 2

The FCN is trying to support the wife of a man with Amyotrophic Lateral Sclerosis (ALS). There has been a slow decline in his ability to function. The wife and husband agree they do not want him to go to a nursing home. Even with the support of the faith community, the wife is tired and the man "just wants to die." He is angry that he does not live in Oregon, where a physician can prescribe drugs that would end his life. His wife is distressed that he would want to commit suicide, since, according to her faith beliefs, suicide is wrong, and he would be damned.

- What are some of the ethical and legal issues the FCN might have to consider in administering care to the client and his wife?

- How would you respond to both of them and their concerns?

Some considerations for Case #2

Careful assessment of the situation may uncover situations or feelings that the couple can discuss with guidance and clarification by the nurse or a counselor. This is a situation where your presence, concentrated listening, and reflection of what is said may help clarify the issues. You may be able to refer them to agencies that could help with the physical and psychological care and provide information and support for this disease, such as the Muscular Dystrophy Association (MDA). In addition, spiritual assessment and support from the spiritual leader is needed.

Expanded Learning Activities

1. **Society's Response to Death.** Arrange to tour two funeral homes. Compare the funeral homes and reflect on the experience. What lessons will be helpful when advising families concerning the care of the deceased and the selection of a funeral home?
   - Explore alternatives to the traditional funeral conducted in a funeral home with burial in a casket. When is embalming required?
   - Discuss "green" funerals and home funerals. What are the legal implications of alternative funerals?

2. **Analyze Standards.** Analyze the *Faith Community Nursing: Scope and Standards of Practice* (2012, 2nd ed.) related to suffering and grief. What are the implications for the nurse?

   The FCN works under the legal guidelines established by the Nurse Practice Act of his or her state and the professional guidelines in the ANA/HMA *Faith Community Nursing: Scope and Standards of Practice*, which refers to the ANA Code of Ethics. These documents help direct the FCN's practice and the evaluation of ethical dilemmas that are frequently part of end-of-life care. As a professional, the nurse collaborates with patients, other nurses, spiritual leaders, physicians, family members, members of the faith community, and members of the general community to develop plans of care to relieve suffering and support people who are mourning. That collaboration can be a daunting process when values and opinions conflict. The nurse needs to be well aware of the regulations that guide the practice, and the support available to help clarify his or her role.

3. **Documentary DVD.** Purchase the DVD documentary, *After the End: A Journey through Loss to Hope* (79 minutes, aftertheendmovie.com). Discuss the issues addressed in the video and how the FCN can incorporate this information while caring for others through their grief.

References

Required Textbook

American Nurses Association and Health Ministries Association. (2012). *Scope and standards of practice: Faith community nursing* (2nd ed.). Silver Spring, MD: Nursesbooks. org.

References

American Nurses Association. (2012). *Code of ethics for registered nurses with statements.* Washington, DC: American Nurses Publishing.

American Nurses Association and Health Ministries Association (2012). *Faith community nursing: Scope and standards of practice* (2nd ed.). Silver Spring, MD: Nursesbooks.org.

American Nurses Association Leadership Institute. (2013). *Competency model.* Retrieved June 6, 2014 from http://www.analeadershipinstitute.org/Doc-Vault/About-Us/ANA-Leadership-Institute-Competency-Model-pdf.pdf.

Doka, K. & Tucci, A. (Eds). (2011). *Beyond Kubler-Ross: New perspectives on death, dying and grief* (2nd ed.). Washington DC: Hospice Foundation of America.

Dyregrov, K., Dyregrov, A. & Johnsen, I. (2013). Participants' recommendations for the ideal grief group: A qualitative study. *Omega, 76*(4), 363–377.

Gamino, L. & Ritter, R. (2012). Death competence: An ethical imperative. *Death Studies, 36*(1), 23–40.

Greenwood, N., Mabibi, R., Mackenzie, A., Drennan, V. & Easton, N. (2013). Peer support for careers: A qualitative investigation of the experiences of careers and peer volunteers. *American Journal of Alzheimer's Disease & Other Dementias, 28*(6), 617–26. doi: 10.1177/1533317513494449.

Kübler-Ross, E. (1969). On death and dying. New York: Macmillan.

Locock, L., & Brown, J. B. (2010). All in the same boat? Patient and carer attitudes to peer support and social comparison in motor neuron disease (MND). *Social Science Medicine, Oct; 71*(8), 1498–1505. doi: 10.1016/j.socscimed.2010.06.043.

Neimeyer, R. (2012). *Techniques of grief therapy: Creative practices for counseling the bereaved.* NY, NY: Routledge.

Neimeyer, R., Harris, D., Winokuer, H., & Thornton, G. (2011). *Grief and bereavement in contemporary society: Bridging research and practice.* New York: Routledge.

Shepherd, B., & Shepherd, R. (2013). *Taking steps in loss and life: A grief support group manual.* CreateSpace Independent Publishing Platform.

Sofka, C., Cupit, I. & Gilbert, K. (2012). *Dying, death, and grief in an online universe: For counselors and educators.* New York: Springer Publishing.

Winokuer, H. & Harris, D. (2012). *Principles and practice of grief counseling.* New York: Springer Publishing.

Wolfelt, A. D. (2012). *Companioning you! A soulful guide to caring for yourself while you care for the dying and the bereaved.* Fort Collins, CO: Companion Press.

Wright, L. M. (2005). *Spirituality, suffering, and illness: Ideas for healing.* Philadelphia: F.A. Davis.

Wright, N. (2006). *Recovering from losses in life.* Grand Rapids, MI: Fleming H. Revell.

Additional References

Corr, A. C., Nabe, C. M., & Corr, D. M. (2009). *Death & dying, life & living.* Belmont, CA: Wadsworth.

Doka, K. (2013). *Counseling individuals with life-threatening illness.* New York: Stringer Publishing Co.

Dominick, S., Irvine, A., Beauchamp, N., Seeley, J., Noel-Hoeksema, S., Doka, K., & Bonanno, G. (2009). An internet tool to normalize grief. *Omega, 60*(1), 71–87.

Dyregrov, A. & Johnsen, I. (2013). Positive and negative experiences from grief group participation: A qualitative study. *Omega, 68*(1), 45–62.

Fiorelli, R. & Jenkins, W. (June, 2012) Cultural competency in grief and loss. *AHNA Beginnings, 32*(3), 10–12.

Isgandarova, N. (May 2010). The concept of compassionate engagement in Islam. T*he Yale Journal for Humanities in Medicine.* Retrieved November 25, 2013 from http://yjhm.yale.edu/essays/nisgandarova20100302.htm.

Lewis, C. S. (1983). *A grief observed.* New York: Bantam.

Mann, D. (2010). Understanding and surviving grief. *Enrichment Journal.* Retrieved May 17, 2014 from http://enrichmentjournal.ag.org/201003/201003_060_Unders_Grief.cfm.

McConnell, S., Moules, N., McCaffrey, G. & Raffin-Bouchal, S. (2012). The hidden nature of death and grief. *Journal of Applied Hermeneutics, 27*(9), 1–7. from http://jah.journalhosting.ucalgary.ca/jah/index.php/jah/article/viewFile/28/pdf.

Morris, R. & Morris, P. (2012). Participants' experiences of hospital-based peer support groups for stroke patients and carers. *Disability and Rehabilitation Journal, 34*(4), 347–354.

Nelson, J, & Aaker, D. (2009). The bereavement ministry program: A comprehensive guide for churches. Notre Dame, IN: Ave Maria Press.

Perrin, K., Sheehan, C., Potter, M., & Kazanowski, M. (2011). *Palliative care nursing: Caring for suffering patients.* Burlington, MA: Jones & Bartlett Learning.

Schotanus-Dijkstra, M., Havinga, P., van Ballegooijen, W., Delfosse L, Mokkenstorm J, & Boon B. (2014). What do the bereaved by suicide communicate in online support groups? A content analysis. *Crisis, 35*(1), 27–35.

Smucker, C. (2009). *Faith community nursing: Developing a quality practice.* Silver Spring, MD: Nursebooks.org.

Swartwood, R., Veach, P., Kuhne, J., Lee, H., & Ji, K. (2011). Surviving grief: An analysis of the exchange of hope in online grief communities. *Omega, 63*(2), 161–81.

Thirsk, L. & Moules, N. (2013). "I can just be me": Advanced practice nursing with families experiencing grief. *Journal of Family Nursing, 19*(1), 74–98. Online publication. doi: 10.1177/1074840712471445.

Vatga, M. A., & Paulus, T. M. (2014). Grieving online: Newcomers' constructions of grief in an online support group. *Death Studies, 38*(7), 443–449.

Walsh, K. (2011). *Grief and loss: Theories and skills for the helping professions.* New York: Pearson.

Westberg, G. (2011). *Good grief.* Minneapolis, MN: Fortress Press.

Wolfelt, A. D. (2010). *Eight critical questions for mourners: And the answers that will help you heal.* Fort Collins, CO: Companion Press.

Wolfelt, A. D. (2014). *The depression of grief: Coping with your sadness and knowing when to get help.* Fort Collins, CO: Companion Press.

Wolfelt, A. D. (2014). *Healing your grief strikes: 100 practical ideas for coping after a tornado, hurricane, flood, earthquake, wildfire, or other natural disaster.* Fort Collins, CO: Companion Press.

Worden, J. W. (2009). *Grief counseling and grief therapy: A handbook for the mental health practitioner.* New York: Springer Publishing.

Yoder, G. (2012). *Companion the dying: A soulful guide for caregivers.* Fort Collins, CO: Companion Press.

Online Resources

Aging with Dignity: http://www.fivewishes.org

American Association of Retired Persons: http://www.aarp.org/home-family/caregiving/grief-and-loss/

Association for Death Education and Counseling: www.adec.org

Helpful information of Jewish practices and rituals: http://www.myjewishlearning.com/life/Life_Events/Death_and_Mourning.shtml

Hospice Foundation of America: www.hospicefoundation.org An interactive tool to help uncomplicated grievers: http://thegrieftoolbox.com

An internet community of persons dealing with grief, death, and major loss: http://www.griefnet.org

The Jewish Way in Death and Mourning: http://www.chabad.org/generic_cdo/aid/266275/jewish/Death-Mourning.htm

Means of keeping family and friends informed: http://www.caringbridge.org

National Funeral Directors Association: www.nfda.org

National Hospice & Palliative Care Organization: http://www.nhpco.org

Palliative care information: http://www.getpalliativecare.org/

Sudden infant death syndrome: http://www.mchlibrary.org/suid-sids/index.html

DVD/Video and Online Resource

Morgan, Andrew (Director) & Ross, Michael (Producer) (2013). Documentary. *After the End: A Journey Through Loss to Hope* [DVD. $20.00]. Available from http://aftertheendmovie.com/.

The Pallium Project; Clinical Communication in Hospice Palliative Care instructional video series (2008). Talking About End of Life Care [Video online. Free]. Retrieved November 25, 2013 from http://www.youtube.com/watch?v=Qo5mCB9gbfY.

PBS: The Emotional Life. *Born on a Sunny Day.* [two-minute online video. Free.] Retrieved on November 28, 2013 from http://www.pbs.org/thisemotionallife/video/born-sunny-day.

Watchwellcast. *The Grieving Process: Coping with Death.* [four-minute online video. Free.] Retrieved on November 28, 2013 from http://www.youtube.com/watch?v=gsYL4PC0hyk.

Resources from the Center for Loss and Life Transition

http://www.centerforloss.com/bookstore/home.php
3735 Broken Bow Road, Fort Collins, Colorado 80526, Phone: (970) 226-6050

DVDs

Wolfelt, A. D., "A Teen's View of Grief" (40-minutes, $29.95).
Wolfelt, A. D., "A Child's View of Grief" (30-minutes, $29.95).

Books

Maloney, R. and Wolfelt, A. D., (2013). *Healing your grieving heart after stillbirth: 100 practical ideas for parents and families,* $11.95.

Wolfelt, A. D., (2013). *Educating the families you serve about the WHY of the funeral* (manual), $99.95.

Wolfelt, A. D., (2013). *Finding the words: How to talk with children and teens about death, suicide, funerals, homicide, cremation and other end-of-life matters,* $14.95.

Wolfelt, A. D., (2013). *The mourners book of faith: 30 days of enlightment,* $15.95.

Wolfelt, A. D., (2014). *Healing a grandparent's grieving heart: 100 practical ideas after your grandchild dies.* $11.95.

Wolfelt, A. D., (2014). *The depression of grief: Coping with your sadness and knowing when to get help,* $14.95.

Wolfelt, A. D., (2014). *Healing your grief when disaster strikes: 100 practical ideas for coping after a tornado, hurricane, flood, earthquake, wildfire, or other natural disaster,* $11.95.

Wrap-Up and Evaluation

Measuring Competency

This chart can be used to assess the individual outcomes in this module.

- A copy of this chart is attached to the Participant Module, so that each participant can complete this short evaluation.
- Have participants read each outcome and then place an X in the box that best matches their opinion about the objective being met.
- Encourage each participant to write a short reflection about this module in the space provided at the bottom of this chart.
- Use this data to make any necessary changes.

Outcome	Not Met	Somewhat Met	Met
1. Define life issues and terms related to loss, suffering and grief.			
2. Apply the basic tenets and theories related to suffering, grief and mourning in faith community nursing practice.			
3. Engage in activities that support and facilitate the transition of life events for individuals in the faith community.			
4. Apply the competencies of faith community nursing to professional development that supports working in the field of grief and loss.			
Reflection: *In one paragraph, write a reflection on this module.*			

Appendix A

Organizations

Association for Death Education and Counseling
111 Deer Lake Rd., Suite 100
Deerfield, IL 60015
847-509-0403
www.adec.org

ADEC is a professional organization that promotes excellence and diversity in death education, grief counseling, and research in thanatology. Information, support, and resources are provided to its membership and to the public.

Hospice Foundation of America
1621 Connecticut Ave., NW, Suite 300
Washington, DC 20009
800-854-3402
www.hospicefoundation.org

HFA exists to help those who cope personally or professionally with terminal illness, death, and the process of grief and bereavement.

National Funeral Directors Association
13625 Bishops Dr.
Brookfield, WI 53005
800-228-6332
www.nfda.org

The NFDA is dedicated to serving the public by providing advocacy, education, information, products, and services.

National Hospice and Palliative Care Organization
1731 King St., Suite 100
Alexandria, VA 22314
703-837-1500
Helpline: 800-658-8898
www.nhpco.org

NHPC is committed to improving end-of-life care and expanding access to hospice care with the goal of profoundly enhancing quality of life for people dying in America and their loved ones. Provides free consumer information and hospice care and links the public to hospice programs.

Self-Help Organizations

Compassionate Friends
P.O. Box 3696
Oak Brook, Illinois 60522
877-969-0010
www.compassionatefriends.org

Compassionate Friends is a self-help organization that provides support to families toward the positive resolution of grief following the death of a child of any age and to provide information to help others be supportive.

Parents of Murdered Children
100 E. 8th St., Suite 202
Cincinnati, OH 45202
888-818-7662
www.pomc.com

POMC provides support and assistance to all survivors of homicide victims while working to create a world free of murder.

Appendix B

Suggested Scriptures Pertaining to Grief

When all the congregation saw that Aaron had died, all the house of Israel mourned for Aaron thirty days.
—Numbers 20:29

The LORD is my shepherd, I shall not want.
He makes me lie down in green pastures;
  he leads me beside still waters;
he restores my soul. He leads me in right paths
  for his name's sake.
Even though I walk through the darkest valley,
  I fear no evil; for you are with me; your rod and
  your staff—they comfort me.
You prepare a table before me in the presence of
  my enemies; you anoint my head with oil; my
  cup overflows.
Surely goodness and mercy shall follow me all
  the days of my life, and I shall dwell in the
  house of the LORD my whole life long.
—Psalm 23

Like vinegar on a wound
is one who sings songs to a heavy heart.
Like a moth in clothing or a worm in wood,
sorrow gnaws at the human heart.
—Proverbs 25:20

Then Jesus went with them to a place called Gethsemane; and he said to his disciples, "Sit here while I go over there and pray." He took with him Peter and the two sons of Zebedee, and began to be grieved and agitated. Then he said to them, "I am deeply grieved, even to death; remain here, and stay awake with me." And going a little farther, he threw himself on the ground and prayed, "My Father, if it is possible, let this cup pass from me; yet not what I want but what you want."
—Matthew 26:36–39

When Jesus saw her weeping, and the Jews who came with her also weeping, he was greatly disturbed in spirit and deeply moved. He said, "Where have you laid him?" They said to him, "Lord, come and see." Jesus began to weep.
—John 11:33–35

Rejoice with those who rejoice, weep with those who weep.
—Romans 12:15

Listen, I will tell you a mystery! We will not all die, but we will all be changed, in a moment, in the twinkling of an eye, at the last trumpet. For the trumpet will sound, and the dead will be raised imperishable, and we will be changed. For this perishable body must put on imperishability, and this mortal body must put on immortality. When this perishable body puts on imperishability and this mortal body puts on immortality, then the saying that is written will be fulfilled: "Death has been swallowed up in victory." "Where, O death, is your victory? Where, O death, is your sting?"
—1 Corinthians 15:51–55

We do not want you to be unaware, brothers and sisters, of the affliction we experienced in Asia; for we were so utterly, unbearably crushed that we despaired of life itself. Indeed, we felt that we had received the sentence of death so that we would rely not on ourselves but on God who raises the dead.
—2 Corinthians 1:8–9

Bear one another's burdens, and in this way you will fulfill the law of Christ.
—Galatians 6:2

But we do not want you to be uninformed, brothers and sisters, about those who have died, so that you may not grieve as others do who have no hope. For since we believe that Jesus died and rose again, even so, through Jesus, God will bring with him those who have died.
—1 Thessalonians 4:13–14

Unit IV
Community

Unit IV: Community

Assessment

Assessment

Introduction

Learning Outcomes

Upon completion of this module, the participant will be able to:

1. Examine various approaches for assessing geographical communities.
2. Use appropriate evidence-based assessment techniques and instruments in collecting pertinent data as a basis for wholistic care.
3. Synthesize available data, information, and knowledge relevant to the situation to identify patterns and variances in individuals, families, and groups, or the faith community as a whole.

Description

This module introduces strategies that will assist the faith community nurse (FCN) in assessing individuals, families, faith communities, and broader communities. A wholistic assessment is pivotal to successful beginnings and continued success of established health ministry programs within the faith community. It is like a compass giving direction to the health ministry team. The faith community assessment can guide decisions about which wholistic health needs are priorities.

Hours: 2

Research

Addressing spiritual needs and concerns in clinical settings is critical to enhancing quality of life. The National Consensus Project for Quality Palliative Care includes spiritual care as one of the eight clinical practice domains. There are very few standardized spirituality history tools. Lucchetti, Bass, and Lucchetti (2013) conducted a systematic review of 25 instruments used to assess spiritual history; FICA, SPIRITual History, FAITH, HOPE, and the Royal College of Psychiatrists were the most commonly used instruments.

Faith Tradition

Jesus placed a particular emphasis on care for the sick and outcast, such as lepers. His apostles also went about curing and anointing the sick. Jesus identified so strongly with the sick and afflicted that he equated serving them with serving him. Promoting the health of individuals and families in the faith community and caring for the sick are responsibilities of the FCN. Assessing the needs of the faith community is a prerequisite to meeting those identified needs. Faith communities that have healthy individuals and families will have more effective ministries.

Key Terms

Health risk appraisal (HRA): a questionnaire that examines a person's health-related behaviors and health history in order to provide an assessment of the person's preventable health risks

Spiritual history: a set of questions designed to invite patients to share their religious or spiritual beliefs in order to help identify spiritual issues. It is to be patient-centered and guided by the extent to which the patient chooses to disclose his or her spiritual needs (Borneman et al., 2010)

Windshield survey: any process by which an individual is guided or directed to a resource or service

Reflection

"Is there no balm in Gilead?
Is there no physician there?
Why then has the health of
my poor people
not been restored?"
—Jeremiah 8:22

Assessment

Content Outline

OUTCOME 1

Examine various approaches for assessing geographical communities.

Assessment of the geographical community that surrounds the faith community can provide valuable information to the FCN striving to meet the needs of faith community members. Performing an assessment of the greater community prior to an assessment of the faith community provides baseline data about resources and gaps in resources available to meet the needs of individuals and groups within the faith community. Having this information will provide direction for the FCN to identify needed resources from within the faith community.

Assessing communities begins with understanding the types of communities that exist and how they may benefit from health services.

- A **geographical** community is defined by geographic boundaries and physical characteristics of the region.
- A **geopolitical** community is defined by both geographic boundaries and political boundaries, such as interactions between schools, social services, and governmental agencies and by their ability to solve problems. Some examples are school districts, townships, and counties.
- A **phenomenological** community forms around common values or interests.
- A **circumscribed** community includes aspects of both geopolitical and phenomenological communities.
- An **aggregate** community is a collection of individuals who have in common one or more personal or environmental characteristics (Stanhope and Lancaster, 2014).

Dimensions of Community Health

Community health has three common dimensions: status, structure, and process. Each dimension reflects a unique aspect of community health.

Status

The **biological** or **physical** part of community is measured in these ways.
- total population demographics
- age distribution in years
- marital status
- racial and ethnic composition
- morbidity and mortality rates
- life expectancy indexes
- risk factor profiles
- birth and death rates
- maternal and infant death rates
- incidence of low birth weight
- number of teen births
- causes of death

The **emotional** part of a community is measured in these ways.
- consumer satisfaction
- mental health indices
- communicable disease incidence, and behavioral risk factors

The **social** part of community is measured in these ways.
- crime rates
- systems functional levels
- system literacy level
- homeless rate
- educational achievement levels

Biological, physical and emotional factors all contribute to measures of
- worker absenteeism
- infant mortality rates

Structure

This category of community assessment includes services and resources, service use patterns, treatment data from various health agencies, provider-to-client ratios, health manpower, health planning groups, and partnerships.

Health and social services include these services.
- availability of acute care hospitals
- mental health services
- long-term and rehab services
- number of physicians, dentists and registered nurses
- home health services, complementary and alternative health providers
- accessibility of Social Security, Medicaid and Medicare offices
- child protective services
- shelters for the homeless
- services for victims of domestic violence

REMEMBER THREE ES

Stanhope and Lancaster (2014) suggest these measures of assessing a community.

1. **Economics***: employment and unemployment rates; average annual household income; number of families below the poverty level; number of individuals or families on public assistance such as Medicaid, Special Supplemental Nutrition Program for Women Infants and Children (WIC), and food stamps; percentages of white collar, blue collar, and agricultural workers; and major employers.*
2. **Education:** *high school graduation rate; dropout rate; percentage of graduates going to college; percentages of school-age population attending public and private schools.*
3. **Environment:** *air and water quality in area; percentage of homes with lead-based paint; value of real estate; adequacy of housing.*

- meal delivery services
- respite care for children and adults with special needs
- adult day care
- substance abuse programs

Transportation assessments measure these factors.
- amount of travel to and from work
- method of transportation to and from work
- accessibility to public transportation
- taxi services
- transportation services for the elderly
- method of transportation that might affect the ability of members of the faith community to attend worship services or receive health care services

Spiritual resource assessments look at these considerations.
- number and diversity of places of worship
- spiritual activities in the area
- types of other health ministries, religious coalitions or collaborations existing in the community (Lucchetti et al., 2013).

Process
Assess processes that may indicate that the community can function effectively in these areas.
- collaboration between community groups
- community problem identification
- community consensus on goals, priorities, and strategies
- community links to the rest of the world through radio, television, Internet
- availability of Internet services to homeowners and general public (Stanhope and Lancaster, 2014)

Methods for Assessment
Generate data by using various methods.
- **Windshield survey.** This is the motorized equivalent of simple observation. It involves driving or walking through an area and making organized observations. It is more than just observing the main street. Using this assessment approach will provide an initial descriptive assessment. Windshield surveys uncover information that may require further investigation. The following elements should be considered (Stanhope & Lancaster, 2014).
  - housing and zoning
  - open space
  - boundaries
  - commons
  - transportation
  - service centers
  - stores
  - street people

KEY TERM

A **windshield survey** *is driving or walking through an area and making organized observations.*

- signs of decay
- race
- ethnicity
- religion
- health and morbidity
- politics
- media
- Participant **observation**
- Informant **interviews**
- **Statistical data**, public documents, minutes from meetings
- Collection of **reported data**
  - Collect information from census data.
  - Compare data from faith community to regional and state statistics. This comparison may give relevance and meaning for the faith community (Stanhope and Lancaster, 2014).

Assessment of the Faith Community's Administrative Staff

An eventual ongoing health ministry has developmental phases. A key element prior to getting a health ministry off the ground is to first be accepted as a faith community ministry. It needs to be very clear to the faith community just what this ministry is going to do and how it will be done. Also it is vital that there is significant support from the spiritual leader, administrative staff, and board members for this ministry to be successful (MacNamara, 2014).

Assess the **structure** of the faith community.
- Who comprises the ministry staff, and what is the hierarchy?
- Who are the faith community leaders (official and unofficial)?
- What areas of responsibility does each staff member have?
- Do both men and women serve in all roles, or are roles gender-based?
- Is there an existing committee structure? Does it include a health ministry? If so, what services does it currently provide?
- Are the human and financial resources adequate to meet community needs?

Assess the process of how the faith community functions.
- What is the mission of the faith community?
- What is the governing body of the faith community?
- Are lay leaders elected or appointed by the clergy?
- Who are decision makers in the faith community?
- Who must be consulted to approve plans and programs?
- Who develops and manages the faith community budget?

> **Critical Thinking**
>
> Why is the comparison of data from your faith community to census bureau and local health department data valuable?
>
> How will determining community assets support health in the community at large?

OUTCOME 2

Use appropriate evidence-based assessment techniques and instruments in collecting pertinent data as a basis for wholistic care.

The assessment process offers the FCN the opportunity to identify the information he or she needs to know about the faith community in order to provide health ministry. Then the FCN can determine the best methods for gathering this information.

What to Assess

HELPFUL RESOURCE
See Appendix A for a brief faith community survey tool.

Assessing the faith community includes these key categories.
- What are the **member demographics?**
  - What births and deaths have occurred?
  - What age groups are heavily represented in the faith community?
  - What attributes, gifts or strengths do members have?
  - Have any members been trained as emergency first responders?
  - Have members been trained as health promoters?
- Are members **willing to participate** in these ways?
  - transportation
  - cooking and preparing meals for families in need
  - lawn care
  - home calls, e-mail messages, sitters, hospital companions
  - leadership of volunteer activities (The FCN should not take responsibility for volunteer coordination if someone else is available for this role.)
- What are the **predominant health concerns**? The FCN could ask these questions of individuals.
  - What are some of the things about your health or your family's health that concern you at this time?
  - When you are not feeling well, with whom do you usually speak?
  - Do you believe the faith community has a role in helping meet the health needs of members? How important is this?
  - What types of services would you like to see the faith community and the FCN establish to help you better meet your health needs?
  - What day and time works best for attending educational programs?
- What are some **evident dynamics** within the faith community?
  - What is the relational community—the sense of connection between members?
  - What is the shared history of the faith community?
  - Is it a safe place for collective memories, hopes, and dreams?
  - Are there shared emotional connections?

- What is the best method to **assess spirituality** of the congregation and individual members?
  - When individuals begin to question the meaning of an illness or the purpose of life, there may be spiritual distress or a need to be further investigated. The FCN can explore an individual's faith or beliefs and the influence of such on their health and illness.
  - The FCN will determine the status of spiritual well-being versus spiritual distress.
  - Spiritual assessment leads the FCN in the direction of screenings that are needed.

As the FCN understands the individual's faith and beliefs, he or she can then recognize the influence those beliefs have on the individual's view of health and illness.

- Borneman et al. (2010) define **spiritual history** as a set of questions designed to invite patients to share their religious or spiritual beliefs to help identify spiritual issues.
- It is to be patient-centered and guided by the extent to which the patient chooses to disclose his or her spiritual needs.

According to The Joint Commission on Accreditation of Healthcare Organizations (TJC), practitioners should conduct an initial, brief spiritual assessment with clients in many settings, including hospitals and behavioral health organizations providing addiction services. TJC does not specify what needs to be included in a spiritual assessment but suggests consideration of the following questions directed to the patient or his or her family (http://www.jointcommission.org/standards_information/jcfaqdetails.aspx?StandardsFaqId=290&ProgramId=47).

- Who or what provides the patient with strength and hope?
- Does the patient use prayer in his or her life?
- How does the patient express spirituality?
- How would the patient describe his or her philosophy of life?
- What type of spiritual or religious support does the patient desire?
- What is the name of the patient's clergy, ministers, chaplains, pastor, or rabbi?
- What does suffering mean to the patient?
- What does dying mean to the patient?
- What are the patient's spiritual goals?
- Is there a role of church or synagogue in the patient's life?
- How does faith help the patient cope with illness?
- How does the patient keep going day after day?
- What helps the patient get through this health care experience?
- How has illness affected the patient and his or her family?

Spiritual Assessment Instruments

Lucchetti, Bassi, and Lucchetti (2013) conducted a systematic review of instruments designed for spiritual assessment. The following five were rated the highest for quality.

KEY TERM

Spiritual History *is a set of questions designed to invite patients to share their religious or spiritual beliefs in order to help identify spiritual issues.*

1. **FAITH** (Neely et al., 2009). This instrument analyzes five dimensions (Faith/spiritual beliefs, Application, Influence/ importance, Talk/terminal events, and Help) and proposes 16 questions. It is easy to use, broad, and can be used in all settings.

2. **FICA** (Puchalski et al., 2000). This instrument analyzes four dimensions (Faith or beliefs, Importance and Influence, Community, and Address) and proposes 11 questions. Health professionals in all settings can use it.

3. **SPIRITual History** (Maugans, 1996). This instrument analyzes six dimensions (Spiritual belief system, Personal spirituality, Integration with spiritual community, Ritualized practices and restrictions, Implications for medical care, and Terminal events) and proposes 22 questions.

4. **HOPE** (Anandarajah, and Hight, 2001). This questionnaire asks questions that cause the participant to examine his or her sources of hope, the influence of organized religion on his or her life, personal spirituality and practices, and effects on medical care and end-of-life issues.

5. **Royal College of Psychiatrists** (Culliford et al., 2006). This instrument was developed by psychiatrists for mental health professionals. It analyzes different dimensions such as meaning, major losses, coping, and support. It analyzes the relationship between spirituality and religious aspects in the past, present, and future of the patient's life.

Health Assessment Tools

The FCN can create a unique health assessment form or adapt one from a standard **health risk appraisal**, a questionnaire that examines a person's health-related behaviors and health history in order to provide an assessment of the person's preventable health risks. This information allows a person to begin to take control of his or her own health and make the necessary changes to prevent health conditions from developing. Inclusion of qualitative and quantitative data is important for complete assessment information.

A **Family Health Assessment**, including the following areas, can help health care professionals provide better care. Assessment of the following areas should be considered:

- cultural or ethnic background
- religious identification
- family's recreational or leisure activities
- developmental stage and history of family
- environmental data: characteristics of home, neighborhood and larger community, family's social support network
- family's communication patterns, power and role structure, family values
- family functions such as nurturance, closeness
- socialization function, such as child rearing practices, value of children in family

KEY TERM

*A **health risk appraisal** is a questionnaire that examines a person's health-related behaviors and health history in order to provide an assessment of the person's preventable health risks.*

- health care function, such as family's health beliefs, values, dietary practices, sleep and rest habits, drug habits, and role in self-care practices, dental health practices, perceptions regarding health services
- family stress and coping, such as coping strategies and dysfunctional adaptive strategies utilized

The **Friedman Family Assessment Model (2003)** includes the following identifying data:
- family name
- address and phone number
- family composition (genogram)
- type of family form
- cultural and ethnic background—extent of acculturation
  - stated ethnic background
  - language spoken at home
  - country of origin
  - family social network from same ethnic group
  - family residence—ethnically homogeneous or blended neighborhood
  - religious, social, cultural, recreational activities within cultural group
  - dietary habits and dress—traditional or westernized
  - cultural influences on home decor
  - traditional or modern family roles and power
  - portions of the community that the family frequents— territorial complex in ethnic community
  - use of health care services and practitioners—folk practitioners, folk remedies, traditional health beliefs
- religious identification
  - family religion
  - family members differing in religious beliefs and practices
  - how actively involved the family is in church, temple, mosque, or other religious organizations
  - religious practices the family engages in
  - religious beliefs and values central in family life
- social status—occupation, education, income
  - estimated family social class
  - identity of income earners
  - source of supplementary income or assistance
  - whether the family considers the income adequate
- social class mobility

A **Family health history** (accessed at https://familyhistory.hhs. gov/fhh-web/home.action) can help identify whether individuals have higher risk for some diseases. It can help the FCN look for early warning signs of disease and guide recommended actions for reducing personal risk of disease.
- The Surgeon General's "My Family Health Portrait" is an Internet-based tool that makes it easy to record family health history.

HELPFUL RESOURCE

Assessment tools for adults, children, and families are available on the Getting to Know You *CD that can be obtained from the Church Health Center online bookstore. Brief Health Assessment Form (Smucker, 2009).*

- The tool is easy to access on the web and simple to fill out. It assembles information and makes a "pedigree" family tree that users can download.
- It is private. It does not store information automatically.
- It gives a health history that can be shared with family members or sent to a health care provider.

Data Collection

Developing a therapeutic relationship is crucial.
- Talk in a nonthreatening environment.
- Establish trust, rapport and presence.
- Listen to the individual's perception of illness and potential strategies to solve the problem.

Methods of data collection include the following.
- questionnaires
  - Only ask for information that will be used and have direct relevance for the FCN.
  - Put the questions in a positive tone by asking people what they want to learn more about rather than about their needs (Hickman, 2006).
  - Open-ended questions encourage more information.
- one-on-one interviews
- key informants of the faith community
- home visits

Home visits are a primary tool for assessing an individual or family's needs and gathering information in order to meet those needs.

A home visit requires **appropriate planning** ahead of time.
- Who initiated the visit? The faith community's spiritual leader, a family member, a friend, or the person you are visiting?
- Who is the reason for the visit? Is it to welcome a new baby? Has an older member just been discharged from the hospital and is in need of assessment for home health services?
- Has the individual recently lost a loved one or a beloved pet?
- Is this someone with whom you have a relationship, or is this a "cold" visit?
- Is it in a safe location? Do you need to be concerned with pets?
- Have you scheduled the visit for a time that is convenient for the family?

On the day of **implementation**, remember that you are a guest and need to honor that boundary.
- Maintain a relaxed environment.
- Maintain privacy and confidentiality. Always ask the client before revealing information to a family member. Never assume information is common knowledge just because people live in the same home.
- Use your observation skills. Ask questions about pictures

you see. Everyone, especially seniors, enjoys sharing their story. Listening will provide great insight into beliefs and values.

- Invite the person to show you the home. As you walk and talk observe safety issues (throw rugs, dangling cords, frayed wires). Is the home cluttered and in need of handyman services? Is there leftover food out on the counter? Is the milk in your tea spoiled? Use your senses of touch and smell as well.
- You are not there to spy on the person but to assess his or her needs, determine resources and, as appropriate, connect the individual with resources within the faith community and the greater community.
- Ask them what their needs are. Does the person need assistance with shopping, cooking or transportation to doctor's appointments? What meds does the client take? Does he or she need help filling the med containers? Is there any concern about paying for their meds?
- If you are visiting a family, how often do they have dinner together?
- Be respectful and courteous; this will hopefully be the first of many visits.
- Recognize that as FCNs we receive the gift of being invited to journey with members of our faith communities. We need to remember that sometimes they are going to make choices we do not necessarily agree with. We still journey with them, encouraging them, being present to them and delighting in watching the way our Lord is working within all of our lives!

WHEN IS THE RIGHT TIME?

If you are gathering information from the faith community as a whole, consider which methods are most likely to yield results in your setting. For instance, you might distribute a survey to individuals attending worship on designated days. Bulletin inserts might be returned at the end of the worship service. With the cooperation of spiritual leaders, gathering data during regularly planned activities may bring more responses—Bible study groups, midweek dinners, youth group gatherings, and so on.

Mailing surveys can be expensive and may have a poor return rate. Tools such as Survey Monkey that allow individuals to respond at their convenience and confidentially may be a better investment. No matter which method you use, avoid distributing surveys around major holidays.

Critical Thinking

When do you think it would be necessary to do a comprehensive individual health assessment?

What are some important aspects that the FCN should assess when making visits?

OUTCOME 3

Synthesize available data, information, and knowledge relevant to the situation to identify patterns and variances in individuals, families, and groups, or the faith community as a whole.

Design programs to address health-related issues that are most prominent in the faith community. Finalize methods of data analysis before collecting data. Investigate utilizing electronic data collection methods to create a database, collect responses and analyze the data.

As you analyze, **look for common threads** and gaps in programming and service requests. Additional data may need to be collected to fill in gaps.

List assets of the faith community. This assessment can help the focus to become positive and empower the community. It determines what the community can offer to its constituents and what constituents can offer to those providing the services within their community.

At the conclusion of the data analysis, develop a nursing diagnosis. The problem could be an actual, perceived, or potential threat.

- A three-part diagnosis includes **risk of** ... (specific problem or health risk faced by the community) **among** ... (specific client the FCN will be working with in relation to the problem) **related to** ... (some characteristic of the community).
- Example: Risk of *infant malnutrition* among *families in Morris County* related to *knowledge deficit among families about infant-related nutrition and WIC (The Special Supplemental Nutrition Program for Women, Infants, and Children).*
- Example: Risk of *caregiver role strain* among *elderly caregivers in Crystal Faith Community* related to *inadequate social services and lack of custodial care.*

The FCN is responsible for validating the diagnosis or diagnoses with the appropriate group, such as the individual, the family, the faith community, or the ministry team.

Establish **priorities for programming.**

- priority setting—those requests with largest number of respondents
- high priority—those requests that the FCN and health ministry team can most readily and appropriately respond to

Set realistic, individualized, measurable goals and outcomes. Consider these factors for success.

- Early and small successes are important when introducing new programs.
- Evaluation: look at outcomes and goals. How did the community do? What were the costs, both in finances and people? Did any new problems arise? Is there a need for additional funding? (Stanhope & Lancaster, 2014).
- What are your resources?
    - Assess resources and needs in the surrounding community as well as possible future partnerships.
    - National Association of County and City Health Officials (NACCHO) at http://www.naccho.org/ is a helpful website with publications, offering a toolbox at your fingertips with program ideas and suggestions and resources. This site includes funding opportunities too.
- Recognize your personal boundaries. What are your limitations personally and professionally? How will you maintain your boundaries?

Critical Thinking

What are the advantages of a systematic assessment of a faith community?

How will the FCN know if needs of the faith community have been met?

Standards of Professional Performance for Faith Community Nursing

Standard 1. Assessment

The faith community nurse collects comprehensive data pertinent to the healthcare consumer's wholistic health or the situation.

COMPETENCIES

The faith community nurse:

- Collects wholistic data including but not limited to physical, functional, psychosocial, emotional, cognitive, sexual, cultural, age-related, environmental, economic, and spiritual or transpersonal assessments in a systematic and ongoing process, while honoring the uniqueness of the person and placing a particular emphasis on spiritual beliefs and practices.
- Elicits the health care consumer's values, preferences, expressed needs, and knowledge of the healthcare situation.
- Involves the health care consumer, family, group, spiritual leader, other healthcare providers, and others, as appropriate, in wholistic data collection.
- Identifies barriers (e.g., psychosocial, literacy, financial, cultural) to effective communication and makes appropriate adaptations.

- Recognizes the impact of personal attitudes, values, and beliefs.
- Assesses family dynamics and impact on healthcare consumer health and wellness.
- Prioritizes data collection activities based on the healthcare consumer's immediate condition, or the anticipated needs of the healthcare consumer or situation.
- Uses appropriate evidence-based assessment techniques and instruments in collecting pertinent data as a basis for wholistic care.
- Synthesizes available data, information, and knowledge relevant to the situation to identify patterns and variances in individuals, families, groups, or the faith community as a whole.
- Applies ethical, legal, and privacy guidelines and policies to the collection, maintenance, uses, and dissemination of data and information.
- Recognizes healthcare consumers as the authority on their own health by honoring their care preferences.
- Documents relevant data in a retrievable format that is both confidential and secure.

Learning Activities

A Case Study: Care of the Community

Instructions:

1. Have the participants read the case study or read it aloud together.

2. Ask them to be prepared to share their responses to the questions following the scenario.

You are the FCN in a small Methodist church in Clark City, a small town in New Mexico with a population of 3,000. You are new to this faith community and would like to learn more about it and the greater community. Since you are new to the area you decide to do a community assessment before doing a faith community assessment.

Clark City is a small town run by a city council and a mayor. Most of these officials are administrators of the local copper mines or owners of large chicken farms in the area. The town is in a largely rural area, and lies 50 miles from Tucumcari. The surrounding countryside is hot and arid.

The ethnic composition of the town is 80 percent Caucasian of European ancestry and 20 percent Latino, primarily of Mexican descent. Fifty percent of the town's population is under eight years of age. There are very few elderly persons in the community, because Clark City is a relatively new town that grew up around copper mines discovered in the last 20 years. The birthrate is 30 per 1,000 population. Approximately 10 percent of all births are premature, and the neonatal death rate is 50 per 1,000 live births. Only about 10 percent of the women receive prenatal care during their pregnancies.

The major industries in the area are copper mines and chicken farms, which employ approximately 85 percent of the adult men and 50 percent of the women. The majority of the Latino population works on the chicken farms. The remaining 15 percent of the adult men and another 20 percent of the adult women are employed in offices and shops in the town. The unemployment level is 0.5 percent, far lower than that of the state and the nation.

The average annual family income is $8,000, and 75 percent of the population is below the poverty level. Nearly one-third of those below the poverty level receive some form of aid, such as Medicaid.

The predominant religion among the Caucasian population is Methodist (many of whom belong to the church the FCN serves) and among the Latino group, it is Roman Catholic. There are four faith communities in the area; the small Methodist church the FCN serves, a larger Methodist congregation, one Catholic church, and a small Southern Baptist congregation.

Many of the Latino group subscribe to folk health practices. They frequently seek health care from a local *yerbero* (herbalist). They may also drive to a nearby town to solicit the services of a *curandera* (faith healer). Close to one-third of the Latino population speak only Spanish.

The average educational level for the community is tenth grade. For the Spanish-speaking group, however, it is only third grade. Educational facilities in the town include a grade school and a high school. The high school also offers adult education classes at night. There is a Head Start program that enrolls 50 children, but no other childcare facilities are available.

There is a high incidence of tuberculosis in the community, and anemia and pinworms are common problems among the school-age children. Several of the men have been disabled as a result of accidents in the mines.

The only transportation to Tucumcari is by car or by train, which comes through town morning and evening. About half of the families in town own cars.

There is one general practice physician and one dentist in the town. The nearest hospital is in Tucumcari, and the funeral home hearse is used as an ambulance for emergency transportation to the hospital. The driver and one attendant have had basic first aid training. The county health department provides family planning, prenatal, well child, and immunization services one day a week in the basement of the larger of the two Methodist churches. The staff consists of a physician, one licensed practical nurse, a masters-prepared family nurse practitioner, and a nutritionist. The well child and immunization services are heavily used, and immunization levels in the community are high among both preschoolers and school-age youngsters.

Concerned that you might become overwhelmed with all of the above, you decide to first focus on your faith community.

Discussion Questions:

1. How will you determine the priority needs of your faith community?

2. Once you have determined the priority needs of your faith community, what steps will you take to begin meeting those needs?

3. Based on the high incidence of tuberculosis, and anemia and pinworms in school-aged children, what primary prevention interventions (health education programs) and secondary prevention interventions (screenings) are appropriate for this population?

4. Based on the information you have about the availability of health providers in the community, what additional services would be most helpful for residents if they could be added to those provided by the county health department one day a week in the basement of the Methodist church?

Community Assessment

Instructions:
Based on the content on community assessment that is presented in the module, facilitate a discussion among participants using the following questions.

1. What are the critical attributes in the definition of community?

2. The community is considered the client when...

3. What is an indicator of community health structure?

4. What is an indicator of community health status?

5. The process of developing data that do not already exist through interacting with community members is called what?

6. The method of community data collection that involves directed conversation with selected community members is known as what?

7. A nurse who reads the local community newspaper to gather information about the community is involved in what?

8. The nurse wishes to conduct informant interviews in a small community. Who should the nurse contact?

Answers:

1. **People, place, function**

2. **The nurse focuses on the collective good**

3. **Emergency room utilization**

4. **Morbidity and mortality rates, crime rates**

5. **Data generation**

6. **Informant interview**

7. **Participant observation**

8. **Local spiritual leader for faith community information**

Data Collection Matching Exercise

Instructions:

1. Identify the most appropriate method(s) of data collection (first column) for each type of data (second column). There may be more than one answer.

Data collection methods	Type of data
a. Participant observation	_____ 1. Environmental hazards
b. Informant interviewing	_____ 2. Health human resources
c. Reviewing existing records of meetings	_____ 3. Norms about preventive care
d. Analyzing existing vital statistical data	_____ 4. Crime patterns
e. Survey	_____ 5. Incidence of reportable disease

2. Compare and contrast the assessment process as it is applied to an individual and a community.

3. Which two of the following options best illustrate the definition of community? Give a rationale for your answer.

   a. Residents of a small Appalachian hollow
   b. Members of the American Public Health Association
   c. An urban neighborhood of East Asian immigrants
   d. Students enrolled in a faith community nursing course

Answers:
Set 1: 1. b, d; 2. b, e; 3. a, e; 4. a, b; 5. e
Set 3: a (geography, people) and c (common culture, place, possible religion)

Case Study: Community Assessment

Instructions:

1. Have the participants read the case study below or read it aloud together.

2. Answer the questions at the end, either individually or as a group.

> Alan Thompson is an FCN and a member of the health ministry committee. The committee has been assigned to assess the provision of care that will address the health care needs of the aging baby boomers in Duxbury County Church. Alan and his committee are aware that as the baby boomer population ages, health care professionals need to prepare for a rapid increase in the number of people over the age of 65. The committee's purpose is to make suggestions to the County Mayor's Office on Aging, the local health department, and spiritual leaders in the faith community staff about how to prepare for the influx in health services that will be needed for these older adults. Currently, 25 percent of the population at Duxbury County Church is over the age of 65. However, in 25 years this percentage is expected to increase to over 50 percent.
>
> The committee determined that there are currently only five primary care providers in the county, with waiting lists ranging from one to three weeks, and only one of these providers specializes in geriatric care. There is one 54-bed long-term nursing care facility in the northern region of the spacious county. Due to rural roads, there is no public transit system. However, residents may call a hospital shuttle program if they need transportation to a doctor's appointment.

Questions:

1. What are the geographic boundaries of the community of interest?

2. Which people are members of this community?

3. What characteristics do they have in common?

4. What methods of data generation would Alan use to assess the community's knowledge and beliefs, values and sentiments, goals and perceived needs, norms, problem–solving processes, power, leadership, and influence?

5. Write a community diagnosis for the faith community.

6. What recommendations would you make to meet the health care needs of the community?

Answers:

1. county lines

2. 65 and older

3. age and increased health care needs

4. informant interview, participant observation

5. risk of lack of access to health care among individuals 65 years and older in Duxbury County

6. Increase the number of geriatric physicians and primary care providers; increase transportation—determine if local organizations provide free transportation

Church related to inadequate number of health care providers and lack of public transportation

Faith Community Guided Imagery

Instructions:
1. Explain how the use of guided imagery can be used to incorporate a modified windshield survey into the program.

2. Pair participants and ask them to relax and participate in guided imagery as you slowly read the text below.

3. Have pairs discuss how the guided imagery will increase their understanding of the neighborhoods in which their faith communities are located.

4. At the end of the exercise, ask participants to answer the follow-up questions.

Guided Imagery

Sit comfortably in your chair, close your eyes and take a deep breath. As you breathe, envision yourself on the steps of your faith community building. Starting on your left, survey the surrounding environment. What do you see? Is it a rural or country setting? Is the parking lot filled with cars? Are they new or old?

Continue to survey the area. What stands out? Walk around the neighborhood surrounding the church. What do you see? Are there schools nearby? What do the homes look like? Are they single family homes or multi-family dwellings? Are the homes in disrepair or very well kept up? Are there apartment buildings? Are there bus stops?

Is there a hospital or clinic in the neighborhood? Are there corner markets, or is there a larger grocery store? Are you feeling safe as you walk? Is the air filled with pleasant aromas or possibly pungent smells? What are your impressions of the neighborhood? Are they favorable?

Return to the faith community building and enter just as services are beginning. Go up into the balcony and look out over your faith community. What do you see? Are the pews filled with seniors leaning on each other's arms? Or young families? Are there little ones snuggling up next to Dad and infants in Mom's arms? Are there teenagers and school-age children? What is the makeup of your faith community? What is the ethnic diversity of your faith community? What are your impressions of your faith community? Does your faith community reflect the neighborhood it meets in?

Follow-up Questions
1. Divide into pairs and share what you discovered about your faith communities.

2. How might this information influence your practice of faith community nursing?

3. What needs did you encounter? Were there any surprises?

4. Did you find this exercise helpful in gathering information about your faith community?

Expanded Learning Activities

Instructions:
1. Compare findings from the faith community with the census data of the state or nation.

2. Compare findings from the faith community to local health department data and US Environmental Protection Agency data.

References

Required Textbook

American Nurses Association and Health Ministries Association. (2012). *Scope and standards of practice: Faith community nursing* (2nd ed.). Silver Spring, MD: Nursesbooks.org.

References

Anandarajah, G., & Hight, E. (2001). Spirituality and medical practice: Using the HOPE questions as a practical tool for spiritual assessment. *American Family Physician, 63*(1), 81–88.

Borneman, T., Ferrell, B., & Puchalski, M. (2010). Evaluation of the FICA tool for spiritual assessment. *Journal of Pain and Symptom Management, 40*(2), 163–173.

Friedman, M., Bowden, V., & Jones, E. (2003). *Family nursing: Research, theory & practice.* Upper Saddle River, NJ: Prentice Hall.

Lucchetti, G., Bassi, R., & Lucchetti, A. (2013). Taking spiritual history in clinical practice: A systematic review of instruments. *Explore, 9*(3), 159–170.

Maugans, T. (1996). The SPIRITual history. *Archives of Family Medicine, 5,* 11–16.

McNamara, J. W. (2014). *Stronger together: Starting a health team in your congregation.* Memphis, TN: Church Health Center.

Neely, D. & Minford, E. (2009). Spiritual history-taking made easy. *The Clinical Teacher, 6,* 181–185.

Royal College of Psychiatrists. (2013). Spirituality and mental health. Accessed June 20, 2014 from http://www.rcpsych. ac.uk/healthadvice/treatmentswellbeing/spirituality.aspx.

Smucker, C. J. (2009). *Faith community nursing: Developing a quality practice.* Silver Spring, MD: Nursebooks.

Stanhope, M. & Lancaster, J. (2014). *Public Health Nursing: Population-centered health care in the community* (8th ed.). St. Louis, MO: Mosby Elsevier.

Tormoehlen, L. (2014). Survey assessment of the faith community: This may help. *Journal of Christian Nursing, 31* (3), 184-187.

Additional References

Banin, L., Suzart, N., Guimaraes, F., Lucchetti, A., deJesus, M., & Lucchetti, G. Religious beliefs or physicians' behavior: What makes a patient more prone to accept a physician to address his/her spiritual issues. *Journal of Religion and Health, 53*(3), 917–928.

Culliford, L. (2007). Taking a spiritual history. *Advances in Psychiatric Treatment, 13*(3), 212–219, 2007. doi: 10.1192/apt. bp.106.002774.

Hickman, J.S. (2006). *Faith Community Nursing.* Philadelphia: Lippincott Williams and Wilkins.

Nies, M.A. & McEwen, M. (2015). Community/Public health nursing: Promoting the health of populations (6th ed.). St. Louis, MO: Saunders Elsevier.

Otterness, N., Gehrke, P., & Sener, I. (2007). Partnerships between nursing education and faith communities: Benefits and challenges. *Journal of Nursing Education, 46*(1), 39-44.

Online Resources

Centers for Disease Control and Prevention: http://www.cdc.gov/nceh/lead/tools/assessement_tools.htm

National Association of County and City Health Officials http://www.naccho.org/topics/HPDP/index.cfm

Wrap-Up and Evaluation

Measuring Competency

This chart can be used to assess the individual outcomes in this module.

- A copy of this chart is attached to the Participant Module, so that each participant can complete this short evaluation.
- Have participants read each outcome and then place an X in the box that best matches their opinion about the objective being met.
- Encourage each participant to write a short reflection about this module in the space provided at the bottom of this chart.
- Use this data to make any necessary changes.

Outcome	Not Met	Somewhat Met	Met
1. Examine various approaches for assessing geographical communities.			
2. Use appropriate evidence-based assessment techniques and instruments in collecting pertinent data as a basis for wholistic care.			
3. Synthesize available data, information, and knowledge relevant to the situation to identify patterns and variances in individuals, families, and groups, or the faith community as a whole.			
Reflection: *In one paragraph, write a reflection on this module.*			

Appendix A

Faith Community Survey/Faith Community Health Needs Survey

In order to help develop the Faith Community/Health Ministry Program at_____, the Faith Community Nurses and Health Ministry Committee would appreciate your thoughts regarding the following questions. All information will be kept confidential.

1. Your age: ___under 20 ___20–29 ___30–39 ___40–49 ___50–59 ___60–69 ___over 70

2. Health status: Please indicate if you have any of the following conditions. Place C by any current conditions and a P by any past conditions.

   ___High blood pressure   ___Diabetes

   ___Physical disabilities   ___Mental illness

   ___Cancer   ___Depression

   ___Arthritis   ___Overweight

   ___Lung/respiratory disease   ___Other: _____

3. Which of the following topics are of particular interest to you?

   ___Blood pressure   ___Babysitting tips

   ___Know your medications   ___Stress and coping

   ___Cancer   ___Cholesterol

   ___Stroke   ___Healthy eating

   ___First aid safety   ___Weight management

   ___Arthritis   ___Nutrition

   ___Heart disease   ___Medicare update

   ___CPR instruction   ___Caring for aging relatives

   ___Exercise   ___Diabetes

   ___Digestive disease   ___Hospice care

   ___Lung disease   ___Alzheimer's disease/dementia

   ___Parenting   ___Spiritual growth

   ___Advance directives   ___Bereavement

   ___Freedom from smoking   ___Caregiver stress/respite care

   ___Self-esteem   ___Prayer

   Other_____

   Other_____

4. Would you attend sessions on any of the above topics? ___Yes ___No

   If yes, when would be the best time to attend classes?

   ___Weekdays, daytime   ___Weekdays, evening   ___Saturday morning

5. If you would like to serve as a volunteer, include your name and phone number below and then indicate your area of interest.

   _____

6. What ways would you like to see the faith community nurse and health ministry utilized in this faith community?

   ___Health education   ___Visitation of hospitalized, homebound

   ___Personal health counseling   ___Screening programs

   ___Health referrals   ___Advocacy

7. Additional thoughts and comments

   _____

   _____

   _____

Unit IV: Community

Accessing Resources

Accessing Resources

Introduction

Learning Outcomes

Upon completion of this module, the participant will be able to:

1. Explain the rationale for the FCN's role in accessing appropriate resources.
2. Assess individual health care consumer care needs and resources available to achieve desired outcomes.
3. Implement a method to access and evaluate internal and external resources, including Internet resources.
4. Assist the health care consumer and family in identifying and securing appropriate and available resources to address health and spirituality needs across the health care continuum.
5. Use documentation, follow-up and evaluation in the referral process.

Description

The faith community nurse (FCN) utilizes referral skills and knowledge of community resources to guide individuals as they access resources. The nurse, with the client's approval, may act as a liaison and provide referrals to resources or health care providers. This module presents the rationale and method for accessing resources for individuals, families, and the faith community at the local, state and national levels, along with accessing resources electronically. Closely linked with the FCN's role in case management and care coordination, the concept of accessing resources is broadened to include educating and empowering members of the faith community in the use of the resources. Referral and follow-up are necessarily related and will be addressed in relation to documentation and evaluation of resources.

Hours: 2

Research

Healthy People 2020 correlates health outcomes with access to services. The dimensions of access include direct factors, such as the client's financial screening, and indirect factors, such as availability of transportation and schedule conflicts. The FCN must recognize the needs of vulnerable populations and assist them in navigating our complex health care system. Vulnerable populations may include those in poverty, the homeless, non-English-speaking and those who speak English as a second language (Siegrist, 2015). Often the assistance needed involves determining the availability of health care resources within the community, educating the member on how to access and assess appropriate resources, making referrals, and evaluating referrals after they are used.

Jiminez et al. (2014) studied factors associated with early intervention referral and evaluation for children with developmental concerns and found that early referrals lead to increased rates of early evaluation. Lee, Hillier and Harvey (2014) studied the impact associated with a partnership between the Alzheimer's Society and memory clinics, and in particular the impact on access to community-based services on clients with dementia and their caregivers. Findings supported the importance of the integration of community agencies early in the diagnosis. Bair-Merritt et al. (2013) documented the positive impact of community referrals for patients suffering from intimate partner violence. Saburi (2011) conducted a study that demonstrated the reduced stress levels of caregivers of children with epilepsy when they are referred to community resources.

FCNs must also be knowledgeable of resources that include technology to enhance their practice. A growing number of investigators (Mohr et al., 2014; Wayne and Ritvo, 2014) have employed a broad range of technologies, such as mobile phones, the Internet, and sensors, to support users in changing behaviors and cognitions related to health, mental health, and wellness.

Faith Tradition

Christian faith communities honor the scriptural passage from 1 Corinthians in which the apostle Paul reminds readers that the Spirit gives different gifts to different members. The Hebrew and Christian Scriptures include many examples of sharing one's gifts for the benefit of others. In the current age of health care specialization, which emphasizes that quality of care is related to interprofessional collaboration and communication, the FCN recognizes that referrals to various members of the interprofessional team and social services can be essential to meeting the health and spirituality needs of clients, and to providing seamless care across the health care continuum.

Key Terms

Healthy People 2020: a program of nationwide health-promotion and disease-prevention science-based, national goals and objectives with 10-year targets set by the US Department of Health and Human Services to improve the health of all people in the United States

Population-focused health: a wholistic approach and perspective that focuses on the broad range of factors and conditions that have a strong influence on the health of populations

Referral: any process by which an individual is guided or directed to a resource or service

Resources: information, equipment, and services that can promote, maintain, or improve health

Reflection

"Now you are the body of Christ and individually members of it. And God has appointed in the church first apostles, second prophets, third teachers; then deeds of power, then gifts of healing, forms of assistance, forms of leadership, and various kinds of tongues. Are all apostles? Are all prophets? Are all teachers? Do all work miracles? Do all possess gifts of healing? Do all speak in tongues? Do all interpret? But strive for the greater gifts. And I will show you a still more excellent way."
—1 Corinthians 12:27–31

"Do not withhold good from those to whom it is due, when it is in your power to do it. Do not say to your neighbor, "Go, and come again, tomorrow I will give it"—when you have it with you."
—Proverbs 3:27–28

Accessing Resources

Content Outline

KEY TERM

Resources *are information, equipment, and services that can promote, maintain, or improve health.*

KEY TERM

Population-focused health *is a wholistic approach and perspective that focuses on the broad range of factors and conditions that have a strong influence on the health of populations.*

OUTCOME 1

Explain the rationale for the FCN's role in accessing appropriate resources.

Resources are information, equipment, and services that can promote, maintain, or improve health.

Population-focused health is an approach and perspective that focuses on the broad range of factors and conditions that have a strong influence on the health of populations. It is a wholistic approach that considers the total health system, from prevention and promotion, to diagnosis, treatment, and care. A population can be defined by geographic boundaries or by a group of people that have common characteristics such as ethnicity or religion. Population-focused practice:

- focuses on the entire population
- is based on assessment of population health status
- emphasizes all levels of prevention
- intervenes with individuals, families, communities, and systems. (Nies & McEwen, 2011).

A faith community can be considered a population, and the FCN not only focuses on promoting the health of individuals in the faith community but on the health of the faith community as a whole. In order to carry out this responsibility the FCN must be well-informed of the nation's health promotion agenda, Healthy People 2020, which has four overarching goals for population health:

- Attain high quality, longer lives free of preventable disease, disability, injury, and premature death.
- Achieve health equity, eliminate disparities, and improve the health of all groups.
- Create social and physical environments that promote good health for all.
- Promote quality of life, healthy development, and healthy behaviors across all life stages.

Healthy People 2020 is a program of nationwide health-promotion and disease-prevention science-based, national goals and objectives with 10-year targets set by the US Department of Health and Human Services to improve the health of all people in the United States. The program strives toward these goals.

- Identify nationwide health improvement priorities.
- Increase access to health care by increasing the proportion of persons with health insurance for medical, dental, and prescription drug services.
- Increase public awareness and understanding of the determinants of health, disease, and disability and the opportunities for progress. Social determinants of health include availability of **resources** such as housing, food, and energy to meet daily needs; education, economic, and job opportunities; transportation; social support; and language literacy.
- Engage multiple sectors to take actions to strengthen policies and improve practices driven by the best available evidence and knowledge (http://healthypeople.gov/2020/default.aspx).
- In order to meet the 10-year national objectives and achieve the goals, health care consumers must make informed decisions about health care and have access to health care services and resources.
- FCNs must be familiar with Healthy People 2020 objectives and focus on relevant areas while serving diverse individuals across the lifespan in their faith communities.
- Educating individuals and families and assisting them in identifying and securing information about available resources is essential to empowering them toward making informed health decisions.

In relationship to accessing resources, the goals of the FCN are the protection, promotion, and optimization of health and abilities of the faith community.

- **Referral**, any process by which an individual is guided or directed to a resource or service, is one of the primary interventions used by the FCN, who utilizes appropriate resources to plan and provide nursing services that are safe, effective, and financially responsible.
- The FCN must consider the economic impact of the plan on the health care consumer, family, caregivers, or other affected parties and how the faith community resources and local community resources might be of assistance.

KEY TERM

Healthy People 2020 *is a program of nationwide health-promotion and disease-prevention science-based, national goals and objectives.*

HEALTHY PEOPLE EXAMPLE

Older adults are the fastest growing segment of the population and are likely to be the predominant age group in many faith communities. In keeping with the Healthy People 2020 objectives, the FCN might work with older members of the faith community to increase the proportion of older adults who use the Welcome to Medicare Preventive Visit benefit and promote achievement of the objective to increase the proportion of older adults who are up-to-date on a core set of clinical preventive services. Older adults may not be aware of the many resources available to them and may often need the following resources.

- *transportation*
- *personal care (bathing, dressing)*
- *home care (light housekeeping, shopping)*
- *in-home meal service*
- *support services for caregivers*
- *adult day care services*
- *financial resources (pharmacy assistance, medical assistance, and so on)*

FCNs should provide information needed to contact the local departments of aging, social services, and health. These agencies offer many important services to older persons.

KEY TERM

Referral *is any process by which an individual is guided or directed to a resource or service.*

The **Affordable Care Act of 2010 has the following implications on resource utilization.**

1. It moves responsibility for the individual's health from the physician or health care provider to the client or patient.
2. It increases access to health care, though not necessarily providing more health care resources.
3. It addresses the major blocks to accessible health care services.
   - cost
   - health literacy
   - location of services
4. HealthCare.gov is a health insurance exchange website operated by the US federal government under the provisions of the Patient Protection and Affordable Care Act. This site is likely to have the most accurate information about obtaining insurance coverage through the ACA.

OUTCOME 2

Assess individual health care consumer care needs and resources available to achieve desired outcomes.

Assessing needs of members of the faith community includes choosing appropriate methods and identifying both internal and external resources.

Choose appropriate assessment methods, including the following.
- interviews with ministerial staff
- suggestions from the health ministry team
- focus groups by age or special interest
- survey of members as part of the faith community assessment
- member inquiries by the FCN

Identify resources within the faith community, including the following.
- counseling
- support and self-help groups
- hospital visitation program
- caregiver support program
- small connect groups
- benevolence fund
- temporary housing

Locate external resources, including the following.
- urgent care
  - hospitals for emergency care
  - hospital or outpatient ambulatory units
  - "minute clinics"
- health-related programs for people living with chronic illness
  - home care
  - palliative care
  - hospice
  - dialysis centers
  - mental health services

- health care providers
  - physicians
  - nurse practitioners
  - dentists
  - clinical psychologists
  - podiatrists
- health-related social services
  - basic economic help (housing, food, WIC and so on)
  - caregiver support
  - support services
  - counseling services for individuals, couples and families
  - health insurance
  - children's special services
  - public health department (for communicable disease treatment and immunizations)
  - legal services (guardianship vs. conservatorship, power of attorney for financial affairs, advanced directives)
  - disaster relief (local health department, Red Cross)

Critical Thinking

What is the most critical resource need in your faith community? Explain your answer.

How does assisting individuals with accessing resources fit into your faith community's mission?

OUTCOME 3

Implement a method to access and evaluate internal and external resources, including Internet resources.

The Internet has become the first place people go when looking for information on diseases. It provides instant access on almost any topic. People facing serious diseases often use this information to make decisions about their illnesses and treatments. Popular websites may help some users determine whether they need to seek medical care. Some sites are more reliable than others, but it can be hard to tell the difference. When it comes to serious illness, the wrong information can hurt. It is important to remind people to look for medical research rather than simply testimonials and opinions. **Always remember that information found on the Internet should not take the place of medical advice.**

The FCN can play a practical role in steering people toward trustworthy health information on the Internet.

Use the Internet to evaluate available resources for accuracy and currency.

1. Research hospital networks (physicians and services).
2. Connect with FCN networks in a specific geographical location.
3. Invite members of the faith community to suggest or locate resources.
4. Explore health care resource booklets distributed by health insurance companies, such as BlueCross BlueShield.
5. Consult local and national resources for veterans.

HELPFUL RESOURCE

See Appendix B, Evaluation of Resources, for key questions to ask to confirm that an identified resource is accurate and reliable.

HELPFUL RESOURCE

Here are some trustworthy sites to help evaluate online information.
- ◆ *Cancer Information on the Internet:*
  http://cancer.org/cancer/ cancerbasics/cancer- information-on-the-internet
- ◆ *Medline Plus Guide to Healthy Web Surfing:*
  http://www.nlm.nih.gov/ medlineplus/ healthywebsurfing.html
- ◆ *Evaluating Health Information:*
  http://www.nlm.nih.gov/ medlineplus/ evaluatinghealthinformation. html

Critical Thinking

Given the geographic location or demographics of your faith community, accessing which resources would present the greatest challenge?

6. Locate mental health services. Local resources can easily be located by using Google or another search engine. For example, the Mental Health Service Directory for Michigan can be retrieved from http://www.mhweb.org/.
7. Consider having a volunteer from the faith community review the faith community's resource directory on a regular basis, such as every six months, to be sure information is current.

Use the Internet to compile available and appropriate resources.

1. Keep resources in a central location (binder, file box, computer file).
2. Include name of resource, physical or Internet address, phone number, and contact person, if available. (See Appendix A.)
   - services—list type of service provided
   - hours of operation, with attention to evenings and weekends
   - other considerations, such as bilingual, accessibility for people with disabilities
3. Include eligibility criteria for service.
   - demographics—age, sex
   - socioeconomic—free, sliding scale, payment
   - insurance—types accepted with special attention to Medicare and Medicaid
   - self-referral vs. referral by health care provider

Use the Internet to access resources. (See Appendix B.)
A variety of health education materials and resources are available from local, state, and national organizations and agencies.
- Such associations provide helpful information about services, educational materials, and links to support groups and self-help groups.
- Often printed and electronic materials are available for free or a nominal cost.
- FCNs must be knowledgeable about resources in order to assist individuals, families, and faith communities to access information, materials, and services (Meade, 2011).

Local resources. Begin with resources available through your city.
- Locate services provided by the hospital, health department, and community agencies. Most can be located on the agency or organization's website.
- Look for health care providers and agencies, as well as social services agencies.

State resources. These can be located through health websites of state departments.
- For instance in Michigan, go to http://www.mich.gov/ som/0,4669,7-192-29942---,00.html.
- Explore health care navigators by state, such as http:// enrollmichigan.com.

Federal government resources. These would include National Institutes of Health, National Cancer Institute, Centers for

Disease Control and Prevention, National AIDS Clearinghouse, and Office on Smoking and Health, Veteran's Administration, and Centers for Medicare and Medicaid.

Voluntary Agencies and their local affiliates.
- Well known agencies in this category include American Heart Association, American Lung Association, Amyotrophic Lateral Sclerosis Association, American Diabetes Association, Alzheimer's Association, American Dairy Council, and American Council for Drug Disorders.
- Often there is a local chapter to serve a specific community.

It is important to be critical when reading or listening to reports of new medical findings. These questions may help you evaluate health information.
- Was the study in animals or people?
- Does the study include people like you?
- How big was the study?
- Was it a randomized, controlled clinical trial?
- Where was the research done?
- If a new treatment was being tested, were there side effects?
- Who paid for the research?
- Who is reporting the results?
(National Institutes of Health National Network of Libraries of Medicine, 2014)

HEALTHY PEOPLE 2020 AND ELECTRONIC HEALTH INFORMATION

Healthy People 2020 seeks to increase the proportion of online health information seekers who report easily accessing health information.

Consumers rely on online resources for health care information and needs.
- *local health care service providers*
- *medical conditions*
- *drug information, particularly side-effects and cost*

Health care providers likewise rely on the Internet to locate information and resources.
- *support shared decision-making between client and health care provider*
- *locate social support networks*
- *locate resources to address health risks and public health emergencies*

OUTCOME 4
Assist the health care consumer and family in identifying and securing appropriate and available resources to address health and spirituality needs across the health care continuum.

Accessing Appropriate Prevention and Care

Accessing the appropriate level of prevention at the appropriate time is important to health outcomes. The FCN should emphasize the importance of preventive activities to prevent illness or injury rather than having to focus on cure after the illness or injury occurs.

Education includes three levels of prevention.
- **Primary prevention** includes activities such as education and health promotion that occur before the onset of illness. Immunizations and exercise programs are examples.
- **Secondary prevention** includes activities such as health screenings that identify risk factors and lead to early diagnosis and treatment. Mammography and lead screenings are examples.

Critical Thinking

How does the FCN's responsibility in identifying and securing resources relate to health promotion and disease prevention?

How do aspects of this function relate to care coordination?

• **Tertiary prevention** is continuing care after diagnosis to minimize complications and optimize well-being to the degree possible. This includes rehabilitation of those with irreversible diseases such as diabetes and spinal cord injury.

Education includes helping individuals understand that, depending on the illness or injury, they may experience three different levels of care.

• **Primary care** is the first and most generalized level of care. It is preferred because it is less expensive for the health care consumer.
• **Secondary care** is care by a specialist. A primary care provider may refer a patient to a specialist.
• **Tertiary care** is the highest level of care within a hospital. It is expensive and specialized, so it should not be the first recourse. Health care consumers requiring tertiary care are likely to have problems beyond those treated at primary and secondary levels.

Purpose of Services

The number and types of health care and supportive services are increasing exponentially. The FCN can have a positive impact on the health of the faith community by educating individuals and families about the **purposes of various services** that are available.

Health care providers are increasingly specialized, thereby requiring the health care consumer to be knowledgeable about services needed. These services may be provided by various health providers who are members of the interprofessional team.

• physicians
• advanced practice nurses (nurse practitioners, clinical nurse specialists, certified registered nurse anesthetists, and certified nurse midwives)
• physician's assistants

Specialized agencies or facilities provide some services. Members of the faith community will benefit from increased understanding of these times of care and the facilities that provide them.

• home care
• hospice
• palliative care
• extended care
• long-term skilled care
• rehabilitation
• continuum of care for the elderly
• programs for the elderly such as Area Agencies on Aging and innovative programs such as PACE (Program of All-Inclusive Care for the Elderly)

OUTCOME 5

Use documentation, follow-up and evaluation in the referral process.

Health care referrals often include providing information about the client's specific needs that may be met by the health care provider, agency or organization.

The Referral Process

According to Stanhope and Lancaster (2012, p. 197) the purpose of **referral** is to identify and access resources and to prevent or resolve problems or concerns.

The referral process includes these steps.

1. **Investigate** community agencies and assemble a large database of community agencies for appropriate referrals.
2. **Assess** the individual or family with varied agency information in mind.
3. **Discuss** all referral options with the individual or family.
4. **Explore** individual or family receptivity to referral.
   - Past experience with referral may have been positive or negative.
   - Personal values may or may not allow the individual or family to accept help from others.
   - Determine individual's or family's ability to make self-referral.
5. **Refer** individual or family to appropriate resource.
6. **Plan** an evaluation of the referral process.

Documentation of the referral should include the following:
- ◆ **Who**—*individual, family or congregation*
- ◆ **What**—*service required and agency or provider*
- ◆ **Process**—*time frame (how long it took the client to gain access) and accuracy of information (location, eligibility requirements and so on)*
- ◆ **Outcome**—*client satisfaction; document whether client's expectations were met*

Best Practices for Referrals and Follow-up Evaluation

1. The FCN respects the **client's right to refuse** a referral. Unless there is a risk of abuse, neglect, or harm to the individual, the client can choose not to accept any service offered.
2. The FCN develops **referrals that are timely, practical, tailored to the client, and coordinated.**
3. The **client participates in the process**, involving family members as appropriate.
4. The client is **encouraged to make self-referral** unless the client or the resource provider feels that an FCN referral is necessary.
5. The FCN **collaborates** with the interprofessional team.
6. The FCN provides **correct, current, and relevant information** regarding the resource needed.

HELPFUL RESOURCE

See Referral Documentation, Follow-up and Evaluation Form in Appendix C.

Critical Thinking

What are the ethical and legal implications of evaluating resources?

What has changed in your understanding of the FCN's role in regard to accessing resources?

7. The FCN **follows up with the client** after resources or referrals are provided to evaluate effectiveness.

Ethical Issues Related to Referrals

1. Confidentiality is required. (See Appendices D and E.)
2. Autonomy of the individual or family is paramount.
3. Respect for the individual's or family's right to self-determination is evident.
4. The FCN is an objective source of information and encouragement.
5. No referrals are made to persons associated with the FCN who could benefit monetarily from the referral.

Specific Individual or Family Issues

1. All screening programs such as blood pressure screenings conducted in the faith community should have a protocol for referral, an assessment form, a list of available resources, tracking form, and evaluation form. (See Appendix C.)
2. Documentation of acceptance or refusal of referral is critical.
3. If the FCN makes a referral and individual or family information is to be shared with a referral agency (or vice versa), the *Release of Information Form* should be signed by the client and kept in the client record.

Standards of Professional Performance for Faith Community Nursing

Standard 4. Planning

The faith community nurse develops a plan that prescribes strategies and alternatives to attain expected outcomes.

COMPETENCIES

The faith community nurse:
- Considers the economic impact of the plan on the health care consumer, family, caregivers, or other affected parties and how the faith community resources and local community resources might be of assistance.

Standard 5: Implementation

The faith community nurse implements the identified plan.

COMPETENCIES

The faith community nurse:
- Applies available healthcare technologies to maximize access and optimize outcomes for health care consumers.
- Utilizes community and faith community resources and systems to implement the plan.

Standard 15. Resource Utilization

The faith community nurse utilizes appropriate resources to plan and provide nursing services that are safe, effective, and financially responsible.

COMPETENCIES

The faith community nurse:
- Assesses individual healthcare consumer care needs and resources available to achieve desired outcomes.
- Identifies health care consumer care needs, potential for harm, complexity of the task, and desired outcome when considering resource allocation.
- Delegates elements of care to appropriate healthcare workers in accordance with any applicable legal or policy parameters or principles.
- Identifies the evidence when evaluating resources.
- Advocates for resources, including technology, that enhance nursing practice.
- Modifies practice when necessary to promote a positive interface between healthcare consumers, care providers, and technology.
- Assists the health care consumer and family in identifying and securing appropriate and available resources to address health and spiritually related needs across the health care continuum.
- Assists the health care consumer and family in factoring costs, risks, and benefits in decisions about treatment and care.
- Develops innovative solutions and applies strategies to obtain appropriate resources for faith community nursing care.

Learning Activities

Community Resource Identification

Instructions:

1. Locate local resources using the Internet.

2. Compile a list of resources that each participant's faith community might need based on a congregational assessment or individual member requests.

3. Have participants use the Community Resource Identification form in Appendix A to identify and share resources in the local area.

Question:
Which identified resources do you think will be the most useful to your practice? Why?

Community Resource Evaluation

Instructions:

1. Pair participants.

2. Ask each pair to select two of the websites below, or a different website that is of interest to them.

3. Answer the questions in Appendix B, Evaluation of Resources, for selected websites.

> American Cancer Society: www.cancer.org
> Affordable Care Act: http://www.healthcare.gov
> Care for the Caregiver: http://www.lotsahelpinghands.org
> Centers for Disease Control and Prevention: http://www.cdc.gov
> FamilyDoctor.org: http://familydoctor.org/
> HealthFinder: http://www.healthfinder.gov/
> HIV InSite: http://hivinsite.ucsf.edu/
> Homecare Compare: http://www.medicare.gov/homehealthcompare/search.html
> Kidshealth: http://www.kidshealth.org/
> MayoClinic: http://www.mayoclinic.com/
> MedlinePlus: http://medlineplus.gov/
> My Care Compare: http://mycarecompare.org
> National Cancer Institute: http://www.cancer.gov/
> National Center for Complementary and Alternative Medicine: http://nccam.nih.gov/
> National Hospice and Palliative Care Organization: http://www.nhpco.org/
> NetWellness: http://www.netwellness.org/
> NIH SeniorHealth: http://nihseniorhealth.gov/
> Nurse Family Partnership: http://www.nursefamilypartnership.org/
> Red Cross: http://www.redcross.org
> The Health Sherpa: www.thehealthsherpa.com
> Veterans Health Administration: http://www.va.gov/health/

Question:
What features of a website do you find most helpful in evaluating its usefulness?

Case Studies

Instructions:

1. Assign the participants to pairs or small groups to discuss the case studies below.

2. Or, participants may want to offer case studies from their own practices.

3. Use Appendix C for documentation, follow-up and evaluation.

4. If time allows, plan for each group to offer a quick recap to the large group.

Questions:

For each case study, ask:

1. What assumptions can the FCN make?

2. What additional assessment data is needed?

3. What local or national resources can the FCN suggest?

CASE 1
Senior Housing

Javier and Isabel are long-time members of the congregation. Isabel makes an appointment to meet with the FCN for the purpose of locating senior housing for her 83-year-old mother. Javier and Isabel feel her mother is no longer able to live by herself. The mother has been widowed for 10 years and has lived in the same house for 35 years.

CASE 2
Accessing Social Services

Cassie, a 75-year-old woman, is a long-time parishioner who lives alone. She is able to function independently, but needs transportation to her medical appointments and various errands, such as grocery shopping. She asks for information about such transportation services.

CASE 3
Social Isolation

Mr. Carter's son calls the FCN for assistance with his 80-year-old father, who has become increasingly isolated after the death of his wife six months earlier. They had been married for 55 years and have five children, all of whom live out of town. Mr. Carter is able to live alone, does his own cooking and grocery shopping, and is in fairly good health except for severe loss of hearing in one ear.

CASE 4
Accessing Family Housing

Travis, a 35-year-old man with a wife and three children, ages two, four and seven, approaches the FCN to request help in securing housing as his house has been foreclosed. He has a steady job as a store manager at a local market, but his wife does not work due to the needs of their youngest child who has congenital heart disease.

CASE 5
Services for Extended Family

Joanie, a 62-year-old woman who teaches biology at a local public high school, has been participating in the weekly low-impact aerobic sessions at church. After the latest session she asks the FCN to check her blood pressure because she has felt dizzy and had vision problems over the past three or four days. Upon further questioning, she shares that her husband has lost his job and her daughter and son-in-law, who have had to move in with them, have just suffered a miscarriage of their first baby. Currently, no one in the household has health insurance and the financial resources for both couples are limited.

CASE 6
Accessing Food and Clothing

Yu-jin, a 32-year-old mother with four children, ages four to ten, calls the FCN requesting help in accessing food and clothing for her and her children. Her husband sustained a severe injury while overseas with the armed forces. He has been in long-term rehabilitation at a VA hospital in another state for the past six months. Yu-jin quit her job so that she could spend more time with her children, who are suffering from their father's injury and absence.

CASE 7
Community Resources for Independence

Colleen, a 45-year-old member of the faith community, calls the FCN for assistance in locating appropriate resources for her 50-year-old brother, whom she and her husband have taken into their home while he undergoes treatment for severe depression and anxiety related to alcohol and drug abuse. Until a year ago he had held a steady job with benefits. Colleen's goal is to assist her brother to live independently and she is not sure where to start.

Note: The following case studies involve a high level of sensitivity on the part of the FCN. While formulating a response, take into consideration the legal and ethical issues involved.

CASE 8
Sexually Suggestive Approaches

Mrs. Bennington, the mother of a 13-year-old boy in the faith community, comes to the FCN distressed because her son told her that he and several other young male friends have been approached several times by the pastor (a male) to watch movies and play video games after school. Mrs. Bennington's son has told his mother that he felt uncomfortable because the videos were sexually suggestive, and he knows he would not be allowed to watch them at home.

CASE 9
Teen Sexual Activity

Jamie is a 16-year-old girl who is a member of the youth group. She approaches the FCN after Sunday services requesting information on family planning. She shares that she has been sexually active with her boyfriend, who is 21 years old. While her parents like the young man, they would never approve of premarital sex. Jamie does not want to go to her family physician because she is afraid he will tell her parents.

CASE 10
Stress and Emotions

You suspect that the spiritual leader of your faith community is having emotional difficulties. She is late for work on a regular basis, and when she is present she seems preoccupied, unable to concentrate or make important decisions. When you question her, she answers that she hasn't been sleeping well and thinks this is probably related to job stress.

CASE 11
Signs of Abuse

A female member of the faith community has come to services recently looking sad and depressed. The FCN has questioned her about this change in her affect but has not gotten satisfactory answers. Last week the woman came to one of the early services and it was clear that she had bruises on her face and neck. She left immediately after the service so the FCN did not have the opportunity to speak with her.

References

Required Textbook

American Nurses Association and Health Ministries Association. (2012). *Scope and standards of practice: Faith community nursing* (2nd ed.). Silver Spring, MD: Nursesbooks. org.

References

Bair-Merritt, M. H., Lewis-O'Connor, A., Goel, S., Amato, P., Ismailji, T., Jelley, M., Lenahan P., Cronholm, P. (2014). Primary care-based interventions for intimate partner violence: A systematic review. *Preventive Medicine, 46*(2), 188–94.

Benedetti, J., Vargas, K. (2014). Evaluating health websites. National Network of Libraries of Medicine. Retrieved June 8, 2014 from http://nnlm.gov/outreach/consumer/evalsite. html.

Cancer Information on the Internet. (2014). American Cancer Society. Retrieved June 8, 2014 from http://www.cancer. org/cancer/cancerbasics/cancer-information-on-the-internet.

Dieckman, J. L. (2013). Running the show: Referral and follow-up, case management and delegated functions. In M. Truglio-Londrigan & S. B. Lewenson (Eds.). *Public health nursing: Practicing population-based care.* Burlington, MA: Jones & Bartlett Learning.

Hickman, J. S. (2006). *Faith community nursing.* Philadelphia, PA: Lippincott, Williams & Wilkins.

Jimenez, M.E., Fiks, A.G., Shah, L.R., Gerdes, M., Ni, A.Y., Pati, S., & Guevara, J. P. (2014). Factors associated with early intervention referral and evaluation: a mixed methods analysis. *Academy of Pediatrics, 14*(3), 315–23.

Keller, L. O., Strohschein, S., Lia-Hoagberg, B., Schaffer, M.A. (2004). Population-based public health interventions: Practice-based and evidence-supported. *Public Health Nursing, 21*(5), 453–468.

Lee, L., Hillier, L.M., Harvey, D., (2014). Integrating community services into primary care: Improving the quality of dementia care. *Neurodegenerative Disease Management, 4*(1), 11–21.

Meade, C. (2011). Community health education. In Nies, M. & McEwen, M. (Eds.), *Community/public health nursing: Promoting the health of populations* (5th ed.). St. Louis, MO: Elsevier/Sanders.

Mohr, D. C., Schueller, S., Montague, E., Burns, M., & Rashidi, P. (June 5, 2014). The behavioral intervention technology model: An integrated conceptual and technological framework for ehealth and mhealth interventions. *Journal of Medical Internet Research, 16*(6). e146. doi:10.2196/jmir.3077.

Nies, M. & McEwen, M. (2011). Health a community view. In *Community/public health nursing: Promoting the health of populations,* 5th ed. St. Louis, MO: Elsevier/Sanders.

Saburi, G. (2013). Stressors of caregivers of school-age children with epilepsy and use of community resources. *Journal of Primary Care Community Health, 4(3),* 167–117.

Siegrist, B. (2015). Faith community nursing. In Nies, M. & McEwen, M. *Community/Public Health Nursing: Promoting the health of populations,* 6th ed. St. Louis, MO: Elsevier/Sanders.

Stanhope, M. & Lancaster, J. (2012). Public health nursing: Population-centered care in the community. Maryland Heights, MO: Mosby.

Wayne, N., & Ritvo, P. (June 6, 2014). Smartphone-enabled health coach intervention for people with diabetes from a modest socioeconomic strata community: Single-arm longitudinal feasibility study. *Journal of Medical Internet Research, 16*(6), e149. doi:10.2196/jmir.3180. Retrieved June10, 2014 from http://www.jmir.org/2014/6/e149/

Online Resources

Additional websites can be found in Appendix B.

Cancer information on the Internet, American Cancer Society: http://www.cancer.org/cancer/cancerbasics/cancer-information-on-the-internet

Denominational websites

Evaluating health information: Retrieved June 8, 2014 from http://www.nlm.nih.gov/medlineplus/evaluatinghealth information.html

Evaluating health websites. National Network of Libraries of Medicine: http://nnlm.gov/outreach/consumer/evalsite. html

Healthy People 2020: http://healthypeople.gov/2020/about/

Medline Plus guide to healthy web surfing. Retrieved June 8, 2014 from http://www.nlm.nih.gov/medlineplus/healthy websurfing.html

National Network of Libraries of Medicine, Health Ministry Outreach Toolkit: http://guides.nnlm.gov/ministry.

Wrap-Up and Evaluation

Measuring Competency

This chart can be used to assess the individual outcomes in this module.
- A copy of this chart is attached to the Participant Module, so that each participant can complete this short evaluation.
- Have participants read each outcome and then place an X in the box that best matches their opinion about the objective being met.
- Encourage each participant to write a short reflection about this module in the space provided at the bottom of this chart.
- Use this data to make any necessary changes.

Outcome	Not Met	Somewhat Met	Met
1. Explain the rationale for the FCN's role in accessing appropriate resources.			
2. Assess individual health care consumer care needs and resources available to achieve desired outcomes.			
3. Implement a method to access and evaluate internal and external resources, including Internet resources.			
4. Assist the health care consumer and family in identifying and securing appropriate and available resources to address health and spirituality needs across the health care continuum.			
5. Use documentation, follow-up and evaluation in the referral process.			
Reflection: *In one paragraph, write a reflection on this module.*			

Appendix A

COMMUNITY RESOURCE IDENTIFICATION

Agency/Program Name: _____

Website Address: _____

Physical Address: _____

Phone: _____

Fax No: _____

Contact Person: _____

Services Provided: _____

Hours of Service: _____

              Evenings: _____

              Weekends: _____

Geographic Area Served: _____

Handicap Accessible: Yes   No

Mode of Transportation Available _____**Needs Transportation:** _____

Eligibility Criteria: _____

              Demographic: _____

                    Age: _____

                    Sex: _____

             Diagnosis: _____

               Income: _____

Payment: ____Free   ____Medicare   ____Medicaid   ____Sliding Scale

           Insurance: _____

Application Process: ____Self   ____Health care provider only

Narrative Information:

Appendix B

EVALUATION OF RESOURCES

Use these questions to help determine if the website is helpful for the members of your faith community.

Who? Who manages the website? Can they be trusted?

What? What information does the site provide that specifically addresses the needs of your clients?

When? When was the information posted or reviewed? Is it up-to-date?

Where? Where did the information come from? Is it based on scientific evidence? Is it reviewed by experts?

How? How is the website funded? Does the site's information favor the sponsor?

Would you recommend this website to members of your faith community?

- Is the website easy to navigate?

- Are the words used on the site easy to understand?

- Are there pictures to illustrate the information on the site?

- Is the website culturally sensitive? Is it bilingual (English and Spanish)?

- Does it protect your privacy? Does it ask for personal information?

- Is there a contact number or email address for questions?

Appendix C

REFERRAL DOCUMENTATION, FOLLOW-UP AND EVALUATION FORM

Date	Client Name	Referred to	Date of Follow-up	Met Client's Expectations?	Comments

Appendix D

Sample Denominational Direction on Health Ministry

AUTHORIZATION TO RELEASE INFORMATION FROM FAITH COMMUNITY HEALTH RECORD TO THIRD PARTY

Print Client's Name: _____

Daytime Phone Number: _____

I, _____**do hereby authorize**

      Name of Client or Legal Guardian

_____ **to release to** _____

    Name of Faith Community Nurse   *Name of Third Party*

the following information:

concerning the care I received from the faith community nurse from

_____ **to** _____.

  beginning date   *ending date*

I understand that I may revoke this consent at any time in writing.

_____   _____

       Client Signature   *Date*

_____   _____

     Witness Signature   *Date*

Appendix E

AUTHORIZATION FOR RELEASE OF MEDICAL INFORMATION TO FAITH COMMUNITY NURSE

I, _____ , authorize _____

(Name of client/faith community member)   *(Name of physician/health provider)*

to allow_____ , a faith community nurse with my faith community,

(Name of Faith Community Nurse)

_____ , to have access to my private health

(Name of faith community)

information in the following situations. Check all those that apply:

_____ I grant the faith community nurse access to my medical record.

_____ I grant the faith community nurse permission to speak with the physician or other health provider named above about my health condition.

_____ I request the faith community nurse to accompany me to an appointment with the physician or other health provider named above regarding my condition.

_____   _____

Client Signature   *Date*

_____   _____

Witness Signature   *Date*

Appendix F

National Network of Libraries of Medicine

What should you look for when evaluating the quality of health information on websites?

Consider the source. Use recognized authorities. Know who is responsible for the content.
- Look for an "About Us" page. Check to see who runs the site: is it a branch of the federal government, a nonprofit institution, a professional organization, a health system, a commercial organization or an individual?
- There is a big difference between a site that says, "I developed this site after my heart attack" and one that says, "This page on heart attacks was developed by health professionals at the American Heart Association."
- Websites should have a way to contact the organization or webmaster. If the site provides no contact information, or if you can't easily find out who runs the site, use caution.

Focus on quality. All websites are not created equal. Does the site have an editorial board? Is the information reviewed before it is posted?
- This information is often on the "About Us" page, or it may be under the organization's mission statement or part of the annual report.
- See if the board members are experts in the subject of the site. For example, a site on osteoporosis whose medical advisory board is composed of attorneys and accountants is not medically authoritative.
- Look for a description of the process of selecting or approving information on the site. It is usually in the "About Us" section and may be called "editorial policy" or "selection policy" or "review policy."
- Sometimes the site will have information "About Our Writers" or "About Our Authors" instead of an editorial policy. Review this section to find out who has written the information.

Be a cyberskeptic. Quackery abounds on the web. Does the site make health claims that seem too good to be true? Does the information use deliberately obscure, "scientific" sounding language? Does it promise quick, dramatic, miraculous results? Is this the only site making these claims?
- Beware of claims that one remedy will cure a variety of illnesses, that it is a "breakthrough," or that it relies on a "secret ingredient."
- Use caution if the site uses a sensational writing style (lots of exclamation points, for example).
- A health website for consumers should use simple language, not technical jargon.
- Get a second opinion! Check more than one site.

Look for the evidence. Rely on medical research, not opinion. Does the site identify the author? Does it rely on testimonials?
- Look for the author of the information, either an individual or an organization. Good examples are "Written by Jane Smith, R.N.," or "Copyright 2003, American Cancer Society."
- If there are case histories or testimonials on the site, look for contact information such as an e-mail address or telephone number. If the testimonials are anonymous or hard to track down ("Jane from California"), use caution.

Check for currency. Look for the latest information. Is the information current?
- Look for dates on documents. A document on coping with the loss of a loved one doesn't need to be current, but a document on the latest treatment of AIDS needs to be current.
- Click on a few links on the site. If there are a lot of broken links, the site may not be kept up-to-date.

Beware of bias. What is the purpose? Who is providing the funding? Who pays for the site?
- Check to see if the site is supported by public funds, donations or by commercial advertising.
- Advertisements should be labeled. They should say "Advertisement" or "From our Sponsor."
- Look at a page on the site, and see if it is clear when content is coming from a non-commercial

source and when an advertiser provides it. For example, if a page about treatment of depression recommends one drug by name, see if you can tell if the company that manufactures the drug provides that information. If it does, you should consult other sources to see what they say about the same drug.

Protect your privacy. Health information should be confidential. Does the site have a privacy policy and tell you what information they collect?

- There should be a link saying "Privacy" or "Privacy Policy." Read the privacy policy to see if your privacy is really being protected. For example, if the site says "We share information with companies that can provide you with useful products," then your information isn't private.
- If there is a registration form, notice what types of questions you must answer before you can view content. If you must provide

personal information (such as name, address, date of birth, gender, mother's maiden name, credit card number) you should refer to their privacy policy to see what they can do with your information.

Consult with your health professional. Patient-provider partnerships lead to the best medical decisions.

For further information: Visit the MedlinePlus page on Evaluating Health Information (http://www.nlm.nih.gov/medlineplus/evaluating healthinformation.html) and Evaluating Internet Health Information: A Tutorial from the National Library of Medicine (http://www.nlm.nih.gov/medlineplus/webeval/webeval.html).

Unit IV: Community
Advocacy

Advocacy

Introduction

Learning Outcomes

Upon completion of this module, the participant will be able to:

1. Advocate for individuals or groups of vulnerable persons.
2. Associate historical examples of health care advocates.
3. Examine contemporary health care issues related to vulnerable persons.
4. Apply advocacy skills in faith community nursing practice.

Description

Health advocacy is one of the key aspects of faith community nursing. As stated in *Code of Ethics for Nurses with Interpretive Statements* (ANA, 2001, p. 16), the faith community nurse (FCN) "promotes, advocates for, and strives to protect the health, safety, and rights of the patient." In faith community settings, this often includes advocating for appropriate levels of care for vulnerable populations and those with limited access to health care resources. Such advocacy may include initiating referrals for clinical treatment, obtaining home care resources, or assisting with transitional care arrangements. FCNs may promote advocacy for health care consumers with low health literacy skills by accompanying them to provider appointments and providing health education in more readily understood terminology. Although the goal of advocacy is self-efficacy, we must advocate for individuals so that they learn to advocate for self. Advocacy is the first step towards self-management. A percentage of the population will always need advocacy. FCNs advocate for public policy that addresses health disparities and promotes health and wellness (ANA/HMA, 2012). FCNs must advocate for equitable health care that is sensitive to the needs of health care consumers, with particular emphasis on the spiritual needs of diverse populations. This module recognizes historical health care advocates and addresses issues related to vulnerable persons, contemporary health care issues, and advocacy competencies of the FCN. Steps that the FCN should take in advocating for individuals, families, and faith communities are included.

Hours: 2

Research

The *Code of Ethics for Nurses with Interpretive Statements* (ANA, 2001) and the *Faith Community Nursing: Scope and Standards of Practice* (ANA/HMA, 2012) specifically state the nurse's duty to advocate on behalf of the client. A literature review on this topic reveals that while nurses, in general, support the concept of advocacy, there is little educational preparation for the specific role of advocate. In her book *Spirituality in Nursing—Standing on Holy Ground*, O'Brien, (2014) describes advocacy as an essential component of the professional role of the Registered Nurse.

Faith Tradition

Two central themes run through the Bible concerning justice. The first is God's all-encompassing love, concern, and mercy for all human beings. The second is our responsibility to love God's earth and to care for God's people. Many faith communities are organizing to answer God's call to love our neighbors, stand with the marginalized, and work with God for a more just society.

Key Terms

Advocate: to speak on behalf of another; one who pleads the cause of another

Autonomy: the right of patients to make decisions about their medical care without their health care provider trying to influence the decision

Health disparity: inequality or disproportionate difference in health care access or health outcomes

Navigator: one who guides

Nursing advocacy: integrating aspects of individuality, professionalism and experiences of empowering

Paternalism: acting as one thinks best for others regardless of their expressed wishes

Vulnerable persons: people at a greater than normal risk of experiencing abuse

Reflection

"If you close your ear to the cry of the poor, you will cry out and not be heard."
—Proverbs 21:13

"If you offer your food to the hungry and satisfy the needs of the afflicted, then your light shall rise in the darkness and your gloom be like the noonday. The LORD will guide you continually, and satisfy your needs in parched places, and make your bones strong; and you shall be like a watered garden, like a spring of water, whose waters never fail."
—Isaiah 58:10-11

"When he returned to Capernaum after some days, it was reported that he was at home. So many gathered around that there was no longer room for them, not even in front of the door; and he was speaking the word to them. Then some people came, bringing to him a paralyzed man, carried by four of them. And when they could not bring him to Jesus because of the crowd, they removed the roof above him; and after having dug through it, they let down the mat on which the paralytic lay. When Jesus saw their faith, he said to the paralytic, 'Son, your sins are forgiven.'"
—Mark 2:1–5

Question for reflection: Many people lack access to healing. Who will remove the roof for them?

Advocacy
Content Outline

Critical Thinking

What person or group of listed vulnerable persons is present in your faith community?

What, if any, health care disparity do you identify with that person or group of persons?

OUTCOME 1
Advocate for individuals or groups of vulnerable persons.

Vulnerable persons are people who are at a greater than normal risk of experiencing abuse. The FCN must **advocate** for, or speak on behalf of, those who are vulnerable because of a disability, age, illness, or socioeconomic circumstances. These individuals may be unable to take care of or protect themselves against significant harm or exploitation. Vulnerable persons may also experience **health disparity**, an inequality or disproportionate difference in health care access or health outcomes. The FCN can help to close this gap.

Vulnerable groups may include:
- pregnant women
- infants
- persons who are chronically ill and disabled
- persons living with HIV/AIDS
- persons who are mentally ill and disabled
- persons with suicide and homicide-prone behavior
- persons living in abusive families
- persons who are homeless
- immigrants and refugees
- older adults (especially those who are unwell, frail, or confused)
- persons who are incarcerated
- persons who abuse alcohol and other substances
- persons who lack family and social support

OUTCOME 2
Associate historical examples of health care advocates.

Historical examples of health care advocates have a foundation in the Judeo-Christian and other faith traditions, especially in the modern era.

In the **Hebrew faith**, Moses is a primary historical figure. In Exodus 3, we read that he did not feel capable of helping the Israelites in bondage, yet the overarching story of his life is fulfilling his call from God and leading the Israelites out of slavery in Egypt.

Often the work of the prophets was to advocate for the well-being of individuals or the nation. For instance, Elisha advocated for the widow whose two sons were about to be taken into slavery by calling on God for oil she could sell, and he advocated for the life of the Shunammite woman's son who had died (2 Kings 4:1–37).

In the **Christian faith**, Scripture describes Jesus and the Holy Spirit as advocates (John 14:25, 1 John 2:1, Hebrews 7:25). Many healing miracles also show individuals in the role of advocate for other people. For example, Jairus begged Jesus to heal his daughter (Luke 8:40–42, 49–56); the centurion asked Jesus to heal his servant from afar (Matthew 8:5–10); the apostle Paul had a ministry of healing (Acts 28:7–10).

In nursing history, during the nineteenth century, **Florence Nightingale** developed the concept of district nursing and home visitation of the sick.

- She also brought environmental and sanitation issues into the foreground of health care.
- Nightingale advocated for proper care and hygiene of soldiers in the Crimean War and upon their return to their country.
- She developed the St. Thomas Hospital School of Nursing to educate nurses, especially in disease prevention, through proper hygiene.

Lillian Wald is another nineteenth-century nurse, well-known for adopting the settlement house concept as the most effective way to bring health care to poor immigrant populations.

- Nurses lived and worked among the poor.
- Wald emphasized health promotion and political activism in work at the Henry Street Settlement House. She coined the term *public health nursing*.
- Wald obtained payment for visiting nurse services in New York City from the Metropolitan Life Insurance Company, a program that was successful after three months and extended nationwide.
- She lobbied for the first White House Conference on Children, which resulted in the school nursing model.
- Wald convinced the Red Cross to expand peacetime efforts to rural America, leading to the establishment of the Rural Nursing Service.

Modern day advocates described a "future full of hope."

- **Martin Luther King, Jr.** (January 15, 1929–April 4, 1968) was an American pastor, activist, humanitarian, and leader in the African-American Civil Rights Movement. He is best known for his role in the advancement of civil rights using nonviolent civil disobedience based on his Christian beliefs.

- **Desmond Tutu** (born October 7, 1931) is a South African social rights activist and retired Anglican bishop who rose to worldwide fame during the 1980s as an opponent of apartheid. He was the first black Archbishop of Cape Town and bishop of the Church of the Province of Southern Africa (now the Anglican Church of Southern Africa).
- **Mahatma Gandhi** (October 2, 1869–January 30, 1948) was the preeminent leader of Indian nationalism in British-ruled India. Employing nonviolent civil disobedience, Gandhi led India to independence and inspired movements for civil rights and freedom across the world.
- **Pope John Paul II** (May 18, 1920–April 2, 2005) was the 264th pope of the Catholic Church from October 16, 1978 until his death. John Paul II is recognized as helping to end communist rule in his native Poland and eventually all of Europe.

OUTCOME 3

Examine contemporary health care issues related to vulnerable persons.

A range of health care issues contribute to or rise out of vulnerability. FCNs can be aware of more than the clinical setting of health care.

Access to health care—The primary concern is that lack of access to health care will lead to unnecessary illness. Ideally, most individuals want the best possible health care regardless of age, sex, race, or ability to pay (Koch, 2014).

Cost of health care—FCNs must become involved in the economics of health care. They must increase knowledge and awareness of health care funding and policy making in order to advocate for the types of funding that will provide appropriate care for diverse populations.

Inadequate housing—Inadequate housing can involve exposure to environmental hazards.

Homelessness—Homeless individuals have complex physical, mental, social, and spiritual needs and their access to health care is problematic. Homeless children are at risk for poor school performance due to multiple factors, including lack of access to facilities for personal hygiene and lack of school supplies (National Center for Homeless Education, 2014).

Hunger or food insecurity—Hunger and food insecurity is likely to occur in geographic areas where affordable and nutritious food is difficult to obtain, particularly for those without access to transportation. These areas, typically called "food deserts," usually exist in rural areas and low-income communities. Food deserts are sometimes associated with supermarket shortages and food security. Diet-related health problems can be common in affected populations.

Right to Life issues across the life span—FCNs may serve as advocates to support positive, pro-life solutions to human problems, such as alternatives to abortion, euthanasia, infanticide, or other deliberate destruction of human beings.

Violence in the family and in the community—FCNs need to understand the basics about domestic violence, how to access and work alongside secular advocates in their communities, and when to provide spiritual support to a victim seeking safety.

Early discharge from the hospital—FCNs may often be in a position to advocate for clients who are facing early discharge from the hospital. Information about lack of family support may sway the decision; however, in instances of early discharge the FCN can identify and access community resources such as home health care and home-delivered meals as well as resources from the faith community to enhance the transition from hospital to home.

Lack of health insurance—The FCN needs to be aware of a variety of health care assistance programs available to help those who lack health insurance. Knowing about the most common types of health care assistance programs can ensure an FCN gets the best and most affordable health care available for members of the faith community.

Cultural Diversity—It is essential for the FCN to know how cultural groups view life processes, define health and illness, and how traditional healers cure and care for members.

These issues can be overwhelming, and the FCN will not be able to resolve them in every instance. The Serenity Prayer may serve as a guide for the FCN involved in advocacy: "God grant me the serenity to accept the things I cannot change, courage to change the things I can, and the wisdom to know the difference."

> **Critical Thinking**
> *List the health care issues of vulnerable persons in priority of greatest to least in your faith community.*
>
> *Which issue would you consider the most important to address first? How would you approach this issue?*

OUTCOME 4

Apply advocacy skills in faith community nursing practice.

Successful advocacy depends on clear understanding of the process and practical actions. Elements of **nursing advocacy**— integrating aspects of individuality, professionalism, and experiences of empowering—include the following:
- positive nurse-client relationship
- respect for the person's **autonomy**, or the right to make decisions about medical care without their health care provider trying to influence the decision
- respect for the person's self-determination
- affirmation of the person's abilities and resourcefulness

A trained FCN acting as a health care advocate brings several advantages.
- knowledge of accessing health resources

> **KEY TERM**
> **Nursing Advocacy** *integrates aspects of individuality, professionalism, and experiences of empowering.*

> **EXAMPLE OF FCN NURSING ADVOCACY**
> *The FCN may work with hospital discharge planners to promote effective transition to home. Preventing avoidable hospital readmissions has the potential to profoundly improve both the quality of life for patients and the financial well-being of health care systems (Cooper and McCarter, 2014).*

- ability to assist in care coordination
- skills to collaborate with the health care community

Autonomy refers to the right of patients to make decisions about their medical care without their health care provider trying to influence the decision.

Specific health advocacy skills include:
- honesty
- assertiveness
- directness
- risk taking
- effective communication
- negotiation

The FCN must use his or her **power to advocate** for improved health of individuals and families in the faith community. This power comes from several sources.
- expert power—in relation to person, evidence-based practice
- legitimate power—license to practice
- referent power—nurses often rank #1 in public opinion, such as in Gallup polls
- reward power—improved health for faith community members

Effective advocacy is not only about power. It involves careful **listening** to the individuals being served.
- Allow individuals to identify their own situations.
- Assist individuals in clarifying personal values.
- Affirm individuals in selecting options.
- Support individuals in decision-making.

And finally, **knowledge** is essential to the advocacy process.
- knowledge of the person—individual, family, faith community and society
- knowledge of the health care system
- knowledge of nursing practice
- knowledge of relevant legal statutes

Follow these **basic steps for advocacy**—either working alone or with others.
1. Assess the nature and source of the issue to be addressed.
2. Determine the appropriate target for the advocacy intervention.
3. With clients, establish mutual goals that are realistic and practical.
4. Negotiate an action plan with the client.
5. Consider the economic impact of the plan on the client and their family.
6. Determine availability of resources.
7. Assess receptivity to advocacy of all involved with the plan.
8. Serve as a **navigator**, one who guides, while avoiding **paternalism**, acting as one who thinks best for others regardless of their expressed wishes.

9. Establish boundaries—limits and lines of demarcation for your responsibilities and actions.
10. Recognize resilience in previous experiences.
11. Implement the plan.
12. Evaluate outcomes.

Standards of Professional Performance for Faith Community Nursing

Standard 5. Implementation

The faith community nurse implements the identified plan.

COMPETENCIES

The faith community nurse:
- Advocates for health care that is sensitive to the needs of healthcare consumers, with particular emphasis on the spiritual needs of diverse populations.

Standard 5A. Coordination of Care

The faith community nurse coordinates care delivery.

COMPETENCIES

The faith community nurse:
- Advocates for the delivery of dignified and humane care by the interprofessional team.

Standard 7. Ethics

The faith community nurse practices ethically.

COMPETENCIES

The faith community nurse:
- Advocates for equitable healthcare consumer care.

Standard 15. Resource Utilization

The faith community nurse utilizes appropriate resources to plan and provide nursing services that are safe, effective, and financially responsible.

COMPETENCIES

The faith community nurse:
- Advocates for resources, including technology, that enhance nursing practice.

Standard 16. Environmental Health

The faith community nurse practices in an environmentally safe and healthy manner.

COMPETENCIES

The faith community nurse:
- Advocates for the judicious and appropriate use of products in health care.
- Advocates for environmental health and social justice, including a commitment to the health of vulnerable populations.

Learning Activities

Case Studies

Instructions:
1. Read the cases aloud. The cases involve different types of advocacy.
2. Assign the participants to small groups and assign one or more case study to each group.
3. Encourage the participants to discuss the case selected using the questions provided.
4. Reconvene the group and have the groups share their observations.

Question:
Use the appropriate basic steps for advocacy to serve the individual, family, faith community, or entire community in your case study.

CASE 1
Individual

Marian is an 85-year-old widow that the FCN has been visiting for several years in order to provide socialization and spiritual care. Marian has a 55-year-old adopted son who lives with her. The son, Perry, is almost completely deaf and has had little education or work experience due to his mother's overprotective lifestyle. Perry is able to read the newspaper, conduct the banking, and prepare simple meals. He also runs errands and is out of the house independently at least a few hours every day. One day, the FCN stops in to visit unexpectedly and finds that Marian has been in bed for the past three days. She is in a fetal position and is barely able to respond. After attending to Marian's immediate needs for food and elimination, the FCN is faced with whether to leave her in her home with her son or make other living arrangements for her.

- What advocacy skills will be most essential for the FCN working with Marian?
- Who might serve as a resource as you advocate for Marian?

CASE 2
Family

Connie has been the FCN at Central United Methodist Church for the past four years. She makes regular visits to homebound congregation members. One family she visits consists of Dan and Martha, an elderly couple with one daughter who lives out of state. Over the course of the past four years, Dan has become increasingly debilitated from Parkinson's disease and is now in the early stages of Alzheimer's disease. Dan and Martha have become disillusioned with their physician and have told Connie a number of times, "We might as well take care of ourselves. The doctor does nothing, and he doesn't even listen anymore." As Connie continues to make her visits, she realizes that Martha can no longer manage her husband's care alone and does not have the emotional stamina anymore to deal with everyday issues.

- What advocacy skills will be most essential for the FCN working with Dan and Martha?

- Who might serve as a resource as the FCN advocates for Dan and Martha?

- Should the FCN notify the spiritual leader of the faith community? Why or why not?

CASE 3
Faith Community

With the current economic recession, it has come to the attention of the faith community's secretary that more calls are coming in to the spiritual leader requesting assistance with food and utility bills. The faith community has a food pantry, but it has been difficult to keep it stocked due to the increasing demand. Some members of the faith community have expressed a desire to merge their pantry with that of another faith community in the area. Members also feel that it is important to keep the pantry open even if the stock is limited.

- Is there a need for the FCN to become involved?

- If so, what should be the role of the FCN?

- What advocacy skills will be most essential for the FCN working with this faith community?

- Who might serve as a resource as the FCN advocates for this faith community?

CASE 4
Faith Community

The local Jewish synagogue has a large Hispanic population. Many of the members who belong to the synagogue have relatives who are working in the United States but do not have appropriate documented papers. Recently, there was a raid at a local meat-packing house. Many of the workers were jailed, causing families to be separated. There were 150 children impacted by this situation. The nearest FCN is in a neighboring faith community, which is not Jewish. Jim, the FCN, has been asked by community leaders to acquire the help of members from his faith community to assist in lobbying efforts to help impact the law on immigration to stop the raids.

- What should Jim do as the FCN?
- What ethical or legal considerations must he consider?
- Will it make a difference that Jim is a member of a different faith community than the one he serves?

CASE 5
Societal, Systemic or Community

The issue of access to health care is a major issue in the United States. Common estimates suggest about 47 million people are without health care coverage. The FCN's faith community takes social justice issues very seriously. Individual members have asked the FCN to help them organize a group of volunteers who will be trained to assist individuals in the community with the process of enrolling and signing up for health care.

- How could the FCN assist in promoting the efforts of this faith community?
- Who might serve as a resource as the FCN advocates for this faith community?

Expanded Learning Activity

Choose one or more of these expanded learning ideas to use with your group according to your time and resources.

1. Locate one website for your denomination and find resources for advocacy. Present a written report and a short reflection on the website information to the other participants. If a laptop and Internet connection is available, demonstrate how to access denominational advocacy resources during the class period.

2. Divide the participants into small groups. Using additional case studies (based on participant experiences), have the participants discuss each situation in relation to a broader social issue. Report back to the larger group if time allows.

3. Use movie clips from films that are strong on social advocacy, such as *Erin Brockovich*. After viewing the movie clips, the participants could identify the skills of the advocate. Note: some movie clips are readily available on YouTube.

4. Conduct an Internet search for advocacy websites and organizations either in, prior to, or after class, depending on location and format of the course (retreat, weekly, long weekend).

5. Select one particular topic of interest to the group and have participants look up the website for their denominations and determine if there are advocacy tools available.

References

Required Textbook

American Nurses Association and Health Ministries Association (2012). *Scope and standards of practice: Faith community nursing* (2nd ed.). Silver Spring, MD: Nursesbooks.org.

References

American Nurses Association and Health Ministries Association (2001). *Faith community nursing: Scope and standards of practice* (2nd ed.). Silver Spring, MD: Nursesbooks.org.

American Nurses Association (2008). *Code of ethics for nurses with interpretive statements*. Washington, DC: American Nurses Association.

Cooper, J. & McCarter, K. (2014). Management program for older adults. *Public Health Nursing, 31*(1), 36-43.

Koch, M. (2014). Paying for health care in America's rising costs and challenges in Cherry, B. and Jacob, S. (Eds.) *Contemporary nursing: Issues, trends, and management* (6th ed.). St. Louis, MO: Elsevier.

National Center for Homeless Education (March 2014). *Education for Homeless Children and Youths Program Data Collection Summary*. Retrieved June 5, 2014 from http://center.serve.org/nche/downloads/data-comp-0910-1112.pdf.

O'Brien, M. E. (2014). *Spirituality in nursing, standing on holy ground*. Burlington, MA: Jones and Bartlett Learning.

Additional References

Bass, D. (2012). Nurses called upon as advocates for patient empowerment through technology. *Computers, Informatics, Nursing (CIN)*. February, 69–70.

Beckmann, D. (2010). Exodus from hunger. Louisville, KY: Westminster John Knox Press.

de Chesnay, M. (Ed.). (2005). *Caring for the vulnerable*. Sudbury, MA: Jones and Bartlett Publishers.

Fowler, M. (2008). *Guide to the code of ethics for nurses*. Silver Spring, MD: Nursesbooks.org.

Gilbert, J.; Green, E.; Lankshear, S.; Hughes, E.; Burkoski, V.; Sawka, C. (2011). Nurses as patient navigators in cancer diagnosis: review, consultation, and model design. *European Journal of Cancer Care. 20*(2), 228–236.

Hearrell, C. (2011). Advocacy: nurses making a difference. *Journal of Emergency Nursing. 37*(1), 73–74.

Henderson, S.; Princell, C.; Martin, S. (2012). The patient-centered medical home. *American Journal of Nursing. 112*(12), 54–59.

Hoglund, B. A. (2013). Practicing the code of ethics, finding the image of God. *Journal of Christian Nursing. 30*(4), 228–233.

Nykiel, L.; Denicke, R.; et al. (2011). Evidence-based practice and family presence: paving the path for bedside nurse scientists. *Journal of Emergency Nursing 37*(1), 9–17.

Schomus, I. (2013). The consequences of crushing poverty: a nurse fights back. *Journal of Christian Nursing 30*(1), 30–33.

Sullivan, E. (2013). *Becoming influential: a guide for nurses* (2nd ed.) Boston: Pearson.

Online Resources

American Public Health Association: http://www.apha.org

Bread for the World: http://www.bread.org

Evangelical Lutheran Church: www.uss-elca.org/wp-content/uploads/2012/02/Advocacy-ministry.pdf

Network—Catholic Social Action Lobby: http://www.networklobby.org

Nightingale Institute: http://www.nightingaledeclaration.net

Patient Advocate Institute: professionalpatientadvocateinstitute.com

Stephen Ministries: http://www.stephenministries.org

United Church of Christ: http://www.ucc.org/justice/advocacy_resources/

Wrap-Up and Evaluation

Measuring Competency

This chart can be used to assess the individual outcomes in this module.
- A copy of this chart is attached to the Participant Module, so that each participant can complete this short evaluation.
- Have participants read each outcome and then place an X in the box that best matches their opinion about the objective being met.
- Encourage each participant to write a short reflection about this module in the space provided at the bottom of this chart.
- Use this data to make any necessary changes.

Outcome	Not Met	Somewhat Met	Met
1. Advocate for individuals or groups of vulnerable persons.			
2. Associate historical examples of health care advocates.			
3. Examine contemporary health care issues related to vulnerable persons.			
4. Apply advocacy skills in faith community nursing practice.			
Reflection: *In one paragraph, write a reflection on this module.*			

Unit IV: Community

Care Coordination

Care Coordination

Introduction

Learning Outcomes

Upon completion of this module, the participant will be able to:

1. Coordinate care delivery in the faith community.
2. Apply competencies and skills that support successful care coordination.
3. Develop volunteers and support groups for ministry in the faith community.

Description

Care coordination is the deliberate, planned organization of activities to manage patient care, including interprofessional collaboration, advocacy, referral, and case management (ANA/HMA, 2012). The faith community nurse (FCN) coordinates care for individuals and for the faith community as a whole. The FCN's work with the ministerial team provides collaborative partners not found in other health care settings to support people in improving health or coping with difficult health situations. This module emphasizes competencies related to care coordination, such as case management and interprofessional alliances important to the practice of faith community nursing. Collaboration as a mechanism for improving faith community health outcomes is discussed. The participant has the opportunity to explore care coordination from the unique role of the FCN and to develop related skills, including collaboration, working with volunteers, and developing and evaluating support groups.

Hours: 2

Research

Interest in the interprofessional collaboration in health care has increased due to changes in delivery of health care, economics, and other sociological changes. Many studies related to care coordination or case management for specific populations, such as people living with diabetes, or health promotion for specific populations in faith communities document program evaluation.

Atherly and Thorpe (2011) demonstrated significant cost reductions among high cost, chronically ill Medicare patients by using an interprofessional clinical team and nurse care coordination to educate and empower patients. The study revealed that for 2007, the total annual Medicare costs for the study sample was 15.7 percent ($3,240) lower than for the control group.

Dyess and Chase (2012) documented FCN services such as caring and intentional spiritual interventions positively impacted the care of adults living with chronic illness. Results supported the connection between faith and health, and the interventions added by the FCN included helping the patient "live in abundance" though nurturing spirituality. This study found that spiritual nurturing helps individuals gain "a beginning understanding of the importance of meaning and purpose in life and offers an alternative to the 'disease management' model of care" (p. 42).

Faith Tradition

Many faith communities recognize the needs of the people and communities they serve and have policy statements that support health ministries and FCN practice. For example, *Ethical and Religious Directives for Catholic Health Care Services* (4th edition, 2001), published by the United States Conference of Catholic Bishops, recognizes changes and challenges to the twenty-first century church and issues a call to the laity to collaborate in ministry. The US Department of Health and Human Services (http://www.hhs.gov/partnerships) also recognizes the role of churches in improving the health of Americans.

Key Terms

Care coordination: the deliberate organization of patient care activities between two or more participants (including the patient) involved in a patient's care to facilitate the appropriate delivery of health care services (Agency for Healthcare Research and Quality)

Collaboration: exchanging information, altering activities, sharing resources, and enhancing the capacity of another organization, for mutual benefit, and to achieve a common purpose

Coordination: exchanging information and altering activities for mutual benefit and to achieve a common purpose

Cooperation: exchanging information, altering activities, and sharing resources for mutual benefit to achieve a common purpose

Reflection

Implementing the role of care coordinator reminds the FCN of the importance of working with a community of people.

"Then I said to the king, 'If it pleases the king, and if your servant has found favor with you, I ask that you send me to Judah, to the city of my ancestors' graves, so that I may rebuild it.'"... "I told them that the hand of my God had been gracious upon me, and also the words that the king had spoken to me. Then they said, 'Let us start building!' So they committed themselves to the common good ..."
—Nehemiah 2:5, 18

The account of Nehemiah's vision and charge to repair the walls of Jerusalem demonstrates many of the fine points of collaboration. Nehemiah collaborated with all levels of society, even with those who were opposed to him and operated from a different value system. He brought together volunteers with diverse skills and abilities to participate in the project so they too felt fulfilled.

See Appendix D for Sample Denominational Direction on Health Ministry.

Care Coordination

Content Outline

OUTCOME 1

Coordinate care delivery in the faith community.

Defining Care Coordination

Organizations involved in quality health care recognize the value of care coordination and define it in various ways.

The **Agency for Healthcare Research and Quality** (AHRQ) uses the following as a working definition of care coordination: "Care Coordination is the deliberate organization of patient care activities between two or more participants (including the patient) involved in a patient's care to facilitate the appropriate delivery of health care services. Organizing care involves marshaling personnel and other resources needed to carry out all required patient care activities, and is often managed by the exchange of information among participants responsible for different aspects of care" (McDonald et al., 2010, p. 4).

The **National Quality Forum's** definition is: "A function that helps ensure the patient's needs and preferences for health services and information sharing across people, functions, and sites are met over time" (National Quality Forum, 2006, p.1).

In a 2012 position paper titled *Care Coordination and Registered Nurses' Essential Role*, **American Nurses Association** (ANA) affirms the integral role of registered nurses in the care coordination process as a core professional competency. This involvement improves quality of care and outcomes across health care settings.

DeBrew, Blaha, Moore, and Herrick (2011, p. 236) suggest the following skills are needed by FCNs to support successful care coordination:

- communication and interpersonal skills
- clinical skills
- teaching skills
- counseling skills
- critical thinking, problem solving and knowledge of community resources

- group process skills
- collaborative networking skills
- leadership skills
- organizational skills
- research skills

Background and Opportunities

A review of current federal health care reform across states identifies that the focus of the reform is on not only expanding coverage for the uninsured or underinsured persons, but also on reorganizing the US health care system to include key elements in prevention and care coordination.

- The inclusion of both is past due. Federally funded demonstration projects, research projects related to complex care coordination, and the impact of preventative health all decrease the cost of health care and improve the health care status of Americans as a population. While it seems that this should be an easy fix, the opposite is true.
- Fragmentation of care within the US has been documented to be attributed to a lack of care coordination, which has produced increased costs and poor patient outcomes.
- Nurses have a unique set of skills that can contribute to care coordination; however, many of the current models of care coordination fall short of including the important role of the FCN in the success of improving health care outcomes for patients. This may be partially due to how early faith community nursing pioneers envisioned their roles in a new and evolving nursing specialty.

Previously, care coordination was something that the case manager did in health care facilities.

- This person may have been a nurse or a social worker or other individual who focused on select categories of patients, primarily those requiring transitioning to another level of care such as long-term care, rehabilitation, or home with home care or hospice.
- Additionally, little outcome evaluation was performed following the patient's discharge. Leape, Osler, and Davis (2013), reported on past performance by agencies: "Part of the problem is that the consequences of doing a bad job seem to fall on the patients not the provider. Who sees it when you do not do a good job? ... for the poorest or those in the worst health? Well they're not really a vocal bunch are they?" (p. 93).

Changes in health care reform have resulted in the Centers for Medicare and Medicaid Services (CMS) and other third-party payers reconsidering the importance of good case management.

- Especially in individuals with multiple diagnoses or complex care situations there are data that show good **care coordination** can prevent readmissions to the hospital, prevent complications, decrease the number of emergency department

KEY TERM

Care coordination *is the deliberate organization of patient care activities between two or more participants.*

visits, and improve the quality of life (Cesta, 2013).
- The important question: Is the FCN on the list of important community-based services that should be considered when there is a patient discharge, transition in care level, complex care situation, or need for supportive wholistic care?

The reemergence of the "patient-centered medical home" (PCMH) due to health care reform has the potential for becoming either an enhancement or a barrier to faith community nursing practice and the FCN's role in care coordination.
- The PCMH is not a new concept. The American Academy of Pediatrics in 1967 introduced the term "medical home" to explain the necessity for a primary site or location for the medical records of chronically ill children (Arent et al., 2012).
- The concept was later expanded to include all the services required by this population, such as primary care that was "accessible, continuous, comprehensive, coordinated, family-centered, and culturally effective" (Arent et al., p. 434).
- Currently this term indicates a model for many populations of patients that includes not only comprehensive primary care, but care that is coordinated from PCMH, and other supportive and community-based services (Arent et. al., 2012).

Critical Thinking

What is the role of the FCN in relation to other people in the faith community who might participate in coordinated care?

The American Academy of Family Physicians have identified Joint Principles of the PCMH that include:
- a personal physician
- physician-directed services (team of health care providers directed by the MD)
- care coordinated across health care systems, and community-based services
- quality and safety incorporated into all layers of care (using evidence based practices, QI activities, information technology, etc.)
- improved access (open scheduling, expanded hours of service, better ways of communicating between providers)
- payment that is appropriate and valuable to the patient

Essential to the success of this system are the care coordinator and case manager.
- National demonstration projects have shown improved patient outcomes and reduced costs of care when these principles are in place.
- The Geisinger Proven Health Navigator Project (Arent et.al., 2012) involved studying patients with diabetes. The outcomes included an 18 percent reduction in hospital admissions, a 36 percent reduction in hospital readmissions, and a 4.3–7.1 percent savings in health care costs, depending upon the medications prescribed for the patient, and a reduction in diabetes-related foot amputation.
- The Group Health Cooperative reported a 20–30 percent improved patient satisfaction score with services and a decreased provider emotional exhaustion score.

- A related outcome for this study was a 29 percent reduction in emergency department visits and a savings of $10.30 per patient per month.

In this and other examples that rely heavily on care management for program success, faith community nursing is not recognized as an essential, community-based service.

OUTCOME 2

Apply competencies and skills that support successful care coordination.

In this section selected competencies and skills related to successful care coordination are discussed, including collaboration and working with volunteers.

Care Coordination and Collaboration

Obviously successful care coordination requires **collaboration** and is a way to partner with other faith ministries and community groups (Kaye & Crittenden, 2005). Collaboration has many benefits.

- First, collaborating with key professionals and various agencies in the community can legitimize an issue. For example, working with a diverse group of professionals that represent many organizations who have come together to address the same issue can demonstrate the size and importance of the issue.
- Also, with the backing of multiple organizations and stakeholders, the ability to collectively capture the interests of key policymakers in the community can be multiplied. Based on collaborative efforts problems are solved that never may have been solved if each group had decided to work independently on the issue.

Collaborating with Individuals

The FCN has the opportunity for collaboration with individuals and groups, many of which may be unique to the practice setting. According to DeBrew et. al, these include:

- Collaborating **with the spiritual leader**. This is an essential member of the care coordination team. The FCN needs the spiritual leader's respect for his or her knowledge and ability and support for programs, activities and care plans for patients and families. The spiritual leader can best guide the FCN in upholding church policies and doctrine.
- Collaborating **with God**. The FCN also provides for the spiritual needs of faith community members. This is sometimes a challenge for the nurse because it requires that the FCN minister through prayer, and by sharing his or her own spiritual gifts.
- Collaborating **with the faith community**. The FCN must learn about the specific skills and competencies of members of

KEY TERM
Collaboration *is exchanging information, altering activities, sharing resources, and enhancing the capacity of another organization for mutual benefit.*

the faith community. These individuals support care coordination efforts through volunteering, sharing resources, and supporting the efforts of the FCN.

- Collaborating **with the physician**. As a professional nurse it is essential that the FCN work with the physician of the person being served and the entire interprofessional health care team to participate in a planned health regime. This also includes representatives from other services (for example, home care, hospice, durable medical equipment (DME)) needed to meet the patient's needs.
- Collaboration **with other ministries**. Working together prevents duplication of services and contributes to success. This includes working across faith communities with other FCNs. Perhaps another faith community can provide resources not available in one's own community.
- Collaborating **with the individual and family**. The FCN provides care for the entire faith community as well as the individual who requests services. The FCN must follow established guidelines related to confidentiality and documentation to maintain legal and ethical requirements for professional nursing practice. (DeBrew et. al., 2011, p. 223–225).

Collaborating for Synergy

Collaboration often brings synergy that occurs through participating in a group (Kaye & Crittenden, 2005). When brainstorming an issue, ideas and energy create new avenues to address the issue. During the collaboration process, people become energized because each person at the table has a vested interest in finding a solution to the problem. This synergy also may bring about new ideas for additional resources that may be needed.

Collaborating for Grant Funding

Collaboration also might help obtain grant money.

- Collaborative efforts may convince granting sources that the FCN or congregation is committed to their members and the important issues in their congregation.
- The FCN may be in the position to provide information to the grant writing process about the multitude of community resources that parishioners could use to improve or maintain their health.
- It is important to note that some faith community-related projects have been awarded grants based on the number and strength of the collaborations formed. Certain funding guidelines sometimes encourage grantees to expand those collaborations to include all stakeholders involved (Nouwen, 2010).

KEY TERM

Coordination *is exchanging information and altering activities for mutual benefit to achieve a common purpose.*

Barriers to Collaboration

Some perceived barriers to collaboration are:
- "Stranger danger"—a reluctance to share information with others.
- "Needle in a haystack"—the belief that others may have already solved the problem. The question becomes, how do you find them?
- "Hoarding"—the basic premise that people do not want to share their knowledge because they see hoarding their information as a source of real power.
- "Not invented here"—the solution is not a product of the group but comes from outside the group (American Red Cross, 2011).

Differentiating Between Coordination, Cooperation and Collaboration

Coordination is exchanging information and altering activities for mutual benefit to achieve a common purpose.
- Coordination requires more than organizational involvement and networking. It can be an important strategy to implement change.
- Coordination is most effective when all parties affected by proposed changes share in the decisions about the possible consequences of the changes. An example of coordination is when community agencies work together to coordinate transportation services for their children.
- Through coordination, families gain access to transportation services. In addition, unnecessary or duplicative services may be eliminated (DeBrew et al., 2011).

Cooperation means exchanging information, altering activities, and sharing resources for mutual benefit to achieve a common purpose.
- Shared resources may include sharing staff, work space, training, information, funding, and, in some cases, legal arrangements.
- An example of cooperation is when the public transportation system and the private local transportation system (such as a bus company) use the same coordinator to assist families in the event of natural disaster evacuation (Kaye & Crittenden, 2005).

Collaboration is exchanging information, altering activities, sharing resources, and enhancing the capacity of another organization, for mutual benefit and to achieve a common purpose.
- Members of a collaborative effort view each other as partners that are willing to share risks, resources, responsibilities, and rewards.
- A multi-sector collaboration is an alliance of public, private, and nonprofit organizations.

KEY TERM

Cooperation *means exchanging information, altering activities, and sharing resources for mutual benefit to achieve a common purpose.*

• An example of collaboration is illustrated by public and private agencies that are currently working together toward the creation of a disaster preparedness plan.
• All available resources, including community contacts and funding, are fully shared (Engle & Prentice, 2013).

Interprofessional Collaboration

The Interprofessional Expert Panel Report (2011) suggests the following four core competencies for successful interprofessional collaborative practice:

1. Work with individuals of other professions to maintain a climate of mutual respect and shared values.
2. Use the knowledge of one's own role and those of other professions to appropriately assess and address the health care needs of the patients and populations served.
3. Communicate with patients, families, communities, and other health professionals in a responsive and responsible manner that supports a team approach to the maintenance of health and the treatment of disease.
4. Apply relationship building values and the principles of team dynamics to perform effectively in different team roles to plan and deliver patient- and population-centered care that is safe, timely, efficient, effective, and equitable.

Grey & Connolly (2008) explain the benefits of interdisciplinary collaboration. They composed the following list of benefits for clients, health care professionals, and organizations from interdisciplinary collaboration in health care.

Benefits to patients:
• improved patient outcomes
• lower mortality
• increased patient satisfaction (enhanced feelings of security, importance, and respect)
• increased feelings of empowerment

Benefits to health professionals:
• increased job satisfaction
• improved registered nurse (RN) retention
• increased RN involvement in decision-making
• decreased burnout
• improved career potential and career mobility
• increased professional growth
• cross-disciplinary peer review and critique of practice and research

Benefits to health care organizations:
• improved cost effectiveness of care
• improved distribution of resources
• improved productivity of collaborators
• more knowledgeable practitioners
• increased funding for practice and research

Critical Thinking

How does collaboration in faith communities differ from other settings?

Why is interprofessional health care collaboration important?

Identify how you as an FCN can collaborate with other ministries or committees in your faith community.

- acceleration of innovation in health care due to cross-fertilization of creative ideas

Collaboration among professionals is a vital factor in safe, effective health care. Grey & Connolly (2008) inform nurses of the potential results of poor collaboration.
- Patient safety issues often depend on how well health care teams function under pressure at the bedside.
- Lack of teamwork and collaboration leads to error and decreased quality in the care setting.
- Lack of collaboration and coordination produces tension and disrespect among health professionals in the health care setting.
- Skills for interdisciplinary collaboration are not taught in health professional education.
- Lack of collaboration for the client results in exclusion from decision-making about care, engenders feelings of powerlessness, and powerlessness leads to frustration and non-compliance.

OUTCOME 3

Develop volunteers and support groups for ministry in the faith community.

Volunteers (unpaid workers) are a necessity in faith community nursing. In some settings even the FCN is a volunteer. Like many nonprofit organizations, a faith community's health ministry program might not be able to function without the help of volunteers.
- Volunteers assist with a variety of tasks such as helping with health-related programming, completing necessary clerical work, or serving as speakers for certain educational events.
- Volunteers in faith-based organizations may see themselves as God's hand extended. They may feel that they are carrying out God's plan for their lives by helping God's people.
- The FCN must know how to recruit, train, manage, and supervise volunteers.
- Recognizing volunteers is also important. A planned program for sustaining volunteer involvement is also essential (McNamara, 2014).

HELPFUL RESOURCE
See Appendix A, 16 Tips for Recruiting Adult Volunteers.

Working with Nurse Volunteers

Depending upon the model of care an FCN adopts, the FCN may need to recruit RNs to support the practice. Volunteer nurses are bound by state statutes in regard to individual practice. Providing nursing care as a volunteer does not relieve the nurse from liability or malpractice or from following scope of practice. Generally when offering volunteer services as a registered nurse the following guidelines and requirements apply. The RN must:

- possess a current, unencumbered license as a registered nurse in the state in which the services will be offered.
- perform only those duties for which the nurse possesses the necessary skills and competencies, including appropriate intervention and referral for persons at immediate risk for illness or injury.
- perform duties according to nationally recognized standards and in accordance with the requirements of the state's Nurse Practice Act.
- follow policies established by the faith community or governing body. (Ohio Nurse Association, 2009, p. 5)

Volunteer nurses should understand however that the **Federal Volunteer Protection Act of 1997** was passed to encourage volunteers and help protect them from lawsuits. The statute provides that volunteers of nonprofit or governmental agencies are not liable for harm due to acts of omission under these conditions.

- The volunteer was acting within the scope of duties.
- The volunteer was properly licensed, certified, or authorized, if required, for the activities performed.
- Harm was not a result of willful or criminal misconduct.
- Harm was not caused by the volunteer operating a vehicle for which the state requires operator licensure and/or insurance (OHA, 2009, p. 5).

Good Samaritan Acts vary from state to state. The volunteer nurse should understand the laws for his or her state. Generally Good Samaritan Laws do not cover activities that are not related to emergency situations, so they do not apply in an FCN practice.

The Recruitment Process

Where do volunteers come from? The FCN might consider this question before recruiting volunteers, whether other RNs or non-health professionals.

Understanding why certain people may want to work with the FCN may help the FCN recruit the right people. A few reasons that people commonly choose to volunteer are:

- They want to make a difference (contribute to a good cause).
- They hope to develop new skills.
- They want to meet people and make new friends.
- Some combination of these reasons.

The best place to recruit volunteers for the health ministry is within the faith community. Congregation members are considered stakeholders and have alliances within that congregation and community. Additionally, often a word from the pastor or spiritual leader may encourage a volunteer to come forward to serve.

At times the FCN may need more volunteers than the immediate faith community can provide. To find more volunteers the FCN can investigate places such as:

- Corporate volunteer programs that provide opportunities for employees to become involved in service to the community and allow their employees to work with nonprofit organizations during the workday.
- Neighboring churches, synagogues, and other religious institutions with volunteer programs may offer a wealth of volunteer prospects who are motivated by religious and altruistic beliefs to serve the broader community.
- Internship programs at colleges and high schools often provide interns free of charge in exchange for a meaningful volunteer project.
- Career counseling centers can help identify individuals who are changing careers and considering entering the nonprofit sector as volunteers.
- Civic clubs, fraternal organizations, sororities, and fraternities can be great resources for large numbers of volunteers.
- Newspapers, radio, television, and social media are excellent vehicles to promote volunteer needs, and many will allow nonprofit organizations to list volunteer opportunities for free.
- Governmental offices may also be a source of volunteers because some governmental organizations allow employees to leave work for up to one half day a week to serve as volunteers in the community.
- High schools and colleges may have programs that require students to give hours of service to community projects.
- Other nonprofit community organizations can be a tremendous resource in identifying and recruiting volunteers.

In order for volunteers to do the best job possible in the health ministry program, it is important to know the recruits, and the recruits must know what to expect.
- At the same time, volunteers are more likely to stay on board if they are picking up useful skills and if they know exactly what they are getting out of their volunteer experience.
- Volunteer **training is essential**. Get to know the policies that are established related to volunteers in the church.
- Many faith communities require volunteers to have a background check and to be educated on roles and responsibilities.
- Additional training depends upon the volunteer's role in the health ministry.

Volunteer Management

Volunteer retention requires careful management. The management goal is to make volunteers feel successful and appreciated.

10 PRINCIPLES OF VOLUNTEERISM

The American Red Cross (ARC) is an organization primarily governed and operated by volunteers. Included in the ARC Volunteer Handbook are the following principles on the importance of volunteers (ARC, 2011).
1. *We can broaden our nation's volunteer force by removing barriers to volunteering.*
2. *Volunteers are not "free."*
3. *Volunteers contribute more than meets the eye.*
4. *"Volunteer" does not mean "amateur."*
5. *Volunteers and the organization they serve must meet each other's expectations.*
6. *Volunteers must never be exploited.*
7. *Volunteers make excellent middle and senior managers.*
8. *When recruiting volunteers, it is more important to place the right person in the right job than to attract volunteers at random.*
9. *We can help shape government policies on volunteerism.*
10. *Everyone benefits when nonprofit organizations collaborate.*

- Remember, managing volunteers is an ongoing task that involves constantly clarifying volunteers' roles and responsibilities, providing feedback on their work, keeping records of their performance, and keeping the volunteers inspired.
- Matching the right person with the right job is critical for volunteers to be successful. For volunteers to feel appreciated and contribute in a meaningful way, the FCN should ask them to work on projects reflecting their strengths. It is best to identify and create projects based on the volunteers' skills and interests.

Show Appreciation

As is the case with paid employees, some volunteers may feel overburdened with work and have the potential to burn out. The FCN can make sure that the volunteers are not shouldering more than their share and that they are comfortable with and have a mechanism for letting the FCN know if they are working too hard. Showing appreciation may help prevent volunteer burnout. The following methods may be helpful in showing appreciation.

- Invite the volunteers to health cabinet meetings.
- Hold volunteer social events.
- Invite volunteers to special training sessions.
- Give a volunteer of the year award.
- Sponsor a volunteer appreciation luncheon.

Identify Roles, Expectations, Responsibilities and Relationships

One of the greatest challenges for any organization to face is preventing friction among staff, whether paid or volunteer.

- If at the top level of the organization, board members and executive directors disagree on where their responsibilities begin and end, similar problems may arise at other levels of the organization.
- To avoid problems arising from unclear or overlapping responsibilities, clear job descriptions must be written out for every position on your volunteer staff. Good job descriptions should itemize all of the duties of a position and should also specify what days and hours the volunteer will be working.

Assignments for volunteers. Remember to match the task to the volunteers' talents. Volunteers can:

- collect data
- provide professional consultation (in their fields)
- design brochures, newsletters, logos, etc.
- edit documents
- maintain a database (remember to teach them about confidentiality rules)
- visit people in hospitals, homes or care facilities
- conduct online services such as "visits," mentoring or instruction

HELPFUL RESOURCE

See Appendix B for a sample volunteer position description.

Documenting volunteer service. It is important to keep records of volunteer work.

- Adequate documentation helps the FCN make sure the volunteer force is used effectively.
- It also protects the FCN if a volunteer must, for some reason, be dismissed or the position responsibilities be revised.
- Documentation on volunteers does not need to be complicated or voluminous. It can be done on paper or can be included in a computer database. The basic information the FCN needs about new volunteers includes:
  - name, address, telephone number
  - education
  - relevant experience
  - interests and skills
  - availability
  - starting date
  - emergency contact information
  - pertinent medical information
- Proper documentation can help the FCN with:
  - evaluating programs
  - justifying program growth
  - documenting volunteer achievements
  - assuring accountability
  - defining training needs
  - pinpointing gaps in service
  - providing letters of recommendation
  - making long-term plans
- Additionally, the FCN can create a work record log that documents dates, times worked, and the assignments carried out.

Dismissing a volunteer. Occasionally the FCN may have to dismiss a volunteer. In doing so, the FCN should follow the same procedures as for a paid employee. To avoid a difficult situation consider the following suggestions.

- Make sure that all volunteers clearly understand the organization's policies and procedures.
- Utilize the work record log.
- Provide volunteers with honest feedback on their performance.
- Never discuss dismissing a volunteer with other staff people. Only the FCN, FCN's supervisor (if applicable), and the volunteer should know about the termination.
- If termination is imminent, be sure to make it very clear to the volunteer the reasons for the decision.
- Manage personal emotions and be professional and polite.
- Perhaps finding a different position for the volunteer will eliminate the need for dismissal.

Insurance. Once the faith community has decided to involve volunteers, the FCN must make sure that the faith community carries liability insurance and is covered adequately.

The FCN must also check with the faith community to see what its policy is about medical insurance for injuries incurred by volunteers. Since there are few insurance companies specializing in nonprofit coverage, the FCN may have to negotiate special arrangements with the faith community's insurance company to supply covering the volunteers.

The FCN must take into account two key areas when considering insuring volunteers: liability and injury.

Liability. There are various ways that the faith community could be sued due to the actions of its volunteers. Be sure to check the faith community's policies and ensure it is protected against the following possible scenarios.

- If a volunteer injures someone (bodily injury).
- If a volunteer slanders someone (personal injury).
- If a volunteer damages someone's property (property damage).
- If a volunteer abuses/molests a client (sexual abuse & molestation).
- If a volunteer renders an unqualified professional service— nursing, counseling, etc. (professional liability).

Injuries. If a volunteer is hurt while working in the faith community he or she may be entitled to compensation beyond what the volunteer's own insurance already covers. Speak to the faith community's insurance company to discuss possible solutions to this problem. One of these two solutions may be possible.

- Coverage under the faith community's worker's compensation policy. Usually, this means adding a "voluntary" endorsement to the faith community's existing worker's compensation policy. The faith community is then charged based on hours worked by volunteers.
- Coverage under a medical accident policy. These policies can cover anyone injured on the faith community's premises, including volunteers. The policy can also be extended to cover off-site activities, sporting events, or transportation to and from activities (National Mental Health Association, 2009).

Critical Thinking

Evaluate how volunteers are recruited and screened in your faith community. What additional steps do you think are necessary for volunteers involved in coordinated care?

Identify both nurses and non-nurses who seem particularly equipped to provide coordination of care.

Support Groups

In the role of care coordinator, the FCN may refer to existing support groups or facilitate the development of a new support group.

- Support groups, sometimes referred to as self-help groups, are people who gather to share common problems, experiences, illnesses, or life situations.
- The support group is generally made up of peers with a professional or volunteer facilitator, who may be the FCN.
- Generally the most effective groups are small in number (10–15) and attendance is voluntary.

In the US, support groups have filled the gap of traditional health care by empowering people in these ways.

- Members solve their own problems.
- Members learn about conditions, diseases, or situations.
- Groups allow safe environments for people to share or "let off steam" with others who understand through shared experiences.
- Attendance limits isolation.

Support groups generally help some individuals reduce anxiety, improve self-esteem, and improve quality of life.
- Research studies related to breast cancer support groups have found that participating individuals have a longer life expectancy and more successful treatment trajectory.
- 6.25 million Americans use support groups at any given time, and over 15 million have participated at some time (Work Group for Community Health & Development, 2013).

Finding the Right Group
Even though some support groups have a long history (Alcoholics Anonymous is the longest), some have a life span and disband after the group's needs are met. FCNs most often will be referring individuals to existing community support groups.
  Many support groups offer:
- information about medical treatments, research and strategies (through brochures, booklets, websites, telephone help lines, and person-to-person sharing in the group meetings).
- information about public policy, legal resources, privacy laws, and protection from discrimination.
- help finding adequate medical or physiological information.
- ways to find out about financial assistance, grants, stipends, or scholarships.

Support groups can vary in how often they meet, their area of focus, and who facilitates them.
- Some support groups are led by professional facilitators or by specific groups (for example, the American Cancer Society).
- Peer-support groups, which were started by individuals and do not have a professional facilitator, sometimes are called self-help groups.
- Support groups exist for many topics. For example, support groups can be for people:
  - with a specific health condition
  - with a relationship to an affected person, such as a sibling, spouse, or child
  - looking for services such as short-term, stand-in help for caregivers, rehabilitation services, or financial and estate planning
  - dealing with grief and loss

Professionals can contribute information and resources and help with organizational tasks such as planning meetings, setting up the meeting room, sending out messages, and obtaining speakers.

HELPFUL RESOURCE
See Appendix C for a guide to evaluating a support group.

It is important for the individual to find a compatible group.
- Some people prefer groups facilitated by professionals while others prefer a peer environment.
- People with some health conditions often become experts, in that they have researched a great deal about the therapeutic, social, and emotional aspects of having a particular disease.
- They may want to connect with others who can help plan solutions from an "I've been there, too" perspective (Shepherd & Shepherd, 2013).

A faith-based support group has the added advantage of being able to draw on shared beliefs and values related to hope and life's meaning.
- A faith-based support group honors the expression and understanding of the integration of faith into a life experience.
- These groups fulfill the modern role of faith community to build relationships among participants.
- A faith-based support group also helps the faith community regain its position as the place for physical and emotional healing.

What are characteristics of a good support group? When a faith community member is searching for a support group, the most important thing is to remind the person: "If the group doesn't feel right to you or doesn't match your needs, try a different group. There are many options available." *Good* is a value judgment that differs from person to person. However, here are some indicators a well-functioning group will display.
- current, reliable information
- prompt response to inquiries
- regularly scheduled meetings or newsletters
- access to appropriate professional advisors (for example, medical specialists, licensed therapists, counselors, or employment attorneys for workplace discrimination)
- strong leadership
- a clearly stated confidentiality policy
- specific qualities the individual is seeking (for example, a group around a specific condition, or a group for siblings). (Greenwood, 2013)

Prior to referring individuals to an established support group, the FCN should understand the purpose, membership, and leadership of the group.

How often a group meets depends on its purpose and the needs of its members.
- Large groups with many chapters may have local meetings once a month and annual meetings for the whole organization.
- Small groups intended to address a specific issue—for example, behavioral changes around managing smoking cessation or being newly single—may meet once a week for a set number of weeks.

- Some groups are designed to last for only a short time, such as four to eight weeks; other support groups may last for many years.

Support groups meet **where the group members are best served.**
- Hospitals offer support groups, but groups can also meet in an individual's home, churches or temples, libraries, or other community buildings.
- There are also online support groups, which may be especially helpful for people who are homebound, have limited free time to attend meetings, or don't have a group nearby that meets their needs (Varga and Paulus, 2014).

Size varies depending on the purpose of the group and the needs of the members.
- Some groups have fewer than ten members; others may have thousands.
- Groups that have as their goal raising money, influencing public health policy, or educating the public, tend to be very large.
- Emotional support groups, such as ones around grief or loss, typically are small, so that participants can feel safe expressing feelings (Graves, 2012).

Starting a Support Group

Starting a new group is time-consuming and takes much work. Additionally, an established group probably has certain advantages, such as existing informational materials, meeting times and places, and professional contacts. However, in some cases the type of group needed may not exist in the faith community or broader community. Ways to begin a new group include getting the help of a local hospital, health provider, or faith community (Graves, 2012).

Organizing considerations include the following.
- knowledge of the stages of group development: formation, maturation, termination and time limits
- group context: physical environment, place, arrangement of space, temperature control and room environment, and expected behavior of participants
- group structure
- group size
- location of meetings
- length of sessions
- group roles
- leadership: lay or professional

CHOOSING A GROUP

A congregational member looking for a support group might consider these questions.
- *Are you seeking specific information about medical treatment options? Companionship? Peer counseling?*
- *How far can you travel? Do you need help with transportation?*
- *Is the kind of group you want just for someone who is ill, or also for family members? Because of the nature of certain medical conditions, these support groups are often made up of affected individuals and their family members. Some members may be at risk, and others may be providing emotional or physical support for someone who is ill. Will a mixed group work for you?*
- *What about the emotional dynamics of the group? Are you looking for a group where you can openly discuss feelings, or are you primarily interested in finding services to further education and research?*
- *Are you seeking a group run by a professional facilitator or a peer-run support group?*
- *Are you seeking to integrate your faith into your healing process?*

Critical Thinking

What would you say is the first step in determining whether your work as an FCN should involve starting a support group?

After a group is launched, the members may want to consider listing it through the local paper or an associated organization (for example, the American Cancer Society), so that other people can learn about this new resource.

It is important for the FCN to remember that a support group is not therapy. Individuals displaying symptoms of extreme emotional distress, long-term emotional complaints, depression, or suicide should be referred as soon as possible to an appropriate counselor or therapist. Many pastors are certified counselors with specific training in assisting individuals or families. The FCN should explore these issues with the minister or pastor prior to offering services.

Standards of Professional Performance for Faith Community Nursing

Standard 5A. Coordination of Care

The faith community nurse coordinates care delivery.

COMPETENCIES

The faith community nurse:

- Coordinates implementation of a wholistic plan of care.
- Coordinates the healthcare of individuals across the life span using principles of interprofessional models of care delivery and case management.
- Organizes the components of the plan.
- Manages a healthcare consumer's care in order to maximize independence and quality of life.
- Assists the healthcare consumer to identify options for alternative care.
- Communicates with the healthcare consumer, family, and system during transitions in care.
- Advocates for the delivery of dignified and humane care by the interprofessional team.
- Documents the coordination of care.

Learning Activities

Suggested Pre-Class Activities

Instructions:
Choose one or more of these activities to assign to participants to complete before the class meets.

1. Visit the website for your individual faith group's governing body. Explore the policy or vision statement related to health and/or FCNs. Identify the activities related to care coordination for the FCN.

2. Identify resources and collaboration opportunities to support care coordination activities in your faith community. Include actual or potential volunteers or related ministries.

3. Obtain a community resource guide for your home area. This may be through the local chamber of commerce, area hospital, or other community agency. This is a starting point for your care coordination activities.

4. If you are in a paid or unpaid FCN position, review your job description. What care coordination responsibilities are identified in the job description that reflect the ANA standards for this competency?

5. Explore the following reading materials and online resources.
   American Association of Colleges of Nursing, American Association of Colleges of Osteopathic Medicine, American Association of Colleges of Pharmacy, American Dental Education Association, Association of American Medical Colleges, and Association of Schools of Public Health (2011). *Core competencies for interprofessional collaborative practice: Report of an expert panel*. Washington, DC: Interprofessional Education Collaborative.
   Clinch, T. (2012, July). The need for high-level care coordination. *Nursing News, 36*(3)14.
   Nutt, M., & Hungerford, C. (2010). Nurse care coordinators: Definitions and scope of practice. *Contemporary Nurse, 36*(1–2), 71–81.

Plan a Collaborative Activity

Instructions:
1. Assign participants to small working groups.

2. Ask each group to brainstorm a creative activity that would promote collaboration for health promotion in a faith community.

3. In addition to the activity idea, groups should answer these questions: Who will you involve from within your faith community and the external community (such as agencies and health care providers)? What would be your role as the FCN in implementing this collaborative activity?

4. Allow a few minutes for quickly sharing ideas with the large group.

Question:
What might be a barrier to collaboration for care coordination in your setting, and what might be the first step to removing the barrier?

Preparing to Recruit Volunteers

Instructions:
1. Ask participants to form small working groups.
2. Guide groups through working on Parts A, B, and C at a pace that fits your time frame.
3. Bring everyone back to the large group for a final discussion.

Question:
What did you discover from this exercise about the process of involving volunteers in your cause?

Part A: The Cause
Why and how does your organization represent a good cause? Take a moment to answer the questions below.
- Whom does your organization help? Consider special communities—ethnicities, socioeconomic levels, age levels.
- How does your work help your local community?
- How does your work help a larger community?

Part B: The Volunteer
Now think about what's in it for the volunteer. Make a list of what volunteers can get out of working for your organization. Your list might include personal rewards such as the satisfaction of helping people or more concrete returns such as developing particular skills.

Part C: The Announcement
Consider the answers to the questions in Part A and Part B. Now design a recruitment announcement that indicates:
- How your organization contributes to the community.
- How volunteers can benefit from working with your organization.

Why Am I Here?

Instructions:
1. Explain that training should be an ongoing process. Volunteers should initially be taught how to manage their duties, and they should also be given the opportunity to continue to learn and expand their skills as they work within the organization.
2. Encourage participants to brainstorm ways to include your volunteers in the broader activities of your organization so that they remain enthusiastic about their involvement. Effective volunteers know exactly what they are getting out of their volunteer work.
3. This exercise will prepare FCNs to help volunteers clarify for themselves what they wish to accomplish in working for an organization.
4. In pairs, have participants role-play interviewing volunteers. They should ask each other in detail why they are giving time to the organization.

Question:
What is important to ask volunteers about their motivation for working with your ministry?

References

Required Textbook

American Nurses Association and Health Ministries Association. (2012). *Faith community nursing: Scope and standards of practice* (2nd ed.). Silver Spring, MD: Nursesbooks.org.

References

American Association of Colleges of Nursing, American Association of Colleges of Osteopathic Medicine, American Association of Colleges of Pharmacy, American Dental Education Association, Association of American Medical Colleges, and Association of Schools of Public Health. (2011). *Core competencies for interprofessional collaborative practice: Report of an expert panel.* Washington, DC: Interprofessional Education Collaborative.

American Nurses Association and Health Ministries Association (2012). *Faith community nursing: Scope and standards of practice* (2nd ed.). Silver Spring, MD: Nursesbooks.org.

American Red Cross. (2011). *American Red Cross: Volunteer handbook.* Retrieved from http://www.redcross.org/images/MEDIA_CustomProductCatalog/m13740313_2012_OKC_Volunteer_Handbook.pdf.

Arent, J., Tsang-Quinn, J., Levine, C., & Thomas, D. (2012). The patient-centered medical home: History, components, and review of the evidence. *Mt. Sinai Journal of Medicine, 79*(450), 433–450.

Atherly, A., & Thorpe, K. E. (2011). Analysis of the treatment effect of Healthway's Medicare health support phase 1 pilot on Medicare costs. *Population Health Management, 14*(1), 23–28.

Cesta, T. (2013, November). Centers for Medicare & Medicaid Services—new interpretive guidelines for the conditions of participation for discharge planning—part 1. *Hospital Case Manager, 21*(11), 151–154.

Clinch, T. (2012, July). The need for high-level care coordination. *Nursing News, 36*(3) 14.

DeBrew, J., Moore, L., Blaha, S., & Herrick, C. A. (2010). New trends in the evolution of case management: Faith community nursing. *Introduction to care coordination and nursing management,* Fero, L.J., Herrick, C.A. & Hu, J. (Eds.) 218–239. Sudberry, MA: Jones & Bartlett.

DeBrew, J., Blaha, S., Moore, L., & Herrick, C. (2011). Philosophy of faith community nursing. In Fero, L., Herrick, C. & Hu, J. eds. *Introduction to care coordination and Nursing management.* Sudbury, MA: Jones and Bartlett.

DeWitt, G. (2003). Why nurses? Nurses and volunteering: A perfect match. Retrieved from www.serviceleader.org

Dyess, S. M., & Chase, S. K. (2012). Sustaining health in faith community nursing practice: Emerging processes that support the development of a middle-range theory. *Holistic Nursing Practice, 26*(4), 221–227.

Engle, J. & Prentice, D. (2013). The ethics of interprofessional collaboration. *Nursing Ethics, 20*(4), 426–435. doi: 10.1177/0969733012468466

Graves, D. (2012). *Setting up and facilitating bereavement support groups: A practical guide.* London: Jessica Kingsley Publishers.

Grey, M. & Connolly, C. (2008). Coming together, keeping together, working together: Interdisciplinary to transdisciplinary research and nursing. *Nursing Outlook, 56*(3), 102–107.

Greenwood, N., Mabibi, R., Mackenzie, A., Drennan, V. & Easton, N. (2013). Peer support for careers: A qualitative investigation of the experiences of careers and peer volunteers. *American Journal of Alzheimer's Disease & Other Dementias, 28*(6), 617–26. doi: 10.1177/1533317513494449.

Kaye, L., & Crittenden, J. (2005). Playing well with others—interdisciplinary collaboration at a center on aging. *Social Work Today, 3*(5), 34–39.

Leape, L., Osler, D. & Davis, A. (2013, August). What makes for good care coordination? *Case Management Advisor, 24*(8), 93–94.

McDonald, K., Sundaram, V., Bravata, D., Lewis, R. et al. (2007, June). *Closing the quality gap: A critical analysis of quality improvement strategies, care coordination.* Agency for Healthcare Research and Quality, 7. Retrieved from http://www.ahrq.gov/research/findings/evidence-based-reports/caregap.pdf

McNamara, J. W. (2014). *Stronger together: Starting a health team in your congregation.* Memphis, TN: Church Health Center.

National Mental Health Association (2009). *Working with volunteers.* Retrieved from http://www.ncstac.org/content/materials/volunteer.pdf

Nouwen, H. J. (2010). *A spirituality of fundraising.* Nashville, TN: The Upper Room.

Nutt, M., & Hungerford, C. (2010). Nurse care coordinators: Definitions and scope of practice. *Contemporary Nurse, 36*(1–2), 71–81.

Ohio Nurses Association (2005). The nurse as a volunteer. *Ohio Nurses Review, 84*(2) 1–5.

Rydholm, L. Moone, R. Tornquist, L., Alexander, W., Gustafson, V., & Speece, B. (2008, April). Care of community-dwelling older adults by faith community nurses. *Journal of Gerontological Nursing, 34*(4), 18–29.

Shepherd, B., & Shepherd, R. (2013). *Taking steps in loss and life: A grief support group manual.* CreateSpace Independent Publishing Platform.

Tahan, H. A. (2005). The role of the nurse case manager. In Cohen, E. L. & Cesta, T. G. (Eds.) *Nursing case management: From essentials to advanced practice applications.* St. Louis, MO: Elsevier.

United Methodist Council of Churches. (2013). Health & wholeness. Retrieved from http://www.umc.org

US Council of Catholic Bishops. (2001). Catholic Health Care Services. Ethical and religious directives for Catholic health care. Retrieved from http://www.usccb.org/bishops/directives.shtml#partone

Varga, M. A., & Trena, M. Paulus. (2014). Grieving online: newcomers' constructions of grief in an online support group. *Death Studies,* (38)7.

White, P. & Hall, M. (2006, April). Mapping the literature of case management nursing. *J Med Libr Assoc, 94*(2), E99–E106.

Workgroup for Community Health and Development at the University of Kansas. (2013). The community tool box. Retrieved from http://ctb.ku.edu/en/table-of-contents/implement/enhancing-support/peer-support-groups/main

Additional References

Hedtke, L. (2012). *Bereavement support groups: Breathing life into stories of the dead.* Ohio: Tao Institute Publications.

Lamb, G. (2014). *Care coordination: The game changer—How nursing is revolutionizing quality care.* Silver Spring, MD: Nursesbooks.org.

Online Resources

www.nursingworld.org

Wrap-Up and Evaluation

Measuring Competency

This chart can be used to assess the individual outcomes in this module.
- A copy of this chart is attached to the Participant Module, so that each participant can complete this short evaluation.
- Have participants read each outcome and then place an X in the box that best matches their opinion about the objective being met.
- Encourage each participant to write a short reflection about this module in the space provided at the bottom of this chart.
- Use this data to make any necessary changes.

Outcome	Not Met	Somewhat Met	Met
1. Coordinate care delivery in the faith community.			
2. Apply competencies and skills that support successful care coordination.			
3. Develop volunteers and support groups for ministry in the faith community.			
Reflection: *In one paragraph, write a reflection on this module.*			

Appendix A

16 Tips for Recruiting Adult Volunteers

Recruiting the right people for the right program requires a commitment of time, energy, creativity and persistence, as well as a well-considered plan.

According to the Center for Intergenerational Learning at Temple University, effective practices include:

1. **Decide on the characteristics you want your volunteers to have.**

    Think about the goals of your project, the strengths and needs of the population it will be serving, and the activities the volunteers will be engaged in with families and youth. Consider the physical and time demands of your program. Factor in the requirements of grants that may be funding your program, including possible time limits on age, gender or place of residence.

2. **Develop a checklist of the most important requirements.**

    The checklist you develop for your volunteer requirements will probably contain similar categories. When writing the volunteer job description, you might not choose to include all of the items you have checked off on your list. However, you should develop an application and interview process that helps you assess whether potential volunteers meet all the requirements.

3. **Identify the barriers that may deter people from volunteering, which may include:**

    - Cultural myths and perceptions that old age is a time for relaxation, not learning or contribution.
    - Lack of confidence in their ability to contribute—inability to translate their life experiences and skills to a particular program's needs.
    - Fear about safety, such as having to use public transportation, go into a stranger's home, and concerns about drugs and crime associated with teens or low-income populations.
    - Physical limitations, such as illnesses or lack of energy.

    - Financial issues, including concerns that expenses associated with volunteering may strain their already limited financial resources.
    - Difficulties with transportation.
    - Competition for volunteers is yet another obstacle; it is likely that many other organizations are trying to recruit the same "volunteer-minded" older adults that you may be targeting. In addition, baby boomers are staying in the workforce longer, or returning to it after retirement, thus limiting the time they have available to volunteer.

4. **Think about what could motivate elderly people to volunteer for your program.**

    Identify ways to address some of the barriers and encourage older adults to volunteer. For example, they might be interested in volunteering because it will give them the opportunity to:

    - Increase their satisfaction with life by participating in an enjoyable and rewarding experience.
    - Increase their sense of connection to the community.
    - Feel productive.
    - Address a social issue in a way that is consistent with personal values.
    - Use their skills and share their experiences, interests and knowledge.
    - Learn new skills.
    - Learn more about youth.
    - Make new friends through the volunteer experience.
    - Leave a legacy for the younger generation.
    - Also identify ways to address logistical barriers such as transportation and the perceived expense of volunteering. Will volunteers be serving in a location that is easily accessible to their homes? Can the

program provide any financial incentives to help cover the volunteers' out-of-pocket expenses?

5. **Develop a recruitment message that "sells your program."**
What is it about your program's mission, goals and population of participants that you can "sell" in order to attract volunteers? In developing your message, consider:
  - Motivations for volunteering.
  - Volunteers' roles and responsibilities (including the length of time they will be expected to participate).
  - Benefits of serving in your program. These could range from benefits to society (making a difference, strengthening a community) to the volunteers' self-interest (learning new skills, acquiring new knowledge, meeting new people) to stipends (if any). Be sure to include information about the training and ongoing support volunteers will receive.

6. **Create recruitment materials that will catch people's attention.**
A recruitment message can be adapted for a wide range of materials, from flyers and brochures to videos and websites. Be sure your print and other media materials reflect the feel and quality of your program:
  - Make sure all materials convey the sense of professional expertise and purpose appropriate to the project. Use attractive graphics that draw attention to the materials, and include your agency logo.
  - Consider the audience when creating materials. Use language that is familiar to them. Make sure fonts are large enough for older adults to read comfortably. Choose colors that will be inviting to your target recruits. When appropriate, translate posters and materials into languages other than English (and be sure a fluent speaker carefully checks the translation).
  - When possible, use photographs and narratives to convey a sense of the program participants and volunteers. However, don't use images or stories that are sad or discouraging. Portraits of your program should be inviting, and convey a sense of

excitement, hope, and purpose. Be sure the photographs reflect the diversity of the pool of potential volunteers.
  - To ensure that your materials are appropriate and appealing, always have someone who is representative of the people you are targeting for recruitment review a draft and give you feedback.

7. **Plan presentations that put a personal "face" on your program.**
When giving presentations to recruit volunteers use some of the following strategies to make your program less anonymous and the potential recruits less able to "hide" behind their own anonymity.
  - Let people see the problem their volunteer work will address. People want to make a difference and are often motivated by their heart to volunteer. Use videos, success stories, and photographs to show the social problems the volunteers will address.
  - Bring along an articulate, older volunteer who can share his or her experiences. If your program is just starting up, but is modeled after another program, you may be able to have a volunteer in that program accompany you to some presentations and convey his/her excitement.
  - Conduct smaller, more intimate presentations. Though in some ways less efficient, presentations to small groups (fewer than 20 individuals) often work better than large group presentations because they reduce the possibility of anonymity among members of the audience.
  - Actively involve your audience. Engage potential recruits in dialogue, asking questions such as "How many of you are parents or grandparents?" "How many of you have ever known a child with a disability?" "How many teens in this city, would you guess, can't read a newspaper?" You can also engage the audience in brief activities, perhaps an example of one you use in training. This kind of interaction helps get people away from the "anonymity trap."
  - Have materials that people can take home with them. These should include volunteer

job descriptions, flyers/posters, application forms, general agency literature, and copies of any local or national news articles about the project.

- Allow time after presentations to interact informally with the people who have attended. Have refreshments available; it encourages people to stay and talk.
- Give people something to remember you by. For example, a pencil, key chain, or refrigerator magnet imprinted with the name of your agency or organization.
- Never walk away from a meeting where you have given a talk without getting the names and contact information of those who are interested. Pass around an attendance sheet for people to sign who want to receive more information.
- If possible, take applications and ask those who know they are interested to complete them on the spot. Be sure you get back to interested applicants within a week.

8. **Use a range of recruitment strategies to reach volunteers.**

Strategies for recruiting range from the uncomplicated and cost-free to the more complex and relatively inexpensive. These include:

- Word of mouth.
- Direct mail. Have personal letters written by your agency sent through other organizations such as local civic associations, community groups, and local chapters of the American Association of Retired Persons (AARP).
- Information tables at community events.
- Presentations to community groups.
- Recruitment meals. These could be potluck dinners or breakfasts that include presentations about your program.
- Flyers, posters and brochures. Be sure the flyers are 8 1/2" by 11" so that they can be easily mailed or posted on bulletin boards.
- Articles or press releases in local and community newspapers. Take advantage of the fact that community newspapers are understaffed and are looking for good copy. Write a one- or two-page press release describing your program and the need for volunteers, and include a high-quality

black and white photograph.
- Other organizations' newsletters. Ask religious institutions and relevant local agencies and organizations to run your press release in materials they send out to their members.
- Presentations on local cable television shows. Look for programming that is aimed at the particular audience you are trying to reach.
- Public service announcements (PSAs). Send television stations a ready-made clip, 30 seconds to one minute long. Create radio PSAs that are 20, 30, 45, or 60 seconds in length, and send them to stations or programs that your potential volunteers or their relatives are likely to listen to.
- Web pages. During recruitment drives, have your message posted on websites that are likely places to be visited by older adults or their relatives. Possibilities include the AARP website or a local daily paper's sites. Be sure your recruitment message is marked "New!"

9. **Start with what's in front of you.**

Recruitment is all about relationships. Think about who you already know. Brainstorm with co-workers about strategies for recruitment. Survey staff, board members, and volunteers to find out what organizations they are or have been involved with—as members or board members or in some other capacity—that might be a good connection for your recruitment efforts.

Think of everyone connected to your program as an assistant recruiter. Staff, volunteers, board members, trainers and consultants all have seen the program at work, and, with prompting, will translate their enthusiasm for the project into recruitment of senior friends and family members.

Current volunteers can be your most effective recruiters. Ask them to talk to their peers about the benefits they have received by being part of the program, and make sure they have the resources (such as extra program materials) they need to recruit. You can formalize this approach by giving them "assignments" such as generating one new volunteer applicant every six months.

You can also find recruiters outside of your program. Have the clergy at your church, synagogue or mosque—or the clergy of your volunteers—make a statement of support for the program. Use your wider social network. Enlist your relatives, friends and professional acquaintances, especially those who work at social service agencies or those who have connections to your desired group of volunteers.

10. **Cast a wide net.**
Do broad outreach to raise awareness of your program in the community. Developing connections with organizations that have credibility with the groups you are targeting can help your program gain visibility and access to those groups.

11. **Target your recruitment efforts.**
Identify the specific community agencies, institutions, and other groups that are most likely to help connect you with potential volunteers. The following steps can help you build on these initial contacts:
   - Take the time to establish relationships with the most promising agencies and institutions. Request assistance from appropriate agency staff on the best way to publicize the project to their older constituents. One way to get them actively involved is to obtain commitments from them to provide a certain number of volunteers from their membership and to identify them as "partners" in all publicity. This approach can help you recruit groups of volunteers, but be aware that some "turf" issues may surface if your agency or program is "competing" with your potential partner agency to provide similar services.
   - Meet with formal and informal community leaders, including block captains, activists, clergy and local politicians. "Sell" the program to them. Invite them to an event or to be part of the program advisory board.
   - Target geographically to neighborhood senior centers or high-rises and housing projects where many seniors live. Offer to give a talk as part of a committee or governance meeting.
   - Request that a church or synagogue "adopt" your program. If that occurs, and a

significant percentage of your volunteers are from that congregation, you can hold trainings and program events in its building. Be sure to give the church or synagogue public recognition for its "adoption."
   - In addition, target mailing and outreach efforts to populations that are already interested in doing the work of your program, or working with the population you are serving, or are generally interested in volunteering.

Other Issues to Consider:
12. **Recruit more people than you actually need.**
Assume that approximately 25 percent of the people who show some interest in your program will not follow through, that a significant number of those who do will not be appropriate for the program, and that some of those who are appropriate will drop out during training.

13. **Pay attention to timing.**
Recruitment may need to be ongoing throughout the duration of the program if attrition is high. (Some attrition is normal in all volunteer programs.) However, most recruitment is likely to be accomplished during one or two major drives each year. Fall and spring are usually the best times for recruitment drives, but what is most important is to minimize the lag between recruitment and program start-up—otherwise you may lose interested applicants. Once people are recruited and screened, begin training with little delay, and get the new volunteers involved in program activities as soon as possible.

14. **Be sure your agency is ready to provide good customer service.**
While recruiting volunteers, be sure your organization is ready to respond to the people who are interested enough to contact you for more information or to apply. Your agency should always be prepared to respond to inquiries from potential volunteers, even during periods when you may not be actively recruiting. Therefore:
   - Have someone on your staff who is specifically responsible for responding to initial telephone inquiries.

- Develop guidelines for the staff member to follow.
- Have materials ready to mail to people who call.
- Be ready to follow up. If a caller completes and returns an application, be prepared to take the next steps.

15. **Avoid the first "warm body" syndrome.**
It is tempting to accept every applicant who wishes to volunteer for your program, but it would be a mistake. Not everyone will meet the requirements you have identified as necessary for serving effectively. Use a screening process that includes tools such as
   - A written application
   - A face-to-face interview
   - References
   - Criminal record and child abuse checks (required in many states for anyone who works with children or youth)

Some programs also use their training sessions as a part of the screening process, particularly because the trainings present an opportunity to see how potential volunteers interact in a group setting. Depending upon the project, a physical examination might also be part of the screening. When the screening process reveals that an applicant is not appropriate for a particular project, offer that person another volunteer assignment in your agency, or encourage the volunteer to apply at a partner agency that would welcome the person's particular skills.

16. **Be patient and persistent.**
Recruiting is almost always a challenge—talking to dozens or even hundreds of people may only result in a few recruits. Don't take the frustration personally. Continue to be diligent and creative in your recruitment efforts. And also be sure to get support for yourself from other staff and peers.

Context: The decision to volunteer is usually a two-step process—a person thinks generally about becoming a volunteer and then a "trigger event" transforms this general thought into concrete action. The trigger is often something very simple: someone they know asks them to volunteer in a specific role, or they learn about an opportunity through an organization to which they belong. This two-step process suggests that it is important to create broad local visibility and name recognition, so that when people are ready to volunteer they will know who you are, and to target your recruitment, so you are asking people who are ready to volunteer.

From World Volunteer Web (http://www.worldvolunteerweb.org/resources/how-to-guides/manage-volunteers/how-do-i-manage-volunteers-additional-reading/doc/16-tips-in-recruiting.html).

Appendix B

Sample Volunteer Position Description

Title: Parish Visitor

Purpose

To offer encouragement and support through the expression of care, concern, and Christian fellowship to a growing number of Immanuel members, homebound living in their own residences or care facilities. To maintain contact with homebound members and their families to remind them they are not forgotten, though they are unable to attend worship or other church activities.

Term

Appointed by the church council in consultation with the pastors and faith community nurse to serve a term of one year, beginning February 1 through January 31.

Expectations

Parish visitors make brief visits (15–20 minutes) once a month to one or more members who are homebound due to frail health or chronic illness. Some parish visitors may be available to visit hospitalized members. As representatives of Immanuel Church, these ministry volunteers embody Christ's love and demonstrate Immanuel cares about each member of the faith community. Parish visitors are encouraged to participate in programs as planned by the Called To Care committee for the development of their caring ministry skills, and to attend the annual gathering of parish visitors for the purpose of feedback, planning, and evaluation of the visitation ministry.

Accountability

At the beginning of each month, the coordinators of our Visitation Ministry contact all parish visitors with names and information about the homebound members to be visited. Assignments are made depending on the volunteer's availability. Parish visitors may agree to see one member or several, during the day or evening, on a weekday or weekend. The parish visitor is expected to contact the assigned member to set up a convenient time to visit. We encourage couples or two friends to visit together. This is usually more comfortable and enjoyable for the homebound member as well as the parish visitors. Before taking along children or pets to visit, parish visitors should check with the visitation coordinators or faith community nurse (as well as the homebound member and their caregivers). Parish visitors are expected to respect designated visiting hours of care facilities and to wear nametags that identify them as "official" parish visitors from Immanuel United Church of Christ. Within 24–48 hours after completing visits, parish visitors are to contact the visitation coordinators to report that the visits were made and offer a brief update on the status of the homebound members. The coordinators will report any changes in health status or other concerns to the pastors and/or the faith community nurse, especially if a pastoral contact is requested or seems appropriate.

Qualifications

This volunteer ministry position requires a person with genuine compassion and respect for older adults and their caregivers. Ability to listen and relate well with older adults is important. A current driver's license, auto insurance, and ability to drive one's own car is very helpful; non-drivers are encouraged to "buddy" with another parish visitor that can drive. A brief orientation to this ministry by the coordinators and/or faith community nurse is required before making the first visits.

Support and Resources

Parish visitors can expect timely notification of monthly visit assignments from the visitation coordinators. These caring ministry volunteers can expect to receive counsel, support, and information on request from the pastors, faith community nurse, or other staff person with primary responsibility for Immanuel's Caring Ministries. Devotional materials, cards, and other special gifts specially prepared for homebound members can be found in the church library or by checking with the faith community nurse. Other resources (for example, The Called to Care Handbook for Lay Caregivers) are available, in the church library or from the FCN, to help prepare for visiting by learning more about certain health conditions.

Immanuel United Church of Christ, Ferguson, MO. Used with permission.

Appendix C

Support Group Resource Guide

1. What is the goal of this group?

2. What are the criteria for membership?

3. Who is the leader of this group?

4. What are the criteria for selecting the leader?

5. How are new members referred and screened for membership?

6. Is there a set minimum or maximum number of members?

7. Where does this group meet?

8. When does this group meet?

9. How long is each meeting?

10. Will this group have a planned ending or will it be ongoing?

11. How is group effectiveness determined?

Appendix D

Sample Denominational Direction on Health Ministry

The US Council of Catholic Bishops charges congregations and parishioners to actively participate in health care ministry.

> While many religious communities continue their commitment to the health care ministry, lay Catholics increasingly have stepped forward to collaborate in this ministry. Inspired by the example of Christ and mandated by the Second Vatican Council, lay faithful are invited to a broader and more intense field of ministries than in the past. By virtue of their baptism, lay faithful are called to participate actively in the Church's life and mission. Their participation and leadership in the health care ministry, through new forms of sponsorship and governance of institutional Catholic health care, are essential for the Church to continue her ministry of healing and compassion. They are joined in the Church's health care mission by many men and women who are not Catholic (US Council of Catholic Bishops, 2012, No. 29).

The United Methodist Church (UMC) provides direction related to the need for integration of health ministries into church activities by explaining the importance of health.

> Health is the ultimate design of God for humanity. Though life often thwarts that design, the health we have is a good gift of God. When God created humankind, God declared it to be very good (Genesis 1:31). Among Jesus' statements on the purpose of his presence is the statement that he came that we might have abundant life (John 10:10). Every account of Jesus' ministry documents how Jesus saw restoration to health as a sign of the Kingdom of Heaven becoming present amongst us. When John the elder wrote to Gaius (3 John 1:2), he wished for him

physical health no less than spiritual. The biblical narrative is filled with stories of God's healing presence in the world. This includes spiritual, psychological, emotional, social, as well as physical healing (UMC, *Health and Wholeness*).

UMC further directs its churches to do the following:

- Organize a Health and Wholeness Team as a key structure in the congregation. Among the team's responsibilities would be to seek each member to develop their spiritual gifts in order that the body of Christ be healthy and effective in the world. The apostle Paul commented that "many are sickly and die among you" (1 Corinthians 11:27–29, NRSV). We suggest that this may have resulted not simply from failing to discern the body of Christ present in the communion bread, but from failing to discern the body of Christ as the congregation. When church members are not allowed to use their spiritual gifts, they stagnate or die spiritually and the spiritual affects the physical health of the individual. The spread of health and wholeness should be discerned clearly as a guiding factor in why it is that we make disciples.
- Accept responsibility for educating and motivating members to follow a healthy lifestyle reflecting our affirmation of life as God's gift.
- Become actively involved at all levels in the development of support systems for health care in the community.
- Become advocates for a healthful environment; accessible, affordable health care; continued public support for health care of persons unable to provide for themselves; continued support for health-related research; and provision of church facilities to enable health-related ministries (UMC, *Health & Wholeness*).

Become a FCN Friend

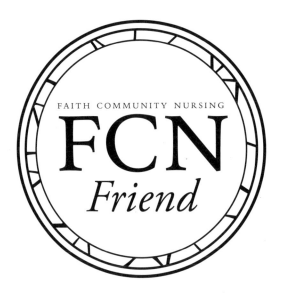

The Church Health Center is proud to announce our new subscription service, the FCN Friends program.

This is a modification of the Friends of the Center program that provides additional benefits to your new or previously existing FOC membership. The FCN Friends program is a subscription service that enables you to:

- Commit to the support of faith community nursing around the world.
- Subscribe to *Perspectives: A Newsletter for Faith Community Nurses*, the quarterly publication about faith community nursing.
- Receive special offers, items, logos and digital downloads exclusively only to FCN Friends, including the Model for Healthy Living Program Packet and FCN Friend Stationary Set
- Receive an FCN Friend subscriber card, decal and new FCN Friend lapel pin.

Subscription rates include:
- One year - $45
- Two years - $75
- Five years - $150
- Lifetime Subscription - $500

To subscribe visit, www.store.churchhealthcenter.org